Advancing Frontiers in Alzheimer's Disease Research

Advancing Frontiers in Alzheimer's Disease Research

Edited by

George G. Glenner, M.D., and Richard J. Wurtman, M.D.

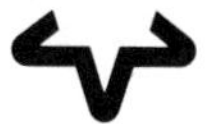 University of Texas Press, Austin

Published in association with Mind Science Foundation, San Antonio

Printed in the United States of America

First Edition, 1987

Library of Congress Cataloging-in-Publication Data
Advancing frontiers in Alzheimer's disease research.
Proceedings of a symposium held June 9–10, 1986 in San Antonio, Tex., and sponsored by the Mind Science Foundation.
Includes bibliographies and index.
1. Alzheimer's disease—Congresses. I. Glenner, George G., 1927- .II. Wurtman, Richard J., 1936- . III. Mind Science Foundation (San Antonio, Tex.) [DNLM: 1. Alzheimer's Disease—congresses. 2. Research—congresses. WM 220 A244 1986]
RC523.A34 1987 618.97'683 86-24928
ISBN 0-292-77602-0

Cover Image

The cover image was obtained using single photon emission computed tomography (SPECT) and the blood flow tracer ^{123}I-N-isopropyl-p-iodoamphetamine (IMP). The study was performed on the Donner Laboratory Cleon 810 SPECT instrument, with a resolution of 14mm full-width at half-maximum after an injection of 5 mCi of IMP. The image was obtained in a plane parallel to the canthomeatal line and 5 cm above the external auditory meatus. It represents 20 minutes of data accumulation and contains 2.8 x 10^6 counts. The patient is a 72 year old female who had a two to three year history of progressive memory loss and the clinical diagnosis of Alzheimer's disease of mild severity. The image demonstrates the characteristic lesion of diminished blood flow in the temporal lobes bilaterally. Frontal lobes and subcortical structures are less affected. Further discussion of technical and clinical factors in SPECT imaging in dementia can be found in chapters 12 and 14. Photo courtesy of Donner Laboratory.

For reasons of economy and speed this volume has been printed from camera-ready copy.

Contents

Preface

With the increasing public awareness of the incidence and extent of Alzheimer's disease and its devastating effects, increasing numbers of research investigators are attempting to decipher the nature and cause of this disease and ultimately to develop intelligent, directed therapy that will lead to its cure.

If, as it is conceded by many, understanding of the brain's function is still in an inchoate stage, then the nature of diseases engrafted upon this is even less apparent. With the exception of infectious processes, the nature and cause of only a few cerebral disorders, mainly those caused by inherited enzyme deficiency states, *e.g.* Tay-Sachs disease, have been determined. To ascertain the nature and cause of Alzheimer's disease is not only a scientific, but also a public health challenge and the ever increasing numbers (three million victims and 40 billion dollars for care costs per year) are too great for further temporizing.

The accelerating interest in Alzheimer's disease has led to numerous recent symposia on the whole or various aspects of the subject. The Mind Science Foundation sponsored the Symposium in June, 1986, from which this book resulted. The Foundation recruited from around the world renowned experts in almost all conceivable aspects of Alzheimer's disease research, and asked them to present and discuss in closed session the results of their most recent investigations. We hoped such an atmosphere would produce cross-fertilization of ideas, crystallization of research approaches and frank discussions of controversial subjects.

Indeed new theories about the cause of Alzheimer's disease, new and previously unpublished significant research results and approaches were presented at this Symposium in a highly amicable atmosphere. Interchanges between scientists in such diverse disciplines as nuclear medicine and neuropathology occured and provocative suggestions for improvement in methodology, changes in interpretation of data and new research tools were offered.

A major focus was the increasing potentiality of a specific diagnostic test for Alzheimer's disease which in turn could shed light on therapeutic approaches. We believe that the participants of this Symposium returned to their countries and laboratories with not only new information revelant to their respective fields, but also a broader view of the scientific attacks being made to unearth the nature of Alzheimer's disease.

This book, therefore, presents the findings reported at the Symposium sponsored by the Mind Science Foundation, in San Antonio, Texas. There was a general feeling at the conclusion of this meeting that seems best exemplified by the statement of Sir Winston Churchill after the Battle of El Alamein:

"This is not the end,
It is not even the beginning of the end,
But it is the end of the beginning."

Perhaps to be consistent with due scientific conservatism it might be best to rephrase that last line to read "this *probably* is the end of the beginning."

The editors wish to express their gratitude and indebtedness to the Elizabeth Huth Maddux Foundation for its grant supporting the Symposium; Mr. and Mrs. E. Bruce Street and The Scott Petty Foundation for matching grants to publish these proceedings, and the the Mind Science Foundation and its director, Catherine Nixon Cooke, for organizing and coordinating the Symposium and publication, and *sine qua non*.

George G. Glenner, M.D.
Senior Editor and Symposium Chairman

Acknowledgments

The Mind Science Foundation wishes to thank George G. Glenner, M.D. for his excellent job as Chairman of its 1986 Alzheimer's Disease Symposium, which included identifying and inviting the outstanding contributors to this publication; Richard J. Wurtman, M.D., for his inspiring keynote address and help with the Symposium and book; Bruce Street, the Foundation Research Partner who first suggested a symposium on this important subject; Elizabeth Huth Maddux, for both her financial and intellectual support of the Symposium; Mr. and Mrs. E. Bruce Street, O. S. and Edwina H. Petty, and Scott and Eleanor Petty for their matching grants to publish these proceedings; and the Foundation's Research Partners and other contributors who make it possible for MSF to explore the mysteries of the human mind.

Special thanks are due as well to Judith Bronson for her fine medical copyediting and to Gennice Dunn for her long, careful hours of typesetting and production.

1. Use of Choline in Cholinergic Neurons to Form Acetylcholine and Membrane Phospholipids: Possible Implications for Alzheimer's Disease

RICHARD J. WURTMAN, M.D.

Department of Applied Biological Sciences
Massachusetts Institute of Technology Cambridge, MA 02139

JAN K. BLUSZTAJN, Ph.D.,* PAMELA G. HOLBROOK, M.S.,* MICHAEL LAKHER, M.S.,* MORDECHAI LISCOVITCH, Ph.D.,* JEAN-CLAUDE MAIRE, Ph.D.,† CHARLOTTE MAURON, B.S.,* U. INGRID RICHARDSON, Ph.D.,* MARIATERESA TACCONI, Ph.D.‡

ABSTRACT: Studies on cholinergic neuron-derived cells maintained in cell culture have demonstrated that the neurons are able to use the choline in membrane phospholipids (like phosphatidylcholine; PC) to synthesize acetylcholine. This property — which is unique to cholinergic neurons — might cause the neurons to become vulnerable in situations where too little free choline is available to meet the cell's needs for acetylocholine synthesis: The neuron might then "autocannibalize" some of its membranes, or synthesize membrane PC (from available choline) at too low a rate. Evidence bearing on this hypothesis is discussed, as is its possible relevance to the pathogenesis and amelioration of Alzheimer's disease.

Introduction

Some of the choline within cholinergic neurons is derived from the circulation: free choline is able to cross the blood-brain barrier via a facilitated diffusion mechanism that is unsaturated at normal plasma choline levels (1). Additionally, some choline can be synthesized *in situ* by the sequential methylation of phosphatidylethanolamine (PE) and hydrolysis of the resulting phosphatidylcholine (PC; also called lecithin) (2).

* Department of Applied Biological Sciences, Massachusetts Institute of Technology, Cambridge; † Departement de Pharmacologie, Centre Medical Universitaire, Geneva, Switzerland; ‡ Instituto di Ricerche Farmacologiche Mario Negri, Milan, Italy.

Within cholinergic neurons, choline can undergo two kinds of biotransformation: it may be acetylated by choline acetyltransferase (CAT), a low-affinity, low-capacity enzyme, to form the neurotransmitter acetylcholine (ACh), or it may be incorporated into choline phospholipids (Ch-PL), (PC, sphingomyelin, and the plasmalogens, which are the principal lipid components of all biological membranes) via the CDP-choline, Kennedy *et al.* (3) or base-exchange pathways, Porcellati *et al.* (4) and Abdel-Latif *et al.* (5). The enzyme that initiates its incorporation via the CDP-choline pathway, choline kinase, is of high affinity and high capacity, so conversion to PC is probably the favored pathway for the utilization of choline in cholinergic neurons.

We hypothesize that a dynamic equilibrium exists between choline's reversible fluxes into and out of ACh and Ch-PL, and that these fluxes are well regulated, allowing both adequate ACh synthesis and maintenance of the functional integrity of the cell's membranes. (Ch-PL are the major lipid components of all biological membranes.) However, under some circumstances—for example, when a neuron is persistantly firing frequently, or when its supply of free choline is inadequate for ACh synthesis—there may be a net flux of choline from intraneuronal Ch-PL to ACh synthesis. If the rate at which the Ch-PL are hydrolyzed exceeds the rate at which they are resynthesized, there may be "autocannibalism" of the neuronal membranes, impairing their remodeling and ultimately threatening the neuron's viability.

The choline obtained by such autocannibalism could be derived generally from the neuron's Ch-PL or perhaps from a pool specifically mobilized for that purpose. Membrane phospholipids such as PC are nonhomogeneous and are differentiated in at least three ways; *i.e.*, by their subcellular location, their fatty acid composition, and the pathway through which they were synthesized; that is, methylation of PE *vs* incorporation of pre-existing choline via the CDP-choline or base-exchange pathways. Initially, the excessive destruction of membrane PC resulting from the hypothetical autocannibalism would be most likely to occur in cholinergic nerve terminals, because these structures both synthesize acetylcholine in relatively large quantities and remodel their membranes by Ch-PL breakdown and resynthesis.

This article describes some of the relationships between choline, ACh and Ch-PL in neurons, presenting evidence derived from experiments on brain slices, synaptosomes and cultured cells. It also suggests ways in which the hypothesized autocannibalism might participate in the pathophysiology of Alzheimer's disease (AD) or the other neurodegenerative diseases that afflict cholinergic neurons.

Neuronal Activity, Acetylcholine Release and Phospholipid Turnover

Because CAT has a low affinity for choline and is highly unsaturated with this substrate *in vivo* (6, cf. 7), ACh synthesis and release can be increased by treatments that elevate extracellular choline levels. The effect of the choline is enhanced if cholinergic neurons are firing frequently (cf. ref. 7). For example, we measured ACh release from rat striatal slices superfused with or without choline (8). In the absence of free choline, ACh was released spontaneously at a mean rate of 7.5 ± 1.3 (S.D.) pmol/mg of protein per minute. Electrical field stimulation (15 Hz for 30 min) accelerated this release (25.6 ± 5.9 pmol/mg protein per minute), and addition of 20 μm choline to the superfusate significantly enhanced both the spontaneous (22.7 ± 5.7 pmol/mg of protein per minute) and the electrically evoked (37.4 ± 6.7) pmol/mg protein per minute) release of the transmitter. Although the amount of ACh in the tissue did not depend on extracellular choline concentration within this range of choline concentrations, tissue choline content did increase when the choline concentration in the superfusate was raised.

The breakdown of membrane PC in neurons can, like ACh synthesis, be accelerated by frequent firing, especially when extracellular choline is unavailable. This was first shown by Parducz *et al.* (9), who electrically stimulated the preganglionic trunk of the cat's superior cervical ganglion in the presence of hemicholinium-3 and observed that the number of synaptic vesicles decreased to 18% that of controls, whereas ganglionic PC concentrations fell to 69% of controls. Other phospholipids were not affected. These observations indicate that when adequate extracellular choline is not available; *e.g.*, after inhibition of its uptake by hemicholinium-3, vesicular PC is used to supply choline for ACh synthesis. We have made similar observations using a striatal slices preparation: in the absence of exogenous choline, the combined efflux of choline + ACh into the superfusate was 75 pmol/mg of protein per minute, whereas the decrease in choline + ACh within the tissue was only 16 pmol/mg of protein per minute (8). Thus, an endogenous pool of choline, present within a larger molecule, must have provided the free choline to sustain ACh synthesis and tissue choline and ACh levels. The only known compounds whose pool sizes would be sufficient for this purpose are the Ch-PL.

Evidence that these compounds are indeed the source of the free choline is provided by the finding that the amount of phosphate in the phospholipids of the slices also decreased (by 23%) when the slices were stimulated, suggesting that neuronal activity accelerated the metabolic degradation of phospholipids (Mauron and Wurtman, in preparation).

Addition of 20 mM exogenous choline to the superfusate prevented the loss of phospholipid phosphate from stimulated slices. This result suggests either that the apparent acceleration in phospholipid degradation reflected an increased need for choline for ACh synthesis, which was met by shifting the equilibrium between ACh, choline and Ch-PL toward ACh, or that there was a general increase in phospholipid turnover related to neuronal firing. In the former case, the exogenous choline presumably was used to maintain high ACh synthesis, thus preventing the shift in the equilibrium; in the latter, the choline presumably provided sufficient substrate to allow the rate of PC synthesis to catch up with its accelerated degradation. Preliminary data suggest that when slices are stimulated in the absence of exogenous choline, the rate of PC synthesis by the *de novo* methylation pathway (see below) is increased (Lakher and Wurtman, unpublished data). Perhaps this result reflects a mechanism for sustaining membrane PC levels; *i.e.*, when PC degradation is accelerated by frequent neuronal firing, or one to maintain the appropriate PE/PC ratio within the membrane. PC degradation would tend to increase this ratio; PE N-methyltransferase (PeMT) activation would decrease it by converting PE to PC.

Relations Between Acetylcholine and Choline Phospholipid Synthesis in a Cholinergic Cell Line, NG108-15

We have studied the relations between Ch-PL and ACh levels in a purely cholinergic cell line, the neuroblastoma × glioma hybrid, NG108-15 (10). The synthesis of ACh in these cells varied with the extracellular choline concentration. When the cells were inclubated for 1 hr in the presence of various [^{3}H-methyl]choline concentrations, the accumulation of [^{3}H-methyl]ACh exhibited saturable kinetics, with an apparent K_m of 193 ± 34 μM, and V_{max} of 268 ± 23 pmol/mg of protein per hour. At the same time, incorporation of the labeled choline into phosphocholine, an intermediate in PC synthesis, proceeded at a much higher rate (apparent V_{max} = 16.8 ± 1.2 nmol/mg of protein per hour) and had a lower apparent K_m (14.9 ± 5.4 μM). Thus choline was more likely to be used in these cells for PC than for ACh synthesis because choline kinase was more likely than CAT to attack the choline. It was hypothesized that a treatment that inhibited choline kinase activity in the cells might enhance their formation of ACh, and it was subsequently shown that addition of 0.5 μM ethanolamine to the incubation medium suppressed the formation of phosphocholine and PC in a competitive fashion (apparent K_i = 180 μM) and concurrently enhanced the labeling of [^{3}H-methyl]ACh. These data demonstrate that the dynamic equilibrium between ACh, choline and

Ch-PL can be shifted toward ACh when choline's utilization for Ch-PL synthesis is slowed.

Choline Synthesis in Neurons

Choline is synthesized *de novo* in brain neurons by a multienzymatic pathway. The terminal steps in this pathway, catalyzed by PeMT, involve the stepwise methylation of PE to PC, using S-adenosylmethionine (SAM) as the methyl donor. This newly formed PC is hydrolyzed to free choline by a variety of phospholipases and other hydrolases. We found that free choline constituted 23% of the total PC synthesized by synaptosomal PeMT from [^{3}H-methyl]SAM during a 30-min incubation period. Furthermore, the enrichment of the free choline pool with newly formed [^{3}H]-choline was 50-fold greater than that of the PC pool by newly formed [^{3}H]PC (2). Thus, the relatively small amount of PC synthesized in nerve terminals *de novo* may have a considerably faster turnover than the bulk of synaptosomal PC. One might expect that the hypothetical PC pool which preferentially provides free choline for ACh synthesis would turn over more rapidly than "storage" PC. Perhaps this pool has a special fatty acid composition. The bulk of synaptosomal PC contains mainly (77%) fatty acids with 0-2 double bonds. However, the PC newly synthesized by PE methylation has a high proportion (up to 97%) of polyunsaturated (4-6 double bonds) fatty acids, partially reflecting the fatty acid composition of its precursor PE (11). Synaptosomal ^{3}H-PC newly synthesized from existing choline either by the CDP-choline or base-exchange pathways* also contains a higher proportion of polyunsaturated fatty acids (65%) (12) than the unlabeled steady-state PC (25%) in membranes (12,13).

Although it had thus been shown that brain could synthesize choline molecules *de novo* both *in vivo* and *in vitro*, it was not certain that this process actually occurred within cholinergic neurons, given the cellular heterogeneity of brain tissue. We therefore used a culture of purely cholinergic cells, the human neuroblastoma line LA-N2, to address this issue. When the LA-N2 cells were incubated with [^{14}C]-ethanolamine for 24 hr, most of the radioactivity in the cells was recovered in [^{14}C]-PE. However, 3%-7% was present in [^{14}C]-PC. Using a newly developed high-performance chromatography method (14), we established that 5%-10% of this PC was apparently hydrolyzed, yielding intracellular [^{14}C]-phosphocholine or free [^{14}C]-choline, which could be recovered from the cell growth medium (15). Thus, cholinergic neurons can synthesize

*Free choline is incorporated into PE or phosphatidylserine (PS) with a concomitant release of free ethanolamine or serine.

choline *de novo* via PE methylation and subsequent PC hydrolysis. Studies now in progress are designed to determine whether this choline is preferentially utilized as a precursor of ACh. We have observed that the cells are capable of converting [^{3}H]-methionine sequentially to [^{3}H]-SAM, [^{3}H]-PC, [^{3}H]-choline and [^{3}H]-ACh.

Autocannibalism and the Pathophysiology of Alzheimer's Disease

An overwhelming consensus now exists among investigators that (a) certain ACh-releasing brain neurons, the septal neurons projecting to the hippocampus and the basal forebrain neurons which innervate the cerebral cortices, invariably degenerate in AD (16-19); (b) other neurons, such as the noradrenergic neurons of the locus coeruleus and cortical somatostatin-releasing or CCR-releasing neurons, also are often afflicted, although to a lesser extent; and (c) many neuronal populations are largely unaffected in the disease. If one or more groups of neurons are invariably damaged in AD, then examination of their biochemical peculiarities may yield insights into the disease's etiology or the pathogenetic process that ultimately causes the neurons to die. Moreover, if the deficient neurotransmitter can be implicated in the abnormal behaviors typical of the disease—such as ACh in memory loss or norepinephrine in the impaired ability to sustain attention—then drugs which substitute for the deficient transmitter or which increase its availability in synapses might be useful in treating the disease.

We propose that the selective vulnerability of cholinergic neurons is related to autocannibalism of their cellular membranes. This hypothesis begs the question of the etiology of the AD, focusing instead on why cholinergic neurons are more likely than others to be damaged by the etiologic factor, and applies equally well whether the etiologic factor is present only in diseased cells or is distributed throughout the brain. The factor that presumably causes the choline deficiency might be a decrease in choline's production by *de novo* synthesis; a decrease in its uptake from the synaptic cleft and extracellular space; or its excessive utilization to form a particular phospholipid. Choline uptake might be impaired if the delivery of oxygen or glucose to the nerve terminals is deficient, perhaps secondary to a diffusion block caused by the perivascular amyloidosis that is characteristic of AD (20). Alternatively, the hypothetical choline deficiency might simply result from its overuse for ACh synthesis, as might happen if the firing frequency of vulnerable neurons is persistently enhanced, or if the presynaptic storage of ACh is impaired. Once cholinergic terminals begin to deteriorate and to release less of the transmitter, it seems likely that surviving, "healthy" terminals might start to release more ACh either because the firing frequencies of their neurons would increase or because release is less subject to presynaptic inhibition. Increased ACh synthesis might also be expected to increase the demand for its precursor, choline, within "healthy" terminals, a process which might ultimately lead to autocannibalism in these terminals as well.

Several pieces of clinical evidence are consistent with the autocannibalism hypothesis of AD:

1. It is the terminals of cholinergic neurons, in the hippocampus and cerebral cortex, and not the perikarya, in the basal forebrain, which apparently degenerate first in AD (21,11). This finding is consistent with the fact that most of the neurons' ACh is formed in the presynaptic terminals.
2. Only long-axon cholinergic neurons are affected by the disease process: the short-axon interneurons in the striatum are spared. Perhaps the short-axon neurons can more easily resynthesize their membranes because Ch-PL are more readily available to them through axoplasmic transport (23,24). This transport would occur over a considerably shorter distance than that separating cholinergic perikarya in the nucleus basalis or septum from terminals in the frontoparietal cortex or hippocampus.
3. Patients with Down's syndrome invariably develop pathological signs (senile plaques and tangles) indistinguishable from those observed in the brains of people with AD (reviewed in ref. 25) as well as a decrease in cortical CAT activity (26). Brain PE and PS purified from autopsy specimens of fetuses affected with this genetic disorder exhibit abnormal fatty acid composition (27), suggesting that abnormal phospholipid metabolism might also be found in the brains of people with AD.
4. PC and PE are metabolized by brain phospholipase A and lysophospholipases to form glycerophosphocholine or glycerophosphoethanolamine, respectively. The amounts of glycerophosphocholine in brain autopsy specimens from patients who died with AD reportedly are 3.6-fold higher than those in samples from normal persons (28). The amounts of PC and PE were found to be unchanged in that study. The increase in glycerophosphocholine is suggestive of increased rates of PC degradation. It is possible that PC degradation is catalyzed by phospholipase A in AD to a higher extent than by phospholipase D (see below), causing a selective increase in glycerophosphocholine. Because phospholipase A might be specific for a different pool of PC; *e.g.*, one containing different fatty acids, than phospholipase B, the net

result might be a change in the molecular species of the surviving PC, which might be pathogenic to membranes.

5. The activities of phospholipase D (the enzyme that catalyzes the hydrolysis of PC to free choline) and of CAT are decreased to a similar extent in autopsy specimens of cortices of patients who died with AD (J. Kanfer, personal communication). It is tempting to speculate that phospholipase D is localized within cholinergic nerve terminals and that the decrease in its activity is a reflection of their degeneration. Alternatively, the decrease in enzymatic activity might reflect a general abnormality in phospholipid metabolism characteristic of AD.

Since the discoveries of cholinergic deficits in AD, several clinical studies have been performed that tested various doses of choline or lecithin as therapeutic agents (reviewed in ref. 19). The rationale for these clinical trials was that the choline, free or liberated in vivo from lecithin, would be used by the surviving cholinergic neurons as the precursor of ACh, restoring some of the cholinergic tone in the brain. It is now apparent that these agents might also increase Ch-PL synthesis and therefore improve the functions of membranes affected by autocannibalism. Although these clinical trials have been only mildly successful at best, and then only when the supplemental choline has been administered for many months; i.e., long enough for the untreated control group to deteriorate further, it should be recognized that people with symptoms of AD probably suffer a cholinergic lesion so severe as to be irreparable. Supplemention with choline or lecithin might be more useful in treating patients with smaller lesions or those who are at risk of getting the disease but do not yet exhibit it. Therefore, it would be highly desirable to develop a diagnostic tool to identify such individuals, to see whether long-term lecithin treatment started early in the course of their illness would slow or halt the progression of AD.

Acknowledgments

These studies were supported by a grant from the National Institute of Mental Health.

References

1. Pardridge, W.M., Cornford, E.M., Braun, L.D. & Oldendorf, W.H. (1979) In: *Nutrition and the Brain*. Vol. 5. (Raven Press, New York) pp. 25-34.
2. Blusztajn, J.D. & Wurtman, R.J. (1981) *Nature* **290**, 417-418.
3. Kennedy, E.P. & Weiss, S.B. (1956) *J. Biol. Chem.* **222**, 193-214.

4. Porcellati, G., Arienti, G., Pirotta, M. & Giorgini, D. (1971) *J. Neurochem.* **18**, 1395-1417.
5. Abdel-Latif, A.A. & Smith, J.P. (1972) *Biochem. Pharmacol.* **21**, 436-439.
6. White, H.L. & Wu, J.C. (1973) *J. Neurochem.* **20**, 297-307.
7. Blusztajn, J.K. & Wurtman, R.J. (1983) *Science* **221**, 614-620.
8. Maire, J.C. & Wurtman, R.J. (1985) *J. Physiol. (Paris)* **80**, 189-195.
9. Parducz, A., Kiss, Z. & Joo, F. (1976) *Experientia* **32**, 1520-1521.
10. Hamprecht, B. (1977) *Int. Rev. Cytol.* **49**, 99-170.
11. Tacconi, M.-T. & Wurtman, R.J. (1985) *Proc. Natl. Acad. Sci. USA* **82**, 4828-4831.
12. Holbrook, P.G., Mauron, C. & Wurtman, R.J. (1985) *Proceedings of the Satellite Meeting of the International Society for Neurochemistry*, Mantova, Italy.
13. Breckenridge, W.C., Gombos, C. & Morgan, I.G. (1972) *Biochim. Biophys. Acta* **266**, 695-707.
14. Liscovitch, M., Freese, A., Blusztajn, J.K. & Wurtman, R.J. (1985) *Anal. Biochem.* **151**, 182-187.
15. Blusztajn, J.K., Richardson, U.I., Liscovitch, M. & Wurtman, R.J. (1986) *Trans. Soc. Neurochem.* **17**.
16. Bowen, D.M., Benton, J.S., Spillane, J.A., *et al.* (1982) *J. Neurol. Sci.* **57**, 191-202.
17. Perry, E.K., Tomlinson, B.E., Blessed, G., *et al.* (1978) *Br. Med. J.* **2**, 1458-1459.
18. Wilcock, G.K., Esiri, M.M., Bowen, D.M. & Smith, C.C.T. (1982) *J. Neurol. Sci.* **57**, 407-417.
19. Wurtman, R.J. (1985) *Sci. Am.* **252(1)**, 62-75.
20. Mandybur, T.I. (1975) *Neurology* (Minneap.) **25**, 120-126.
21. Pearson, R.C.A., Sofroniew, M.V., Cuello, A.C., *et al.* (1983) *Brain Res.* **289**, 375-379.
22. Perry, R.H., Candy, J.M., Perry, E.K., *et al.* (1985) *Neurosci. Lett.* **33**, 311-315.
23. Abe, T., Haga, T. & Kurokawa, M. (1973) *Biochem. J.* **136**, 731-740.
24. Droz, B., Brunetti, M., Di Giambernardino, L., et al. (1981) In: *Cholinergic Mechanisms*, ed. Pepeu, G. (Plenum Press, New York) pp. 377-386.
25. Epstein, C. (1983) In: *Biological Aspects of Alzheimer's Disease, ed. Katzman, R. (Cold Spring Harbor Laboratory, New York) pp. 169-182.*
26. *Yates, C.M., Simpson, J., Maloney, A.J.F., et al.* (1980) *Lancet* **2**, 39.
27. Brooksbank, B.W.L., Martinez, M. & Balazs, R. (1985) *J. Neurochem.* **44**, 869-874.
28. Barany, M., Chang, Y-C., Arus, C., *et al.* (1985) *Lancet* **1**, 517.

2. The Biochemistry of Cortical and Subcortical Neurons in Alzheimer's Disease

DAVID M. BOWEN, Ph.D.
PAUL T. FRANCIS, ALAN M. PALMER

Department of Neurochemistry Institute of Neurology
Queen Square London, WCIN 3BG, U.K.

ABSTRACT: Biochemical and related studies on autopsy and biopsy samples are described which have led to the well-established "cholinergic hypothesis" of Alzheimer's disease. Changes in serotonergic, somatostatinergic and glutamergic neurones also seem to occur and these are discussed in relation to cholinergic changes.

Introduction

Primary cerebral atrophy is one of the commonest causes of dementia in the presenium and the elderly. Alzheimer's disease (AD), a major type of cerebral atrophy, is characterized histopathologically by intense neurofibrillary degeneration (tangles) and senile plaque formation in the cerebral cortex.

Cholinergic Changes

Reductions in the activity of acetylcholinesterase (AChE) in the AD brain, reported in 1964 (1), provided an indication that the cholinergic system is affected in this condition. However, it was not until over a decade later, when large reductions in choline acetyltransferase (CAT) in the neocortex and hippocampus were identified (2-4), that an appreciation of the potential importance of these cholinergic changes began to develop. This enzyme was apparently largely unaffected by postmortem time and the agonal state of the patients (2,5) and thus provided a particularly suitable marker for studies in autopsy tissue. These reductions in CAT activity have been confirmed in all investigations in which the enzyme was measured (reviewed in 6 and 7), and this remains the most consistent neurochemical change so far described in AD. Comparable reductions were also found in samples of neocortex removed at diagnostic craniotomy (8), further confirming the validity of the autopsy studies. The reductions in CAT provided evidence that specific neurotransmitter deficits may underlie the symptoms of the disease and suggested the possibility that these symptoms could be ameliorated by pharmacological manipulation.

CAT is apparently present in large excess over normal requirements for acetylcholine (ACh) synthesis, and its reaction is generally considered not to be the rate-limiting step in this process (9,10; but see also 11). Thus, the effects of the reductions in this enzyme activity on ACh synthesis in intact tissue were not readily predictable. To resolve this issue, the synthesis of [^{14}C]-ACh from [U-^{14}C]-glucose was measured in tissue prisms (minislices) prepared from fresh neocortical tissue samples from patients with dementia (12-14). In this study, as in subsequent investigations of brain biopsy specimens, control values were obtained using apparently normal neocortex removed as a necessary part of surgery, usually to gain access to deep-seated tumors. Samples from demented patients, in which the diagnosis of AD was confirmed histologically, showed markedly lower synthesis of ACh under both resting (5 mM K^+) and K^+-depolarized (31 mM) conditions. Similar reductions were seen whether the samples had been obtained from the frontal or the temporal lobe.

The uptake of high-affinity choline into the prisms was similarly reduced (approximately 55% of control) in the biopsy samples from patients with AD (14). Comparable reductions (approximately 50% of control) in high-affinity choline uptake were also found in synaptosomes prepared from frontal cortex of fresh autopsy brains from AD cases. Synaptosomes prepared from hippocampus showed even less preservation of activity (to approximately 20% of control), suggesting even greater loss of cholinergic function within this region (15).

Several years ago, Whitehouse *et al.* (16,17) reported that in AD, there is a significant loss of large AChE-positive neuronal cell bodies in the nucleus basalis of Maynert, which provide the major cholinergic projection to the neocortex. This observation has been confirmed in a number of studies (18-23).

The identification of reductions in CAT activity led rapidly to attempts to ameliorate the deficits using cholinergic agonists or AChE inhibitors (reviewed in 6 and 24). Such trials were encouraged by early reports that the numbers of muscarinic receptors were similar in AD and control brains (25-28), suggesting that suitable targets for the agonists or an increased ACh signal were available. The recent findings that there may be two or more subclasses of muscarinic receptors, distinguished at present largely by their antagonist-binding properties (29), has led to a re-examination of the status of these receptors in AD. Evidence to date indicates that the high-affinity pirenzapine-binding site (often labeled

M_1) is unaffected in AD, whereas the lower-affinity site(s) is apparently reduced (30,31). One possibility consistent with the observed losses is that the affected (M_2) sites may be primarily presynaptic autoreceptors and are reduced in parallel with other presynaptic markers, but as yet the physiological and anatomical importance of these is undetermined.

Nicotinic receptors are also present in human brain, albeit as only a small proportion of the total cholinergic binding sites. A recent study indicates that binding at these sites is also reduced in AD (32). As with the muscarinic receptor subtypes, the function of these nicotinic sites is poorly defined, and the biological significance of the observed disease-induced alterations cannot at present be predicted.

The available evidence from the effects of drugs and lesions in humans and animals suggests a role for the cholinergic system in memory and cognitive function (33,34), but the specific functions of cholinergic inputs in the limbic system and particularly the diffuse projections to the neocortex remain poorly defined. A correlation between CAT activity in autopsy brain and an overall measure of cognitive function determined within six months prior to death was found for a group of patients presenting with either AD or depression (35). In patients with AD who underwent biopsy, there was also a significant correlation between an overall clinical assessment of the degree of dementia and [^{14}C]-ACh synthesis although not CAT activity (36,37). Among specific psychometric tests (Weschler adult intelligence scales [WAIS], token test and visual reaction time) only the reaction time showed a significant correlation with the rate of ACh synthesis. The observed significant correlations do not allow any conclusions to be drawn as to a cause and effect relation but do indicate that cholinergic deficits and the degree of dementia advance in parallel and are at least consistent with there being a cholinergic contribution to the development of the symptoms of AD.

Serotonergic Changes

Like cholinergic cells, serotonergic neurons innervate large areas of cerebral cortex from discrete subcortical nuclei. However, the integrity of serotonergic neurons has been less thoroughly investigated in AD, largely because of the difficulty of measuring the activity of tryptophan hydroxylase in postmortem brain (38). With the exception of studies of the serotonin (5-HT) carrier (39-41), all estimates of serotonergic neurons in postmortem samples have relied on determination of the concentrations of 5-HT and 5-hydroxyindoleacetic acid (5-HIAA), (8,36,40,42-46). The 5-HT concentration in the neocortex from AD subjects has in general been found to be reduced, whereas 5-HIAA is unaltered except according to one report (42) of reduced concentration.

This discrepancy may be related to postmortem delay, which was shorter in the latter study than in other investigations (43,46). Postmortem changes are known to affect the indoleamines (47), particularly in the cortex (48). Moreover, as oxygen is a cofactor for tryptophan hydroxylase, the terminal hypoxia usually associated with AD may be partly responsible for some of the observed changes.

Problems associated with postmortem material have been circumvented by assessing the integrity of serotonergic varicosities in AD biopsy samples. Uptake of [^{3}H]-5-HT is reduced in such material (40). We have now studied three additional indices of serotonergic neurons: (a) uptake of [^{3}H]-5-HT dependent on a specific 5-HT uptake inhibitor; (b) K^+-evoked release of endogenous 5-HT and (c) concentrations of 5-HT and 5-HIAA (39). All these indices were substantially reduced in AD biopsy samples. This is a selective change, as markers of dopaminergic neurons were not reduced in the same samples. Serotonergic dysfunction was found in patients who probably had had the disease for 2 years or less. The biopsies typically were taken 3.5 years after the onset of symptoms (37,49), which is approximately at the midpoint of the disease (see 50). At this stage, the temporal cortex of the average patient has lost some 60% of each of the markers for serotonergic and cholinergic neurons. The frontal cortex is less affected, as 5-HT and 5-HIAA content and 5-HT release are reduced by less than 50%. Thus the serotonergic lesion is more severe in the temporal cortex, as was found postmortem (46). These findings presumably reflect the spread of the disease process and are consistent with serotonergic denervation occurring in AD as a result of changes in the neocortex. Neurofibrillary degeneration and neuronal loss from the raphe nucleus have been reported (51-53), but it is not known whether the affected cells relate topographically to areas of pronounced neocortical damage.

In contrast to presynaptic cholinergic dysfunction, serotonergic denervation does not correlate with dementia rating. This may be because, unlike in the case of the cholinergic system, the neuropsychological consequences of impaired serotonergic neurotransmission can also involve marked loss of 5-HT receptors, in particular the 5-HT_2 type (Table 1). Alternatively, serotonergic denervation could predispose patients to amnesia, with the increasing severity of dementia being due to other overriding changes within the cortex such as pyramidal neuron loss or cholinergic denervation, both of which correlate with dementia rating (49). A compensatory increase in the rate of 5-HT turnover in the remaining neurons may account for the reported (39) increase in the concentration of 5-HIAA in cerebrospinal fluid (CSF) as the disease intensifies (as measured by the dementia rating). There is other evidence for increased 5-HT turnover in AD (46,47) and for similar changes in dopamine and noradrenaline metabolism in neurodegenerative disease (54), including AD (55).

Indices of serotonergic cells did not significantly correlate with indices of cholinergic neurons, pyramidal cell number or plaque formation. However, in agreement with data from postmortem tissue (39,46), 5-HIAA concentration significantly correlated (negatively) with tangle counts, suggesting that intrinsic cortical change may be a determinant of serotonergic denervation.

The selective loss of serotonergic receptors has been equated with degeneration of cortical neurons containing 5-HT receptors (glutamergic pyramidal or somatostatin neurons) which may then lead to denervation of the ascending 5-HT projection by retrograde degeneration (see 40 and 56-61). The observed correlation between tangle formation, which occurs predominantly in pyramidal cells, and 5-HIAA is consistent with such a mechanism involving the glutamergic neuron. Moreover, increased glucose oxidation, which occurs *in vitro* in AD and correlates with 5-HIAA concentration (13,39), is also likely to be due to alterations in pyramidal neurons, as these are the largest and most abundant type of cortical nerve cell and many have terminal fields within their own and other cortical areas, whereas serotonergic and cholinergic varicosities and somatostatin cells are only minor components of neuropil (40,62,63). As loss of cortical pyramidal neurons correlates with dementia rating (37), investigation of the action of serotonergic drugs on glutamergic neurons may provide a novel therapeutic approach for AD.

Somatostatinergic Changes

Some tangle-bearing cortical neurons stain for somatostatin (64), and a small percentage of normal cortical neurons are thought to contain this peptide (63,65). These cells have received particular attention in AD because of the apparent stability of neuropeptides in autopsy tissue and the consistently found reduction postmortem in the content of somatostatin-like immunoreactivity (SLIR; 66). This change has, in general, not been related to the results of positron emission tomographic and chemicohistopathologic investigations (56,67-69), which indicate that in AD there is not a uniformly diffuse degenerative process in the neocortex. The temporal lobe is always severely degenerate; *i.e.*, always contains numerous senile plaques and tangles and has consistently shown a reduction in the concentration of SLIR (70-74). There is evidence of reduced SLIR content in the parietal cortex (71,72,75), and this lobe often shows pronounced degeneration. In the frequently less-degenerate areas, such as the frontal lobe and anterior cingulate cortex, the content is often not reduced (71-76). Some inconsistency does seem to exist, as the concentration of SLIR is reduced in the motor cortex (72,76), which is only slightly degenerate, and not all investigators report a reduced SLIR content in the parietal lobe (76).

We have measured tissue concentrations and *in vitro* release of SLIR in AD using neocortex obtained at diagnostic craniotomy. Somatostatin-containing neurons have previously been investigated in living demented patients but only indirectly, by assay of lumbar CSF. Such studies have shown a reduced SLIR content in clinically suspected examples of the disease (77-80) as well as in histologically verified cases (81,82).

The concentration of SLIR was not reduced compared with control values in frontal cortex obtained at autopsy from patients with AD (Table 2). This result is in agreement with the reports of Rossor *et al.* (76), Perry and Perry (73) and Tamminga *et al.* (75). Table 2 confirms that in AD the concentration of SLIR is significantly reduced in temporal cortex. The reduction of 39% was similar to that reported by Ferrier *et al.* (72), although losses of more than 65% have been described by Davies and Terry (71) and Beal *et al.* (74). The concentrations of SLIR in both frontal and temporal cortex from AD biopsy samples were not significantly different from control values (Table 2).

Electron microscopic examination of the tissue prisms or minislices used for studying SLIR release reveals that, as for rat brain prisms, these are primarily preparations of intact synaptic endings in the presence of disintegrated cell structures. Thus, as with conventional preparations of synaptosomes, the prisms provide a useful means of determining neurotransmitter functions free from the influence of the cell body (13). Other investigators using synaptosome (83) and slice (84) preparations from rat brain have shown that elevated K^+ concentrations stimulate the release of endogenous SLIR. The present results demonstrate that this response is also a feature of both control and diseased human brain tissue, as the concentrations of SLIR in incubation medium containing 50 mM K^+ were significantly higher than in medium containing 5 mM K^+ (Table 3). The mean value for the K^+-stimulated release of SLIR from tissue prisms prepared from the AD (Table 3) was slightly elevated, 129% of control values, but this effect was not statistically significant.

The concentration of SLIR significantly correlates with scores for WAIS full-scale IQ ($R_S = 0.76$, $n = 9$, $p < 0.02$). Aphasia, reflecting disordered temporal lobe function, seems to relate to SLIR content, as scores for WAIS verbal IQ subscale and the Token Test (a measure of language comprehension) correlate with SLIR (Fig. 1). Counts of tangles, plaques and neurons do not correlate with SLIR content, whereas markers of serotonergic and cholinergic neurons correlate with these parameters (37,39,46).

Discussion

Assay of biopsy samples has provided conclusive evidence of a deficit in cholinergic and serotonergic varicosities in the frontal and temporal lobes in AD. The markers used for these cells include high-affinity uptake of [^{3}H] choline and 5-HT into tissue prisms and the synthesis of ACh by these preparations in media containing either low or high K^+ concentrations, as well as the release of endogenous 5-HT in the presence of high concentrations of K^+. All these measures are reduced in AD, whereas K^+-stimulated tissue prisms of AD patients release at least as much SLIR as controls, so the somatostatin deficit in AD does not seem to be as prominent a change.

The present data for the SLIR content of AD autopsy samples conforms with results of previous studies, which have shown that the peptide is consistently reduced in the temporal lobe but often spared in frontal regions. The other samples we have assayed for SLIR content have been obtained at diagnostic craniotomy (37,49), which is approximately at the midpoint of the disease (see above). At this stage, the AD patients showed no conclusive evidence of a somatostatin deficit, as measurements in samples obtained during diagnostic craniotomy revealed that the content of SLIR in tissue, as well as *in vitro* release of endogenous SLIR, were not significantly different from control values. Thus, in the present study, clear evidence of a somatostatin deficit in demented patients has been found only in a severely affected cortical region at the end point of the AD process; *i.e.*, in temporal cortex postmortem.

The advent of aphasia, which occurred in addition to perceptuospatial and memory disorder in two-thirds of the biopsied patients, is not unexpected, as tangle and plaque formation in the temporal cortex was abundant in most patients. Linguistic dysfunction is reflected by low verbal IQ and Token Test scores (37,49), which correlated with the concentration of SLIR in the temporal lobe, suggesting that somatostatin-containing neurons are involved in the pathophysiology of AD in the temporal cortex. Previously, reduced SLIR concentrations have been found in lumbar fluid obtained during clinical investigation of demented patients, including histologically verified examples of AD. Therefore, there is other evidence that a change in some somatostatin-containing neurons occurs relatively early in the disease. Some of these cells may be located in the parietal association cortex (see 75) and relate to perceptuospatial dysfunction. The present determinations on tissue samples obtained at surgery, moreover, do not eliminate the possibility of altered somatostatin function as a secondary phenomenon, perhaps because of changes in connecting neurons or loss of postsynaptic somatostatin receptors as has been detected in AD postmortem (74).

The cholinergic hypothesis of the pathogenesis of AD (28,36) has shortcomings: (a) cholinergic replacement therapy has not been successful; (b) hypometabolism and cholinergic denervation do not concur (69,75); (c) dementia and Alzheimer histopathologic change can precede major cholinergic denervation (60); and (d) the hypothesis fails to account for neurofibrillary tangles within cortical pyramidal neurons (56) and loss of these cells, which is correlated with dementia (37). Most shortcomings have been equated with somatostatin neurons (75), yet only a few cortical cells stain for the substance. A major type of cortical neuron is the glutamergic pyramidal cell, but there is only indirect evidence of the involvement of these, as no marker suitable for human brain has existed (57). Recently, specific Na^+-dependent binding of [^{3}H]-D-aspartate has been used in preliminary studies to provide an index of these neurons (85,86). There is a lower density of [^{3}H]-D-aspartate binding sites in the temporal cortex of Alzheimer patients postmortem with the affinity unchanged (61). These data are consistent with a loss of glutamergic nerve endings from the temporal cortex, possibly due to the degeneration of corticocortical association fibers (86). We have also assayed a less-degenerate region (Brodmann area 7; 68) and found no change. These data indicate that [^{3}H]-D-aspartate binding may be a useful neurochemical correlate of the degenerate cortical pyramidal neurons. Further investigations are needed to establish whether [^{3}H]-D-aspartate binding provides an index for hypometabolism (69,75), the proposed histopathologic progression of the disease (68) and the cognitive decline (37,49).

References

1. Pope, A.H., Hess, H. & Lewin, E. (1964) In: *Morphological and Biochemical Correlates of Neural Activity*, eds. Cohen, M.M. & Snider, R.S. (Harper and Row, New York) pp. 98-111.
2. Bowen, D.M., Smith, C.B., White, P. & Davison, A.N. (1976) *Brain* **99**, 459-496.
3. Davies, P. & Maloney, A.J.F. (1976) *Lancet* **2**, 1403.
4. Perry, E.K., Perry, R.H., Gibson, P.H., Blessed, G. & Tomlinson, B.E. (1977) *Neurosci. Lett.* **6**, 85-89.
5. McGeer, P.L. & McGeer, E.G. (1976) *J. Neurochem.* **26**, 65-76.
6. DeKosky, S. & Bass, N.H. (1985) In: *Handbook of Neurochemistry*, ed. Lajtha, A. (Plenum Press, New York) pp. 617-649.
7. Perry, E.K. (1986) *Br. Med. Bull.* **42**, 63-69.
8. Bowen, D.M., White, P., Spillane, J.A., Goodhardt, M.J., Curzon,

G., Iwangoff, P., Meier-Ruge, W. & Davison, A.N. (1979) *Lancet* **1**, 11-14.

9. Fonnum, F. (1975) In: *Cholinergic Transmission*, ed. Waser, P. (Raven Press, New York) pp. 145-159.
10. Marchbanks, R.M. (1982) *J. Neurochem.* **39**, 9-15.
11. Tucek, S. (1985) *J. Neurochem.* **44**, 11-24.
12. Sims, N.R., Bowen, D.M., Smith, C.C.T., Flack, R.H.A., Davison, A.N., Snowden, J.S. & Neary, D. (1980) *Lancet* **1**, 333-335.
13. Sims, N.R., Bowen, D.M. & Davison, A.N. (1981) *Biochem. J.* **196**, 867-876.
14. Sims, N.R., Bowen, D.M., Allen, S.J., Smith, C.C.T., Neary, D., Thomas, D.J. & Davison, A.N. (1983) *J. Neurochem.* **40**, 503-509.
15. Rylett, R.J., Ball, M.J. & Colhoun, E.H. (1983) *Brain Res.* **289**, 169-175.
16. Whitehouse, P.J., Price, D.L., Clark, A.W., Coyle, J.T. & DeLong, M.R. (1981) *Ann. Neurol.* **10**, 122-126.
17. Whitehouse, P.J., Price, D.L., Struble, R.G., Clark, A.W., Coyle, J.T. & DeLong, M.R. (1982) *Science* **215**, 1237-1239.
18. Wilcock, G.K., Esiri, M.M., Bowen, D.M. & Smith, C.C.T. (1983) *Neuropathol. Appl. Neurobiol.* **9**, 175-179.
19. Arendt, T., Bigl, V., Arendt, A. & Tennstedt, A. (1983) *Acta Neuropathol.* **61**, 101-108.
20. Candy, J.M., Perry, R.H., Perry, E.G., Irving, D., Blessed, G., Fairbairn, A.F. & Tomlinson, B.E. (1983) *J. Neurol. Sci.* **59**, 277-289.
21. Mann, D.M.A., Yates, P.O. Marcyniuk, B. (1984) *J. Neurol. Neurosurg. Psychiatr.* **47**, 201-203.
22. McGeer, P.L., McGeer, E.G., Suzuki, J., Dolman, C.E. and Nagai, T. (1984) *Neurology* **34**, 741-745.
23. Rogers, J.D., Brogan, D. & Mirra, S.S. (1985) *Ann. Neurol.* **17**, 163-170.
24. Hollander, E., Mohs, R.C. & Davis, K.L. (1986) *Br. Med. Bull.* **42**, 97-100.
25. White, P., Hiley, C.R., Goodhardt, M.J., Carrasco, L.H., Keet, J.P. Williams, I.E.I. & Bowen, D.M. (1977) *Lancet* **1**, 668-671.
26. Perry, E.K., Perry, R.H., Blessed, G. & Tomlinson, B.E. (1977) *Lancet* **1**, 189.
27. Davies, P. & Verth, A.H. (1978) *Brain Res.* **138**, 385-372.
28. Bartus, R.Y., Dean, R.L., Beer, B. & Lippa, A.S. (1982) *Science* **217**, 408-417.
29. Caulfield, M. & Straughan, D. (1983) *Trends Neurosci.* **6**, 73-75.
30. Caulfield, M.P., Straughan, D.S., Cross, A.J., Crow, T. & Birdsall, N.J. (1982) *Lancet* **2**, 1277.

31. Mash, D.C., Flynn, D.D. & Porter, L.T. (1985) *Science* **228**, 1115-1117.
32. Whitehouse, P.J., Martino. A.M., Antuono, P.G., Lowestein, P.R., Coyle, J.T., Price, D.L. & Kellar, K.H. (1986) *Brain Res.* **371**, 146-151.
33. Brimblecombe, R.W. (1974) *Drug Action on Cholinergic System* (Macmillan, London).
34. Drachman, D.A. & Sahakian, B.J. (1980) In: *The Psychobiology of Aging*, ed. Stein, D.G. (Elsevier-North Holland, New York) pp. 347-365.
35. Perry, E.K., Tomlinson, B.E., Blessed, G., Bergmann, K., Gibson, P.H. & Perry, R.H. (1978) *Br. Med. J.* **2**, 1457-1459.
36. Francis, P.T., Palmer, A.M., Sims, N.R., Bowen, D.M., Davison, A.N. Esiri, M.M., Neary, D., Snowden, J.S. & Wilcock, G.K. (1985) *N. Engl. J. Med.* **313**, 7-11.
37. Neary, D., Snowden, J.S., Mann, D.M.A., Bowen, D.M., Sims, N.R., Northen, B., Yates, P.O. & Davison, A.N. (1986) *J. Neurol. Neurosurg. Psychiatr.* **49**, 229-237.
38. McGeer, P.L. & McGeer, E.G. (1981) In: *The Molecular Basis of Neuropathology*, eds. Davison, A.N. & Thompson, R.H.S. (Edward-Arnold, London) pp. 649-666.
39. Palmer, A.M., Francis, P.T., Benton, J.S., Sims, N.R., Mann, D.M.A., Neary, D., Snowden, J.S. & Bowen, D.M. (1986) *J. Neurochem.* (in press).
40. Bowen, D.M., Allen, S.J., Benton, J.S., Goodhardt, M.J., Haan, E.A., Palmer, A.M., Sims, N.R., Smith, C.C.T., Spillane, J.A., Esiri, M.M., Snowden, J.S., Wilcock, G.K. & Davison, A.N. (1983) *J. Neurochem.* **41**, 266-272.
41. Perry, E.K., Marshall, E.F. & Blessed, G. (1983) *Br. J. Psychiatr.* **142**, 188-192.
42. Cross, A.J., Crow, T.J., Johnson, J.A., Joseph, M.H., Perry, E.K., Perry, R.H., Blessed, G. & Tomlinson, B.E. (1983) *J. Neurol. Sci.* **60**, 383-392.
43. Gottfries, C.G., Adolfsson, R., Aquilonius, S.M., Carlsson, A., Eckernas, S.-A., Nordberg, L., Oreland, L., Svennerholm, L., Wiberg, A. & Winblad, B. (1983) *Neurobiol. Aging* **4**, 261-271.
44. Arai, H., Kosaka, K. & Iizuka, R. (1984) *J. Neurochem.* **43**, 388-393.
45. Reynolds, G.P., Arnold, L., Rossor, M.N., Iversen, L.L., Mountjoy, C.Q. & Roth, M. (1984) *Neurosci. Lett.* **44**, 47-51.
46. Palmer, A.M., Wilcock, G.K., Esiri, M.M., Francis, P.T. & Bowen, D.M. (1986) *Brain Res.* (in press).
47. Palmer, A.M., Francis, P.T. & Bowen, D.M. (1986) *Biochem. Soc. Trans.* **16**, 608-609.

48. Goldman-Rakic, P.S. & Brown, R.M. (1981) *Neuroscience* **6**, 177-187.
49. Neary, D., Snowden, J.S., Bowen, D.M., Mann, D.M.A., Sims, N.R., Benton, J.S., Northern, B., Yates, P.O. & Davison, A.N. (1986) *J. Neurol. Neurosurg. Psychiatr.* **49**, 163-174.
50. Sulkava, R., Haltia, M., Paetau, A., Wikstrom, J. & Palo, J. (1983) *J. Neurol. Neurosurg. Psychiatr.* **46**, 9-13.
51. Curico, C.A. & Kemper, T. (1984) *J. Neuropathol. Exp. Neurol.* **43**, 359-368.
52. Mann, D.M.A. & Yates, P.O. (1983) *J. Neurol. Neurosurg. Psychiatr.* **46**, 96.
53. Yamamoto, T. & Hirano, A. (1985) *Ann. Neurol.* **17**, 2573-2577.
54. Scatton, B., Javoy-Agid, F., Rouquier, L., DuBois, B. & Agid, Y. (1983) *Brain Res.* **275**, 321-328.
55. Raskind, M.A., Peskind, E.R., Halter, J.B. & Jimerson, D.C. (1984) *Arch. Gen. Psychiatr.* **41**, 343-346.
56. Pearson, R.C.A., Esiri, M.M., Hiorns, R.W., Wilcock, G.K. & Powell, T.P.S. (1985) *Proc. Natl. Acad. Sci. USA* **82**, 4531-4534.
57. Bowen, D.M. & Davison, A.N. (1986) *Br. Med. Bull.* **42**, 75-80.
58. Cross, A.J., Crow, T.J., Ferrier, I.N. & Johnson, J.A. (1986) *Neurobiol. Aging* **7**, 3-8.
59. Middlemiss, D.N., Bowen, D.M. & Palmer, A.M. (1986) In: *New Concepts in Alzheimer's Disease*, eds. Briley, M., Kato, A. & Weber, M. (Macmillan Press Ltd., London) (in press).
60. Palmer, A.M., Procter, A.W., Stratmann, G.C. & Bowen, D.M. (1986) *Neurosci. Lett.* **66**, 199-204.
61. Procter, A.W., Palmer, A.M., Stratmann, G.C. & Bowen, D.M. (1986) *N. Engl. J. Med.* (in press).
62. Palmer, A.M., Middlemiss, D.N. & Bowen, D.M. (1986) In: *Brain Serotonergic Mechanisms: The Pharmacological, Biochemical and Potential Therapeutic Actions of 8-OH-DPAT*, eds. Dourish, C.T., Ahlenius, S. & Hutson, P.H. (Ellis Horwood Ltd., London) (in press).
63. McDonald, J.K., Parnavelas, J.G., Karamanlidis, A.N., Brecha, N. and Koenig, J.I. (1982) *J. Neurocytol.* **11**, 809-824.
64. Roberts, G.W., Crow, T.J. & Polak, J.M. (1985) *Nature* **314**, 92-94.
65. Hendry, S.H.C., Jones, E.G. & Emson, P.C. (1984) *J. Neurosci.* **4**, 2497-2517.
66. Rossor, M. & Iversen, L.L. (1986) *Br. Med. Bull.* **42**, 70-74.
67. Wilcock, G.K., Esiri, M.M., Bowen, D.M. & Smith, C.C.T. (1982) *J. Neurol. Sci.* **57**, 407-417.
68. Brun, A. (1983) In: *Alzheimer's Disease: The Standard Reference*, ed. Reisberg, B. (The Free Press, New York) pp 37-47.

69. Foster, N.L., Chase, T.N., Fedio, P., Patronas, N.J., Brooks, R.A. & DiChiro, G. (1983) *Neurology* **33**, 961-965.
70. Rossor, M.N., Emson, P.C., Mountjoy, C.Q., Roth, M. & Iversen, L.L. (1980) *Neurosci. Lett.* **20**, 373-377.
71. Davies, P. & Terry, R.D. (1981) *Neurobiol. Aging* **2**, 9-14.
72. Ferrier, I.N., Cross, A.J., Johnson, J.A., Roberts, G.W., Crow, T.J., Corsellis, J.A.N., Lee, Y.C., O'Shaughnessy, D., Adrian, T.E., McGregor, G.P., Baracese-Hamilton, A.J. & Bloom, S. (1983) *J. Neurol. Sci.* **62**, 159-170.
73. Perry, E.J. & Perry, R.H. (1985) *Danish Med. Bull.* **32**, Suppl. 1, 27-34.
74. Beal, M.F., Mazurek, M.F., Tran, V.T., Chatta, G., Bird, E.D. & Martin, J.B. (1985) *Science* **229**, 289-291.
75. Tamminga, C.A., Foster, N.L. & Chase, T.N. (1985) *N. Engl. J. Med.* **313**, 1294-1295.
76. Rossor, M.N., Emson, P.C., Iversen, L.L., Mountjoy, C.Q., Roth, M., Fahrenkrug, J. & Rehfeld, J.F. (1982) In: *Alzheimer's Disease: A Report of Progress*, eds. Corkin, S., Davis, K.L., Growdon, J.H., Usdin, E. & Wurtman, R.J. (Raven Press, New York) pp. 15-24.
77. Oram, J.J., Edwardson, J. & Millard, J.H. (1981) *Gerontology* **27**, 216-233.
78. Wood, P.L., Etienne, P., Lal, S., Gauthier, S., Cajal, S. & Nair, N.P.V. (1982) *Life Sci.* **31**, 2073-2079.
79. Soininen, H., Pitkanen, A., Halonen, T. & Riekkinen, P.J. (1984) *Acta Neurol. Scand.* **69**, 29-34.
80. Steardo, L., Tamminga, C.A., Barone, P., Foster, N., Durso, R., Ruggeri, S. & Chase, T.N. (1984) *Neuroendocrinol. Lett.* **6**, 291-293.
81. Francis, P.T., Bowen, D.M., Neary, D., Palo, J., Wikstrom, J. & Olney, J. (1984) *Neurobiol. Aging* **5**, 183-186.
82. Francis, P.T., Lowe, S.L., Palmer, A.M., Procter, A.W., Stratmann, G.C., Neary, D., Snowden, J.S. & Bowen, D.M. (1986) *Biochem. Soc. Trans.* (in press).
83. Bennett, G.W., Edwardson, J.A., Marcano de Cotte, D., Berelowitz, M., Pimstone, B.L. & Kronheim, S. (1979) *J. Neurochem.* **32**, 1127-1130.
84. Iversen, L.L., Iversen, S.D., Bloom, F., Douglas, C., Brown, M. & Vale, W. (1978) *Nature* **273**, 161-163.
85. Vincent, S.R. & McGeer, E.G. (1980) *Brain Res.* **104**, 99-108.
86. Parsons, B. & Rainbow, T.C. (1983) *Neurosci. Lett.* **36**, 9-12.
87. Cross, A.J., Crow, T.J., Johnson, J.A., Perry, E.K., Perry, R.J., Blessed, G. & Tomlinson, B.E. (1984) *J. Neurol. Sci.* **64**, 109-117.
88. Middlemiss, D.N., Palmer, A.M., Edel, N. & Bowen, D.M. (1986) *J. Neurochem.* **46**, 993-996.

89. Cross, A.J., Crow, T.J., Ferrier, I.N., Johnson, J.A., Bloom, S.R. & Corsellis, J.A.N. (1984) *J. Neurochem.* **43**, 1574-1581.
90. Perry, E.K., Perry, R.H., Candy, J.M., Fairbairn, A.F., Blessed, G., Dick, D.J. & Tomlinson, B.E. (1984) *Neurosci. Lett.* **51**, 353-357.
91. Francis, P.T., Gladwell, R.T. & Holman, R.R. (1984) *Psychoneuroendocrinology* **9**, 69-76.
92. Francis, P.T. & Bowen, D.M. (1985) *Biochem. Soc. Trans.* **13**, 170-171.

TABLE 1. 5-HT Receptors in AD

Brain Region		*AD subjects (significant loss, as a % of corresponding controls)*				*References*
		[^{3}H] 5-HT Binding (5-HT_1 Type)	*[^{3}H] LSD Binding (5-HT_1/ 5-HT_2 Type)*	*[^{3}H]-Ketanserin Binding (5-HT_2 Type)*	*[^{3}H] 8-OH-DPAT* Binding (5-HT_{1_A}. Type)*	
Temporal cortex:						
Whole lobe		-	66	-	-	8
Brodmann area	21	69	-	-	-	40
	21	-	47	-	-	87
	21/22	-	-	-	NS	88
		54	-	36	-	89
		NS†	-	57	-	58
	38	-	-	-	NS	62
Frontal cortex:						
Brodmann area	4	NS	-	NS	-	89
	10	53	-	-	-	40
	10	-	74	-	-	87
	10	-	-	-	NS	62
	11	-	-	58	-	45
	9/46	-	-	-	52	58
Parietal cortex:						
Brodmann area	40	74	-	NS	-	90
	7/40	-	-	-	73	62
Entorhinal cortex:						
Brodmann area	28	-	-	42	-	90
Cingulate cortex:						
Brodmann area	24	NS	-	53	-	89
Hippocampus		60	-	NS	-	89

* 8-hydroxy-2-(di-n-propylamino) tetralin; † NS not significantly different from control.

TABLE 2. Brain tissue concentrations of SLIR (fmoles/mg protein)* in AD patients and controls

Samples obtained	Mean ± S.D. Controls (N)	AD (N)
Autopsy:		
Frontal cortex	164 ± 53 (26)	152 ± 58 (18)
Temporal cortex	456 ± 194 (9)	280 ± 101 (9)†
Neurosurgery:		
Frontal cortex	636 ± 342 (17)	958 ± 415 (4)
Temporal cortex	1363 ± 668 (14)	1034 ± 415 (9)

* SLIR was determined as previously described (81,82); † $p<0.02$ compared to control.

TABLE 3. SLIR (fmol/mg protein) release (mean ± S.D.) from tissue prisms prepared from neocortex obtained at diagnostic craniotomy of AD patients and controls*

K^+ concent. in medium (mM)	Control (N) Temporal Cortex	Control (N) Frontal Cortex	AD (N) Frontal Cortex
5	19 ± 7 (7)	16 ± 11 (7)	22 ± 9 (6)
50	59 ± 31 (8)†	52 ± 38 (7)†	67 ± 38 (6)†

* Incubations were as previously described (91,92) and SLIR was determined as in Table 2; † p at lease <0.05 compared to 5 mM K^+.

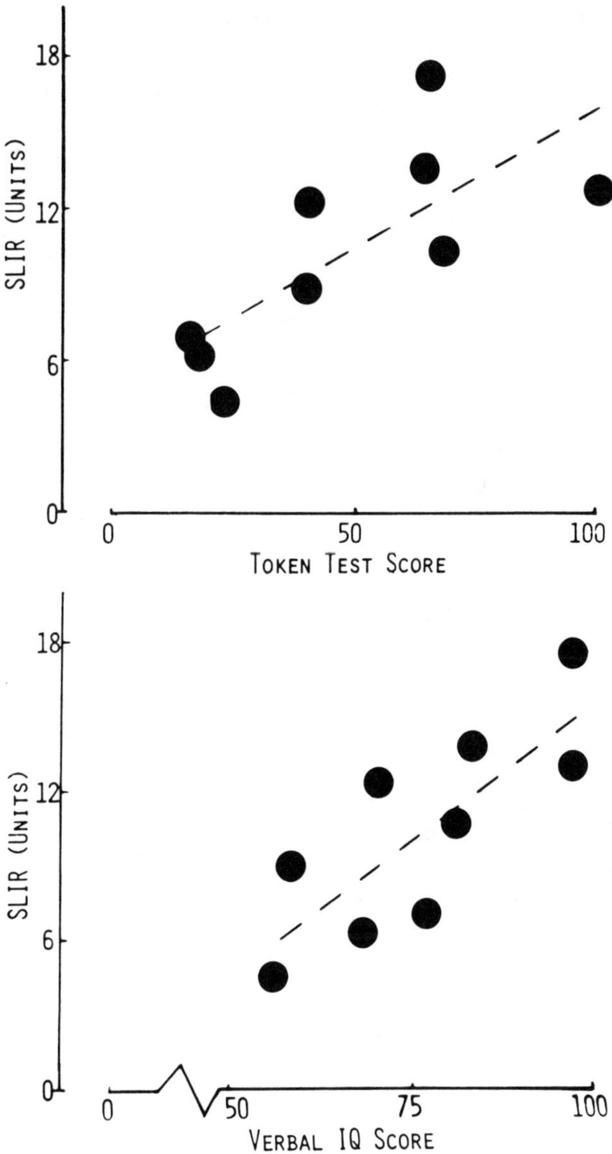

Figure 1. Relation (Spearman's rank correlation coefficient, R_S) between neuropsychological test scores and SLIR measurements on temporal cortex biopsy samples (units = 10^2 x fmoles/mg protein). Token Test score (units 0-100% correct) correlates with SLIR content, R_S 0.70 ($p<0.04$). Verbal IQ score (relative units) correlates with SLIR content, R_S 0.83 ($p<0.01$). Line (linear regression analysis) is for illustrative purposes. SLIR was determined as in Table 2.

3. Disturbances of Monoamine Systems in Brains of Patients with Alzheimer's Disease

CARL-GERHARD GOTTFRIES, M.D.

St. Jorgen's Hospital 422 03 Hising Backa Sweden

ABSTRACT: Twenty-two brains from patients with normal aging and 21 brains from patients with Alzheimer's disease (AD) or senile dementia of the Alzheimer type (SDAT) were investigated. The caudate nucleus and the hippocampus were analyzed for their content of the monoamines, their metabolites, choline acetyltransferase (CAT) and acetylcholinesterase (AChE). Significant correlations were seen between active amines and aging, whereas there were no significant correlations between the monamine metabolites and aging. In the brains from patients with AD or SDAT, concentrations of CAT, AChE, 5-hydroxytryptamine (5-HT) and 5-hydroxyindolacetic acid (5-HIAA) were reduced, and the catecholamines and their metabolites were reduced in some areas of these brains. Concentrations of phospholipids, cholesterol, cerebrosides and sulfatides were significantly reduced in white matter from the brains of patients with organic dementias.

Samples of cerebrospinal fluid (CSF) from patients with AD, SDAT or schizophrenia were investigated for their content of 5-HIAA, homovanillic acid (HVA) and 3-methoxy-4-hydroxphenylglycol (HMPG), and the patients were rated with a geriatric scale. Whereas the schizophrenics had normal levels of these metabolites in their CSF, patients with organic dementias had reduced concentrations of HVA. Significant correlations were found between concentrations of metabolites and the rated variables of mental impairment. It appears that both the levels of HVA and 5-HIAA and the ratio of 5-HIAA to HVA are significantly correlated with rated variables.

Introduction

To make progress in the clincial care of demented patients, it is important to have a relevant classification of the dementia disorders. The present classification is based on findings dating in part from the beginning of this century. It can be assumed that this classification can be improved.

At present, we subdivide dementias into two main groups: the primary degenerative disorders and the cerebrovascular diseases (multi-infarction dementia) (MID). Of the primary degenerative disorders, senile dementia is quantitavely the most important subgroup. Patients with an onset of the disorder after the age of 65 years and a slowly progressing course of the disease are considered to have senile dementia. Presenile dementia, Alzheimer's disease (AD), is a dementia with an onset before the age of 65 and is characterized histologically by senile plaques and fibrillary tangles in the brain tissue. At least some of the patients with senile dementia also have the above-mentioned (Alzheimer) lesions in their brains, and therefore they are said to have senile dementia of the Alzheimer type (SDAT).

Patients with AD and SDAT are often sampled as one group (AD/SDAT), yet it may be unwise to combine groups of patients with these two disorders, as it can be assumed that SDAT at least is a heterogenous group. Certainly the hereditary patterns of the two disorders indicate that they should be separated (1). There are also biochemical findings indicating that the disorders should be kept apart (2,3). We have some preliminary findings indicating that vitamin B_{12} may be of importance for dementia disorders with late onset (4).

Several reports have shown neurochemical changes in brains from patients with AD/SDAT. A disturbance of the cholinergic system has been reported (5), and some authors have given this cholinergic disturbance special etiological importance. There are investigations which have shown disturbances of other neurotransmitter systems as well (3,6).

Membrane lipids have been less studied in brains from demented patients. In 1978, Brun and Gustafson reported white matter degeneration in dementia, not only in patients with a cerebral vascular disorder but also in patients with AD/SDAT (7). The neuropathological picture was considered to indicate incomplete infarctions (8,9). Findings with nuclear magnetic resonance (NMR) in patients with dementia also revealed white matter changes in AD/SDAT and in MID (10).

This article reports biochemical findings from postmortem investigations of individuals with normal aging and of patients with AD/SDAT. Some reports from this work are already published (3,11-15). Some data from cerebrospinal fluid (CSF) investigations in patients with mental impairment will also be reported (16).

Material and Methods

At autopsy, 22 brains from patients with normal aging were dissected. The caudate nucleus and the hippocampus were dissected according to anatomical landmarks. The tissue was deep frozen, and a powder homogenate was formed for chemical analyses. One piece of white matter was taken from the centrum semiovale. Also, one piece of hippocampus and one piece of frontal cortex were taken for histological investigation. Brains from 21 patients with AD/SDAT were dissected in the same way. The diagnosis of AD/SDAT was made according to DSM-III, according to the macroscopic and microscopic findings of the brain tissue and according to dementia ratings made near the time of death by a nurse.

In the caudate nucleus and the hippocampus, 5-HT, 5-HIAA and HVA were determined according to Magnusson *et al.* (17). HMPG was determined according to Andersen *et al.* (18) and dopamine (DA) and noradrenaline (NA) according to Felice *et al.* (19) with some modification. CAT was determined according to Fonnum (20) as modified by Askmark *et al.* (21). Phospholipids, cholesterol, cerebrosides and sulfatides were determined in white matter by the methods of Svennerholm and Vanier (22) and Svennerholm and Fredman (23).

In 13 patients with chronic schizophrenia, 14 patients with AD and 26 patients with SDAT, 12-ml CSF samples were taken. Lumbar puncture was made under local anesthesia at 8:00 a.m. after an overnight bedrest with the patient still in bed. The sample was collected on ice, gently mixed to avoid gradient effects and immediately frozen and stored at -20° C without preservatives until analyzed. The CSF levels of HMPG, HVA and 5-HIAA were measured according to the method described by Andersen *et al.* (18). The patients with schizophrenia had been hospitalized for many years and showed the obvious symptoms of mental impairment usually described as schizophrenic dementia. The diagnoses of the organic dementias were made according to DSM-III, and all of the patients underwent routine laboratory blood testing to exclude other causes of dementia. EEG and cerebral computed tomography (CT) scans were used to exclude the presence of cerebrovascular disorders.

The patients with chronic schizophrenia, AD or SDAT were rated near the time of the lumbar puncture with the GBS rating scale (24). This scale is divided into three subscales measuring motor, intellectual and emotional impairment. It also includes six items measuring different symptoms common in dementia. Every variable has seven scale steps, of which 0, 2, 4 and 6 are clearly defined with 0 being equivalent to normal function or absence of symptoms, while 6 means total loss of function or maximal disturbance.

Group differences were analyzed according to Student's t-test, and the product moment method was used for analyzing the correlation between brain tissue biochemical concentrations and age. Correlations between monoamine metabolites in the CSF and clinical variables were analyzed with Spearman's rank correlation.

Results

The Influence of Age: The mean age of the 22 controls was 75.6 ± 10.5 (S.D.) years. The mean age of the 21 AD/SDAT patients was 79.3 ± 8.7. The difference was not significant. The controls included one patient aged 28 years who was excluded from the statistical analyses of the group differences.

As is evident from Table 1, the product moment correlation (r) between age and biochemical variables in brain tissue from normal aged patients is negative and statistically significant for age and 5-HT in the caudate nucleus, for age and NA in the hippocampus and for age and DA in the caudate nucleus as well as in the hippocampus. AChE activity in the caudate nucleus is also negatively correlated with age, and this correlation almost reaches statistical significance. Of interest is the fact that the metabolites are not significantly correlated with age; *i.e.*, in normal aging, the active amines decrease with age whereas the metabolite concentrations are still normal. If the concentrations of the active amines are related to the number of neurons and the metabolites are related to the release of neurotransmitter, then there are, in the normally aged brain, a loss of neurons but an increased speed of turnover in the remaining neurons (14).

Biochemical Findings in Brains from Patients with AD/SDAT: There was severely reduced (46% to 55%) CAT activity in the AD/SDAT brains (Tables 2 and 3). A disturbance of the cholinergic system was also reflected by reduced AChE activity, which neared statistical significance in the caudate nucleus. (For further information see ref. 12).

In the serotonergic system, there also were disturbances, as reflected by reduced concentrations of 5-HT and 5-HIAA. This also was true in the caudate nucleus and the hippocampus. The disturbance was almost as severe as the disturbance of the cholinergic system.

DA also was reduced, but the reduction did not reach statistical significance in the caudate nucleus. The principal metabolite, HVA, of DA was significantly reduced in the caudate nucleus but not in the hippocampus. NA showed a slight reduction in the two nuclei which was significant only in the hippocampus. HMPG was not reduced in the demented brains. (For further information see ref. 14).

The lipids in white matter were all reduced in the demented brains. Phospholipids and cholesterol were reduced to 75%, cerebrosides to 72% and sulfatides to 63% of the control values (Table 4).

Results from CSF Studies and Ratings: The chronic schizophrenic patients had only slight motor and intellectual impairment, whereas the emotional bluntness in these patients was striking (Table 5). The AD group had significantly less emotional impairment than the schizophrenics, and the SDAT group had significantly more intellectual impairment than the schizophrenics and the AD patients.

In the schizophrenics, the CSF concentrations of HMPG, HVA and 5-HIAA did not diverge from the reference limits of normal in our laboratory. The schizophrenics were divided into a group that had received continous neuroleptic drug treatment and another in which the neuroleptics had been withdrawn weeks before CSF sampling, and no differences were found between these two subgroups in the monoamine metabolites. There was a slight, insignificant reduction of HMPG in the AD group when compared to the schizophrenics, and HVA was significantly decreased in the AD and SDAT groups when compared to the schizophrenics. The AD group had significantly lower HVA concentrations than the SDAT group. Concentrations of 5-HIAA were not significantly reduced in the two groups with organic dementias when compared to the schizophrenics.

When the relations between the ratings and the biochemical variables in the CSF were analyzed, no significant correlations were found in the schizophrenic group. However, comparisons between biochemical variables and the ratings in the patients with organic dementias showed that HVA was negatively correlated with motor, intellectual and emotional impairment (Table 6). The correlation was statistically significant in the SDAT group but did not reach significance in the AD group. A surprising finding was that 5-HIAA in the AD group correlated positively with the rated variables; this correlation borders significance for motor impairment. However, when studying the same variables in the SDAT group, the correlations were in the opposite direction: 5-HIAA correlated significantly and negatively with motor impairment, and the correlation between 5-HIAA and emotional impairment was also negative and bordered significance. When the two groups were combined, all significant correlations between 5-HIAA and rated variables disappeared, and the only significant correlation that remained was the one between motor impairment and HVA.

The ratio between 5-HIAA and HVA also was correlated with the rated variables (Table 6). This ratio correlated better than 5-HIAA or HVA alone with the rated variables, at least in the AD group. It is obvious that motor, intellectual and emotional functioning are dependent, not only on DA and 5-HT metabolism, but also on the balance between these two systems.

Discussion

The data from the postmortem human brain investigations show that in patients older than 60 years there is an accelerated decrease of 5-HT, NA and DA. This decrease has been found in several other investigations (see 25) and indicates that in this age group, there is an involution taking place in the brain. The reduced concentrations of the active amines are not accompanied by a reduction of the metabolites 5-HIAA, HMPG and HVA in normal aging. This means that if the reduced concentrations of the active amines reflect a neuron loss, the remaining neurons have increased metabolism that evidently compensates for the loss.

In patients with AD/SDAT, there are multiple disturbances of neurotransmitters. We were able to confirm the reduced activity of CAT and of AChE. The 5-HT and 5-HIAA reductions indicate that the serotonin system is as severely disturbed as the cholinergic one. Also, the catecholamines are to some extent disturbed in the brains of patients with AD/SDAT. As shown in other investigations, the neuropeptides, somatostatin and substance P also are reduced in brains from patients with AD/SDAT (5).

In the brains from patients with AD/SDAT, there not only are disturbances in gray matter but also in white matter, as shown by reduced concentrations of myelin components. These extensive and multiple disturbances in brains from patients with AD/SDAT indicate that the findings may be secondary to a disturbance on a more basic level, the nature of which still is unknown.

In the brains of patients with AD/SDAT, there seems to be not only a disturbance due to a neuron loss but also a chemical lesion of the remaining neurons. These neurons seem not to be able to respond to feedback mechanisms in the same way as the neurons in the normally aged brain. At least the compensatory mechanism of increasing metabolic speed, as seen in the normally aged brain, does not function in the Alzheimer-demented brain. This finding may explain the disappointing results in pharmacological treatment trials. The neurons in the Alzheimer-demented brain do not respond to pharmacological provocation in the way we expect them to do.

Although the disturbances recorded in the brains from patients with AD/SDAT cannot be considered of primary etiological importance, they may have pathogenetic importance, causing the symptoms which impair the demented patient. In our investigation of CSF, we were able to support this assumption. There are significant correlations between the levels of monoaminergic metabolites in CSF and the rated mental impairment: the levels of HVA and 5-HIAA can be correlated with motor, intellectual and emotional functioning. The correlation is, however, somewhat complicated. It is not only the activity in the two systems that is of importance, but also the balance between HVA and 5-HIAA. The most evident correlations are seen between the ratio 5-HIAA to HVA and the rated variables. A relation between the 5-HT and the DA systems is discussed in other reports (26,27).

The investigation of CSF also shows that patients with chronic schizophrenia who have been hospitalized for many years and show signs of mental impairment do not have changes of their monoamine metabolites in CSF. Thus the reduced concentrations of HVA and 5-HIAA in patients with organic dementia seem not to be due to environmental factors.

Acknowledgments

This study was supported by grants from the Swedish Medical Research Council, King Gustaf Vth and Queen Victoria's Foundation, and the Lundgren's, Osterman's, Hjalmar Svensson's and Thuring's Funds.

References

1. Larsson, T., Sjogren, T. & Jacobson, G. (1963) *Acta. Psychiatr. Scand.* Suppl. 167.
2. Rossor, M.N., Iversen, L.L., Reynolds, G.P., Mountjoy, C.Q. & Roth, M. (1984) *Br. Med. J.* **288**, 961-964.
3. Gottfries, C.G., Karlsson, I. & Svennerholm, L. (1985) In: *Normal Aging, Alzheimer's Disease and Senile Dementia: Aspects on Etiology, Pathogenesis, Diagnosis and Treatment,* ed. Gottfries, C.G. (De l'Universite de Bruxelles, Bruxelles) pp. 111-118.
4. Regland, B. & Gottfries, C.G. (1986) (Submitted).
5. Reisberg, B. (1983) *Alzheimer's Disease: The Standard Reference.* (The Free Press, New York and London).
6. Hardy, J., Adolfsson, R. Alafuzoff, I., Bucht, G., Marcusson, J., Nyberg, P., Perdahl, E., Wester, P. & Winblad, B. (1985) *Neurochem. Int.* **7**, 545-563.
7. Brun, A. & Gustafson, L. (1978) *Arch. Psychiatr. Nervenkr.* **226**, 76-93.
8. Brun, A. (1983) In: *Alzheimer's Disease,* ed. Reisberg, B. (The Free Press, New York and London) pp. 37-47.
9. Brun, A. & Englund, E. (1986) *Ann. Neurol.* **19**, 253-262.
10. deLeon, M.J., George, A.E., Ferris, S.H., Christman, D., Gentes, C.I., Miller, J.D., Fowler, J., Reisberg, B. & Wolf, A.P. (1985) In: *Normal Aging, Alzheimer's Disease and Senile Dementia: Aspects on Etiology, Pathogenesis, Diagnosis and Treatment.* ed. Gottfries,

C.G. (De l'Universite de Bruxelles, Bruxelles.) pp. 199-202.
11. Carlsson, A. (1986) In: *Mental Health in the Elderly: A Review of the Present State of Research,* eds. Heffner, H., Sartorious, N. & Moschell, G. (in press).
12. Danielsson, E., Eckernas, S.A., Westlind-Danielsson, A., Nordstrom, O., Bartfai, T., Wallin, A. & Gottfries, C.G. (1986) In: *Muscarinic receptors and cGMP synthesis: Studies on human and rat tissues.* Danielsson, E., thesis, University of Stockholm.
13. Gottfries, C.G. (1986) *The l986 Sandoz Lectures in Gerontology* (Basle, Switzerland) (in press).
14. Gottfries, C.G., Bartfai, T., Carlsson, A., Eckernas, S.A. & Svennerholm, L. (1986) *Prog. Neuro-Psychopharmacol. Biol. Psychiatr.* (in press).
15. Oreland, L. & Gottfries, C.G. (1986) *Prog. Neuro-Psychopharmacol. Biol. Psychiatr.* (in press).
16. Brane, G., Gottfries, C.G., Gottfries, J., Karlsson, I. & Parnetti, L. (Submitted).
17. Magnusson, O., Nilsson, L.B., & Westerlund, D. (1980) *J. Chromatogr.* **221**, 237-247.
18. Andersen, O., Johansson, B.B. & Svennerholm, L. (1981) *Acta Neurol. Scand.* **63**, 247-254.
19. Felice, L.J., Felice, J.D. & Kissinger, P.T. (1978) *J. Neurochem.* **31**, 1461-1465.
20. Fonnum, F. (1975) *J. Neurochem.* **24**, 407-409.
21. Askmark, H., Aquilonius, S.M., Fawcett, P., Nordberg, A. & Eckernas, S.A. (1982) *Acta Physiol. Scand.* **116**, 429-435.
22. Svennerholm, L. & Vanier, M.T. (1972) *Brain Res.* **47**, 457-468.
23. Svennerholm, L. & Fredman, P. (1980) *Biochim. Biophys. Acta* **617**, 97-109.
24. Gottfries, C.G., Brane, G., Gullberg, B. & Steen, G. (1982) *Arch. Gerontol. Geriatr.* **1**, 311-330.
25. Gottfries, C.G., Adolfsson, R., Aquilonius, S.M., Carlsson, A., Eckernas, S.A., Nordberg, A., Oreland, L., Svennerholm, L., Wiberg, A. & Winblad, B. (1983) *Neurobiol. Aging* **4**, 261-271.
26. Fibiger, H.C. & Miller, J.J. (1977) *Neuroscience* **2**, 975-987.
27. Agren, H., Mefford, I.N., Rudorfer, M.V., Linnoila, M. & Potter, W.Z. (1986) *J. Psychiatr. Res.* (in press).

TABLE 1. Product moment correlation (r) between age and biochemical variables in brains from patients with normal aging

Age vs.:	*Nucleus caudatus* *r*	*No.*	*Hippocampus* *r*	*No.*
5-HT	-0.60*	22	-0.04	22
5-HIAA	-0.06	22	0.22	22
NA	0.20	22	-0.70*	22
HMPG	0.29	22	0.31	22
DA	-0.58*	22	-0.58*	22
HVA	-0.34	22	-0.15	22
CAT	0.27	20	0.32	22
AChE	-0.66‡	9	-0.43	10

* p<0.005; ‡ p<0.10.

TABLE 2. Neurochemical variables in nucleus caudatus from controls and patients with AD/SDAT

	Controls			*AD/SDAT*					
	No.	*Mean*	*S.D.*	*No.*	*Mean*	*S.D.*	*t**	*p*	*%*
5-HT (ng)	21	254	96	20	200	74	2.06	0.05	79
5-HIAA (nmol/g)	21	594	337	20	319	19	3.54	0.002	79
NA (ng)	21	28	16	20	22	19	1.09	>0.20	79
HMPG (nmol/g)	21	0.36	0.22	20	0.36	0.11	-0.01	>0.20	99
DA (ng)	21	1827	754	20	1454	699	1.64	0.11	80
HVA (nmol/g)	21	18.1	5.7	20	12.8	5.0	3.17	0.003	71
CAT (ukat/kg protein)	19	4131	1253	21	2301	981	5.16	0.0001	56
AChE (mU/mg protein)	9	171	134	12	159	74	0.25	>0.20	93

*t = Student's t test.

TABLE 3. Neurochemical variables in hippocampus from controls and patients with AD/SDAT

	Controls			*AD/SDAT*					
	No.	*Mean*	*S.D.*	*No.*	*Mean*	*S.D.*	*t**	*p*	*%*
5-HT (ng)	21	52.05	25.2	19	31.2	15.3	3.26	0.003	59
5-HIAA (nmol/g)	21	288	115	19	164	69	4.16	0.0002	57
NA (ng)	21	19.4	6.2	19	15.2	6.4	2.10	0.05	78
HMPG (nmol/g)	21	0.36	0.16	20	0.39	0.17	-0.56	>0.20	108
DA (ng)	21	20.6	16.0	19	9.1	10.8	2.64	0.01	44
HVA (nmol/g)	21	1.8	0.7	20	1.6	1.3	0.54	>0.20	89
CAT (ukat/kg protein [left])	21	488	329	19	223	206	3.08	0.005	46
CAT (ukat/kg protein [right])	19	504	268	19	241	218	3.32	0.002	48
AChE (mU/mg protein)	10	1291	385	9	927	456	1.89	0.07	72

*t = Student's t test.

TABLE 4. Neurochemical variables in white matter from controls and patients with AD/SDAT

	Controls			*AD/SDAT*					
	No.	*Mean*	*S.D.*	*No.*	*Mean*	*S.D.*	*t**	*p*	*%*
Phospholipids	17	97.0	11.4	13	73.0	14.6	5.08	0.0001	75
Cholesterol	17	122.0	16.2	13	84.3	20.2	4.16	0.0003	75
Cerebrosides	17	39.5	6.4	13	28.3	5.4	5.14	0.0001	72
Sulfatides	14	15.9	4.0	13	10.0	2.6	4.49	0.0001	63

*t = Student's t test.

TABLE 5. Age, rated impairment and CSF variables expressed as means (M) ± standard deviations (SD) in chronic schizophrenics and patients with Alzheimer's disease (AD) and senile dementia of Alzheimer type (SDAT). Group differences according to Student's t-test

	I *AD* *(n=14)* *M* ± SD	*I/II*	*II* *SDAT* *(n=26)* *M* ± SD	*III* *AD/SDAT* *(n=40)* *M* ± SD	*IV* *SCHIZ* *(n=13)* *M* ± SD	*I/ IV*	*II/ IV*	*III/ IV*
Age	63.8 ± 8.7		78.2 ± 6.3	73.6 ± 9.7	76.5 ± 10.1			
GBS scores:								
- motor	1.9 ± 1.9		2.1 ± 1.7	2.0 ± 1.8	1.5 ± 1.1			
- intell.	2.7 ± 1.8	*	3.5 ± 1.6	3.2 ± 1.7	2.2 ± 1.3		*	*
- emotional	2.1 ± 1.8	†	2.9 ± 2.0	2.6 ± 2.0	3.1 ± 1.7	*		
HMPG (nmol/1)	44 ± 12		52 ± 21	49 ± 19	51 ± 15			
HVA (nmol/1)	140 ± 43	*	236 ± 140	202 ± 123	387 ± 147	‡	*	‡
5-HIAA (nmol/1)	95 ± 42		128 ± 48	117 ± 50	150 ± 43			†

* p<0.05; † p<0.10; ‡ p<0.005.

TABLE 6. Spearman's correlation coefficient between rated motor, intellectual and emotional impairment and CSF-levels of HVA, 5-HIAA and the ratio of 5-HIAA/HVA

GBS Scores	*Motor Impairment*	*Intellectual Impairment*	*Emotional Impairment*
AD (No.=14)			
HVA	-0.35	-0.34	-0.27
5-HIAA	0.50†	0.45	0.27
5-HIAA/HVA	0.65*	0.62*	0.40
SDAT (No.=26)			
HVA	-0.48‡	-0.39*	-0.49‡
5-HIAA	-0.40*	-0.26	-0.36†
5-HIAA/HVA	0.40*	0.37†	0.40*
AD/SDAT (No.=40)			
HVA	-0.36*	-0.24	-0.32*
5-HIAA	-0.01	0.11	-0.08
5-HIAA/HVA	0.48§	0.39*	0.37*

* p<0.05; † p<0.10; ‡ p<0.01; § p<0.005.

4. Anatomy and Functions of the Rostral Cholinergic Column: Implications for the Pathophysiology of Alzheimer's Disease

H. C. FIBIGER, Ph.D.
C. L. MURRAY

Division of Neurological Sciences
Department of Psychiatry University of British Columbia
Vancouver, B.C. V6T 1W5, Canada

ABSTRACT: The rostral cholinergic column is a continuous group of cholinergic neurons that extends from the medial septal nucleus rostrally to the nucleus basalis (nBM) caudally. Although most research on cholinergic mechanisms in Alzheimer's disease (AD) has focused on the nBM, the entire rostral cholinergic column degenerates in this condition. Animal studies have been used to determine the extent to which damage to the rostral cholinergic column, particularly the nBM, contributes to the learning and memory deficits seen in AD. Ibotenic-acid lesions of the nBM in rats produce learning and memory impairments on a variety of behavioral tests. Many of these deficits can be rapidly and significantly ameliorated either by acetylcholinesterase (AChE) inhibitors or by muscarinic-receptor agonists. Such studies suggest that damage to the rostral cholinergic column contributes to some of the cognitive impairments as seen in AD. They also indicate that further clinical research on the use of cholinomimetic drugs in the treatment of AD may be worthwhile.

Cholinergic Mechanisms in Alzheimer's Disease

Cholinergic neurons in the basal forebrain form a continuous column of cells delimited by the medial septal nucleus rostrally and the nucleus basalis (nBM) caudally. Satoh, Armstrong and Fibiger (1) have referred to this group of neurons as the "rostral cholinergic column" in order to distinguish it from the caudal cholinergic column, which is located in the brain-stem. There is now a large literature, reviewed elsewhere in this volume, indicating that the cholinergic neurons in the nBM either degenerate or undergo marked shrinkage in Alzheimer's disease (AD).

For reasons that are not clear, much of the research on cholinergic systems in AD has been preoccupied with the nBM; this has had the unfortunate effect of suggesting that cholinergic neurons in the nBM are somehow pivotally involved in the pathophysiology of AD. In fact, there is strong evidence that the whole of the rostral cholinergic column is damaged in AD. For example, in those studies where choline acetyltransferase (CAT) activity has been measured in both the hippocampus and the cerebral cortex, the decrease is generally as great in the hippocampus (which receives most of its cholinergic innervation from neurons in the medial septum and nucleus of the diagonal band) as it is in the cortex (which is primarily innervated by cholinergic neurons in the nBM) (2,3). Therefore, the rostral cholinergic column as a whole appears to degenerate in AD, and at present, there is no evidence to suggest that the nBM, as opposed to the rest of the rostral cholinergic column, is particularly vulnerable in this condition.

The extent, if any, to which the neurons which form the caudal cholinergic column are damaged in AD is not known. These cells also appear to form a continuous group which is delimited by the caudal part of the substantia nigra rostrally and by the laterodorsal tegmental nucleus caudally (1). The ascending projections of these cells include the tectum, thalamus and medial prefrontal cortex (4). Although indirect, evidence indicating that CAT activity is reduced in the thalamus of patients with AD raises the possibility that the caudal cholinergic column is also damaged in this condition (2). Nevertheless, quantitative histological studies of the integrity of the caudal cholinergic column will be required to determine if this cell group contributes to the pathophysiology of AD.

Although neurons of the rostral cholinergic column are reliably damaged in AD, it is becoming increasingly clear that AD cannot simply be considered to be a cholinergic deficit syndrome. Many noncholinergic neuronal systems are also impaired to various degrees. For example, there is evidence that noradrenergic (5,6), serotoninergic (6,7) and somatostatin-containing (8,9) neurons are damaged or lost in AD. In addition, chemically unspecified neurons are lost in both the hippocampus and the neocortex of AD brains (7,10). It is becoming increasingly clear, therefore, that AD is a heteroneuronal disease state. Given this, it is important to determine what symptoms of the disease are specifically associated with impaired cholinergic function and to distinguish them from those that are due to damage to the noncholinergic systems. This is important from both theoretical and clinical perspectives. For example, to date, attempts to treat symptoms of AD with cholinergic precursors, acetylcholinesterase (AChE) inhibitors, or muscarinic-receptor agonists have met with only limited success

(11,12). One reason for this may be that only those symptoms associated with impaired cholinergic function would be expected to be improved by this type of chemical replacement therapy; cholinergic agonists would not be expected to have an effect on those aspects of the syndrome caused by damage to the noncholinergic systems. If the specific symptoms that result from impaired cholinergic function could be delineated, then it might be possible to focus clinical research with cholinergic agonists on those symptoms and thereby more thoroughly assess the potential utility of cholinergic replacement therapy. Furthermore, other pharmacological strategies would have to be developed to deal with those symptoms associated with the loss of noncholinergic systems.

Some Animal Models of Cholinergic Dysfunction

One approach to determining the role of impaired cholinergic function in AD is to study the effects of lesions of cholinergic neurons in the basal forebrain on various behaviors in animals. A neurotoxin that is specific for cholinergic neurons would be ideal for this purpose. Unfortunately, sufficiently specific neurotoxins are not at present available. One early candidate, AF64A (13), has some degree of selectivity for cholinergic neurons but causes an unacceptable amount of damage to noncholinergic neurons when injected directly into brain tissue (Fibiger, unpublished observations). Another approach has been to create electrolytic lesions in regions of the basal forebrain that contain cholinergic perikarya. Unfortunately, much of the rostral cholinergic column is located in fiber-rich regions of the forebrain. For example, in the rat many neurons of the nBM are located between fascicles of the internal capsule (14). Electrolytic lesions of these cells would unavoidably produce extensive damage to this major fiber bundle, thus making interpretation of the behavioral data almost impossible. A third approach has been to use neurotoxins such as kainic acid or ibotenic acid that have only minor, if any, effects on axons passing through the volume of the lesion. Of these two toxins, ibotenic acid is greatly preferred because, unlike kainic acid, it does not result in lesions distant from the injection site (15,16). In fact, in the absence of thorough histological analysis that specifically demonstrates an absence of distant lesions, studies involving kainic acid-induced lesions of the rostral cholinergic column are open to question and of limited value. Data generated by studies using ibotenic-acid lesions are also not without interpretative limitations. For example, noncholinergic neurons are intermixed with cholinergic cells throughout the rostral cholinergic column, and these neurons will also be damaged by ibotenic acid injections in this region. The extent to which resulting behavioral deficits can be attributed to the loss of cholinergic neurons must therefore be carefully considered. If these deficits are reversed by cholinergic agonists, then this increases the probability (but does not prove) that they were the result of damaged cholinergic neurons.

Effects of nBM Lesions on Learning and Memory

Despite the caveats mentioned above, there is growing evidence from animal research that the rostral cholinergic column plays an important role in learning and memory. Most of the recent work using ibotenic-acid lesions has been concerned with the caudal part of the rostral cholinergic column, the nBM. Lesions in this region of the basal forebrain affect both the acquisition and retention of a variety of learned behaviors. For example, either acquisition or retention of the following tasks is impaired by ibotenic-acid lesions of the nBM: passive avoidance conditioning (17-21), win-shift or win-stay spatial alternation in a T-maze (19,22-24), win-shift spatial discrimination in radial arm mazes (19,21,25-27) and spatial navigation in a Morris water maze (28).

Although learning and memory related interpretations have most frequently been applied to explain the effects of these lesions, the possibility that other factors, such as changes in motor function, attention or arousal, may contribute to these findings cannot be ruled out completely. However, the fact that the lesions impair performance on some but not all tasks (22,24,27), and that deficits are seen in tasks that vary in response requirements, type of motivation, reinforcement and response-reinforcement contingency, suggests that the behavioral effects of these lesions are caused by an impairment in learning and/or memory. The exact nature of the learning-memory deficit is somewhat controversial. Some investigators have observed that nBM lesions have their most potent effects on trial-dependent tasks (working memory) (24,27), whereas others have observed that trial-independent tasks (reference memory) are more severely affected (22,25,28). Many procedural factors, including preoperative *vs.* postoperative training, the extent and location of the lesion and the time of testing after lesion creation (21) could account for some of these apparent discrepancies. It is also likely that current conceptualizations concerning (a) different types of learning and memory and (b) the processes that are being measured by different behavioral tasks are inadequate.

Specific examples from this laboratory of the nature and extent of the deficits that can be produced by ibotenic-acid lesions of the nBM are presented below. In all experiments, rats received bilateral, stereotaxically guided injections of ibotenic acid (5 $\mu g/\mu l$) into the region of the nBM. These lesions typically decrease CAT activity in the anterior neocortex by about 40% and in the posterior neocortex by about 15% but do not have significant effects on hippocampal CAT activity (22,25).

Radial Arm Maze

The first study examined the effects of nBM lesions on spatial learning in a 16-arm radial maze. Six weeks after creation of the ibotenic-acid lesions, the animals were food-deprived and maintained at 85% of free-feeding body weight for the duration of the experiment. Each animal was assigned a random set of nine maze arms which served as the baited set. This set remained the same throughout the experiment for any given rat, although it was different for each animal. This controlled for possible directional preferences with respect to external cues, as well as for odor cues, by ensuring that every arm was baited at some point during testing. Prior to training, the animals were accustomed to the cereal "Froot Loops," which was used as the reinforcer, by placing pieces in their home cages for several consecutive days. Froot Loops were also spread liberally around the outside of the maze to further control for odor cues.

The animals were initially adapted by allowing them to explore the maze and eat from the center hub and the arms of the baited set for 15 min on 2 consecutive days. No reinforcement was ever placed at the entrance to or down an arm not in the baited set. On the third day, testing commenced. At the beginning of each daily trial, the rat was placed in the center of the maze and permitted to choose among the arms until it either successfully completed the trial (*i.e.*, obtained all nine rewards) or until 15 min elapsed. An arm choice was defined as all four of the rat's legs crossing an arm threshold. Arm choices, as well as the time required to complete the trial, were recorded. This acquisition phase continued for 35 days. At the end of the 5-week training period, the animals were run for an additional 2 days. On the third day, they received intraperitoneal (i.p.) injections of physostigmine sulfate (0.5 mg/kg) 30 min prior to behavioral testing. This dose may have been too high for the control animals, as they did not move after being placed in the maze. For this reason, testing of the control group was discontinued at this point. This was not the case for the nBM-lesioned animals, and consequently this group continued to receive daily physostigmine injections prior to behavioral testing for 7 days.

At the beginning of the training period, both lesioned and control groups performed at approximately chance levels (Fig. 1). With additional training, the performance of the control animals gradually improved, so that by the fifth week these animals correctly chose the baited arms on 86% of the first nine arm entries. In contrast, the nBM-lesioned group failed to reach this level of performance during the 5-week period, making only 62% correct choices during the last week (Fig. 1). Analysis of variance of the learning scores revealed a significant difference between the performance of the control and nBM-lesioned groups ($p<0.0001$), a significant effect of training ($p<0.0001$) and a significant group x training interaction ($p<0.001$) over the 5-week period. The sigificant interaction indicates that the control group improved at a rate that was significantly greater than that of the nBM-lesioned animals.

The effect of physostigmine on the performance of the nBM-lesioned animals is presented in the right-hand panel of Figure 1. In the statistical analyses (correlated t-tests), the seven daily scores of each animal during the week of physostigmine administration were averaged and compared to the average performance during the 7 predrug days. Analyses of the data from the nBM-lesioned animals revealed a significant improvement when compared to the last week of acquisition ($p<0.001$). Further analyses indicated that this improvement in performance did not change significantly over the 7 days of drug treatment, suggesting that the attenuation of the spatial memory deficit with daily pretreatment with physostigmine was rapid and already fully evident on the first day of physostigmine treatment.

Spatial Alternation in a T-Maze

Other experiments have examined the effect of ibotenic-acid lesions of the nBM on reinforced spatial alternation in a T-maze and the extent to which physostigmine or the muscarinic-receptor agonist pilocarpine could reverse any lesion-induced deficits.

Physostigmine: Rats were accustomed to run for food by placing them in a T-maze with all doors raised and allowing them to eat Froot Loops from along both goal arms and in the food receptacles in the goal boxes for 20 min on each of 2 consecutive days. On the third day, testing commenced, and the rats were trained under conditions of contingent reinforcement for alternation. On each trial, the rat was placed in the start box; the door was raised and then closed after the rat moved out. When the rat entered a goal box, the door of the goal box was closed, and the rat was confined there for approximately 10 sec. On the first trial each day, a response to either the left or the right goal arm was reinforced. On subsequent trials, the rat was rewarded only if it went into the goal arm opposite that entered on the previous trial. Reward consisted of one Froot Loop located in a plastic cup at the end of the goal box. The intertrial interval was as brief as possible—the time required to remove the rat from the goal box and replace it in the start box. Errors were punished by confining the rat in the empty goal box for the same length of time (8-10 sec) as for positive reinforcement. This acquisition period continued for 18 daily sessions of six trials each, or five opportunities to alternate.

At the end of the acquisition period, the number of trials in each session was increased to 10, and the animals were run for an additional 4 days. On the next day, both groups received i.p. injections of methylscopolamine hydrobromide (1.0 mg/kg) 35 min prior to testing and physostigmine sulfate (0.5 mg/kg) 30 min prior to testing. This procedure was repeated for 8 days, following which the animals were tested for 5 days without drug treatment.

Figure 2 shows the alternation scores of both groups during the 18-day acquisition period. A two-way analysis of variance indicated a significant difference between the performance of the two groups ($p<.0001$) and a significant group x days interaction ($p<.05$); however, the overall effect of training was not significant. The significant interaction suggests that the control group learned at a greater rate than the nBM-lesioned group.

The effects of the physostigmine administration are presented in Figure 3. A two-way analysis of variance of the 8 days of drug treatment revealed no difference between the performances of the two groups, no significant group x days interaction and no effect of training. It is apparent that the physostigmine treatment moved the performance of the lesioned animals close to that of the controls.

The findings of this experiment provide further evidence that rats display spatial memory deficits following lesions of the nBM. It was demonstrated that even after 35 days of training in rewarded spatial alternation, rats with nBM lesions were impaired. Physostigmine attenuated the performance deficit observed in the lesioned animals. This is consistent with the results of the drug manipulation in the radial arm maze experiment.

Pilocarpine: The procedure was the same as that in the previous experiment except for the following changes: subjects were given 10 trials in each daily session (nine opportunities to alternate); the acquisition period continued for 17 days; there was a 2-day predrug period following the acquisition period; drug administration consisted of i.p. injections of methylscopolamine hydrobromide (1.0 mg/kg) 20 min prior to testing and pilocarpine nitrate (3.0 mg/kg) 15 min prior to testing and this continued for 7 days; the animals were then tested for an additional 4 days without any drug treatment.

The performance during the 17-day acquisition period is presented in Figure 4. A two-way analysis of variance revealed a significant group difference ($p<.0001$) and a significant effect of training ($p<.0001$). There was no significant group × days interaction. A one-way analysis of variance of the performance of each group indicated that the control animals demonstrated significant learning over the acquisition period ($p < .0001$). The nBM-lesioned animals' performance failed to change significantly over the 17 days of training. Nevertheless, examination of Figure 4 reveals that there was a trend toward improved performance in this group.

Figure 5 presents the alternation scores from the predrug, drug administration, and postdrug sessions. A two-way analysis of variance of the 7 days of pilocarpine administration revealed that there was no difference between the performances of the control and nBM-lesioned group, no group × days interaction and no effect of training. A comparison of the two groups by using each subject's mean alternation scores from the predrug (days 18-19), drug administration (days 20-26), and postdrug sessions (days 27-30) revealed that the performances differed significantly during the predrug sessions (p'.0001); however, the groups did not differ significantly during drug treatment. Inspection of Figure 5 reveals that, whereas the pilocarpine treatment improved the performance of the lesioned animals, it worsened the performance of the controls.

As was the case in the previous experiment, these results show that rats with nBM lesions are impaired on the acquisition of a rewarded spatial alternation task. These animals, in contrast to the controls, failed to demonstrate statistically significant learning, although there was a trend toward improved performance in the latter half of the 19-day acquisition period. The results of the drug manipulation are also consistent with the earlier experiments. Potentiation of central cholinergic tone with pilocarpine significantly and rapidly improved the performance of the nBM-lesioned animals. The decline in the performance of the control group, which was not observed in Experiment 2, may have been the result of excessive stimulation of postsynaptic cholinergic receptors. There is evidence that memory is differentially vulnerable to cholinergic manipulation as a function of the level of training (29), and it has been reported that there exists a narrow range at which augmentation of cholinergic function is beneficial (30). For the control animals, optimal levels of cholinergic activity that were present prior to drug administration may have been exceeded by the pilocarpine treatment.

Discussion

In the three experiments reviewed above, the lesioned animals were immediately and significantly improved by drug treatment. This was observed with both pilocarpine and physostigmine. Such findings suggest that nBM lesions may impair the accessing or retrieval of previously learned information, as opposed to affecting the storage of new information. If a certain level of cholinergic activity is important for certain types of learning to take place and if the drugs served to restore this level of activity, then the nBM-lesioned animals would have been expected to show a gradual improvement in performance across the drug days rather than the highly significant improvement that was already evident on the first day of drug treatment. Studies designed specifically to assess the possible differential effects of nBM lesions on information storage *vs.* retrieval would be of considerable interest.

The finding that the directly acting muscarinic-receptor agonist pilocarpine effectively reversed the deficits produced by the nBM lesions provides an interesting clue concerning the manner in which the nBM-cortical projection normally functions. This result suggests that the temporal pattern of stimulation of postsynaptic muscarinic receptors by acetylcholine is not an important variable in the transfer of information through this system. Rather, it appears that random occupancy of muscarinicreceptor sites is all that is required for adequate functioning of brain regions that are innervated by the nBM. In this respect, the nBM-cortical projection appears to be similar to the nigrostriatal dopaminergic system, where directly acting dopamine-receptor agonists reverse behavioral deficits produced by lesions of these dopaminergic neurons (31-33). This suggests that acetylcholine and dopamine may function more as neurohormones than as true neurotransmitters in projections of the nBM and substantia nigra, pars compacts, respectively. The fact that fetal grafts of dopaminergic neurons transplanted into the striatum (34) or of cholinergic neurons into the hippocampus (35) can reverse some of the impairments caused by lesions of intrinsic dopaminergic and cholinergic neurons, respectively, is consistent with this possibility.

The present findings provide further evidence that the nBM is important in the learning and memory of spatial tasks, and they indicate that degeneration of this structure may be responsible for some of the cognitive deficits manifested by patients with AD. A better delineation of the functions of other cholinergic systems, including the septohippocampal projection, is required to determine the extent to which the components of the rostral cholinergic column specifically contribute to the memory impairments characteristic of AD. The success with which pilocarpine and physostigmine can attenuate the deficits produced by the nBM lesions would seem to justify continued clinical research with cholinomimetics in patients with AD.

References

1. Satoh, K., Armstrong, D.M. & Fibiger, H.C. (1983) *Brain Res. Bull.* **11**, 693-720.
2. Davies, P. (1979) *Brain Res.* **171**, 319-327.
3. Rossor, M.N., Rehfeld, J.F., Emson, P.C., Mountjoy, C.Q., Roth, M. & Iversen, L.L. (1981) *Life Sci.* **29**, 405-410.
4. Satoh, K. & Fibiger, H.C. *J. Comp. Neurol.* (in press).
5. Bondareff, W., Mountjoy, C.Q. & Roth, M. (1982) *Neurology* **32**, 164-168.
6. Adolfsson, R., Gottfries, C.G., Roos, B.E. & Winblad, B. (1979) *Br. J. Psychiatr.* **135**, 216-223.
7. Bowen, D.M. (1983) *Banbury Rep.* **15**, 219-231.
8. Rossor, M.N., Emson, P.C., Iversen, L.L., Mountjoy, C.Q. & Roth, M. (1984) In: *Alzheimer's Disease: Advances in Basic Research and Therapies,* eds. Wurtman, R.J., Corkin, S.H. & Growdon, J.H. (Center for Brain Sciences and Metabolism Charitable Trust) pp. 29-37.
9. Davies, P., Katz, D.A. & Crystal, H.A. (1982) In: *Alzheimer's Disease: A Report of Progress in Research,* eds. Corkin, S., Davis, K.L., Growdon, J.H., Usdin, E. & Wurtman, R.J. (Raven Press, New York) pp. 9-14.
10. Ball, M.J. (1977) *Acta Neuropathol.* **37**, 111-118.
11. Bartus, R.T., Dean, R.L., Beer, B. & Lippa, A.S. (1982) *Science* **217**, 408-417.
12. Terry, R.D. & Katzman, R. (1983) *Ann. Neurol.* **14**, 497-506.
13. Mantione, C.R., Fisher, A. & Hanin, I. (1981) *Science* **213**, 579-580.
14. Fibiger, H.C. (1982) *Brain Res. Rev.* **4**, 327-388.
15. Guldin, W.O. & Markowitsch, H.J. (1982) *J. Neurosci. Methods* **5**, 83-93.
16. Stewart, D.J., MacFabe, D.F. & Vanderwolf, C.H. (1984) *Brain Res.* **322**, 219-232.
17. Flicker, C., Dean, R.L., Watkins, D.L., Fisher, S.K. & Bartus, R.T. (1983) *Pharmacol. Biochem. Behav.* **18**, 973-981.
18. Haroutunian, V., Kanof, P. & Davis, K.L. (1985) *Life Sci.* **37**, 945-952.
19. Hepler, D.J., Wenk, G.L., Cribbs, B.L., Olton, D.S. & Coyle, J.T. (1985) *Brain Res.* **346**, 8-14.
20. Altman, H.J., Crosland, R.D., Jenden, D.J. & Berman, R.F. (1985) *Neurobiol. Aging* **6**, 125-130.
21. Bartus, R.T., Flicker, C., Dean, R.I., Pontecorvo, M., Fiogueiredo, J.C. & Fisher, S.K. (1985) *Pharmacol. Biochem. Behav.* **23**, 125-135.
22. Murray, C.L. & Fibiger, H.C. (1986) *Behav. Neurosci.* **100**, 23-32.
23. Salamone, J.D., Beart, P.M., Alpert, J.E. & Iversen, S.D. (1984) *Behav. Brain Res.* **13**, 63-70.

24. Hepler, D.J., Olton, D.S., Wenk, G.L. & Coyle, J.T. (1985) J. *Neurosci.* **5**, 866-873.
25. Murray, C.L. & Fibiger, H.C. (1985) *Neuroscience* **14**, 1025-1032.
26. Dubois, B., Mayo, W., Agid, Y., LeMoal, M. & Simon, H. (1985) *Brain Res.* **338**, 249-258.
27. Knowlton, B.J., Wenk, G.L., Olton, D.S. & Coyle, J.T. (1985) *Brain Res.* **345**, 315-321.
28. Wishaw, I.Q., O'Connor, W.T. & Dunnett, S.B. (1985) *Behav. Brain Res.* **17**, 103-115.
29. Deutsch, J.A. (1971) *Science* **174**, 788-795.
30. Bartus, R.T. (1982) In: *Alzheimer's Disease: A Report of Progress in Research*, eds. Corkin, S., Davis, K.L., Growdon, J.H., Usdin, E. & Wurtman, R.J. (Raven Press, New York) pp. 271-280.
31. Lenard, L.G. & Beer, B. (1975) *Pharmacol. Biochem. Behav.* **3**, 887-893.
32. Ljungberg, T. & Ungerstedt, U. (1976) *Physiol. Behav.* **16**, 277-283.
33. Marshall, J.F. & Gotthelf, T. (1979) *Exper. Neurol.* **65**, 398-411.
34. Bjorklund, A., Stenevi, U., Dunnett, S.B. & Iversen, S.D. (1981) *Nature* **289**, 497-499.
35. Dunnett, S.B., Low, W.C., Iversen, S.D., Stenevi, U. & Bjorklund, A. (1982) *Brain Res.* **251**, 335-348.

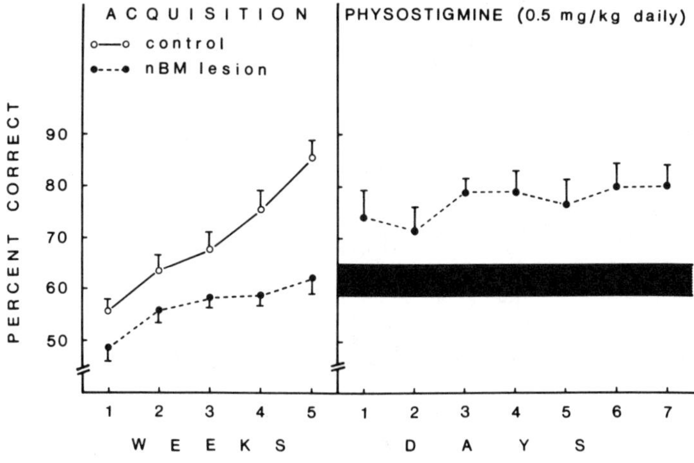

Fig. 1. The effects of ibotenate-induced lesions of the nBM on the acquisition (left panel) of a radial arm maze spatial-memory task. Data are expressed as the per cent of entries into food-containing arms (*i.e.*, correct entries) out of the first nine entries and reflect a general measure of performance. The effects of physostigmine sulfate given 30 min prior to each daily session are shown in the right panel. The shaded area indicates the average performance (± S.E.M.) of the nBM-lesioned animals during the 3 days prior to the first physostigmine injection. Data represent X ± S.E.M. of 9 or 10 animals in each group. (Reprinted from reference 25 with permission.)

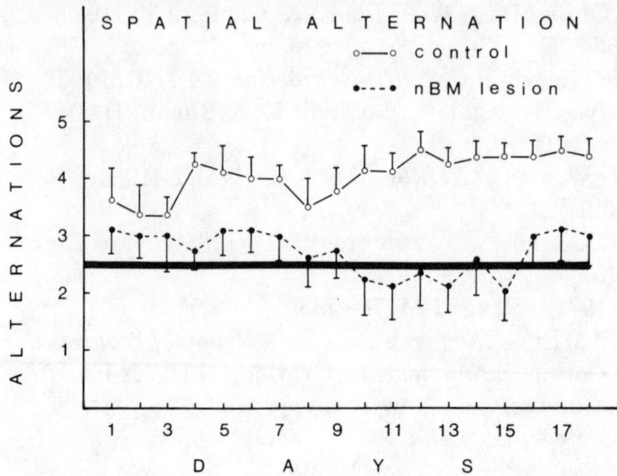

Fig. 2. Effects of ibotenate-induced lesions of the nBM on the acquisition of rewarded spatial alternation. Data are mean correct responses (alternations); vertical bars indicate S.E.M. The dark horizontal line indicates chance (50%) performance. The maximum number of possible alternations is 5. (Reprinted from reference 22 with permission.)

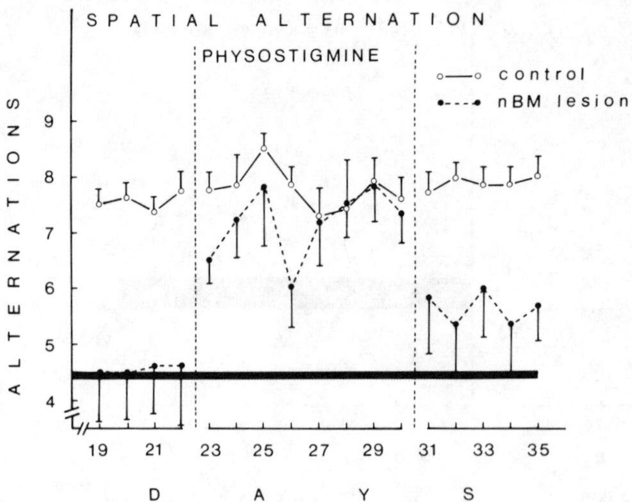

Fig. 3. Effects of physostigmine sulfate (0.5 mg/kg) administered 30 min prior to each test session on spatial alternation deficits produced by lesions of the nBM. Data are mean alternated responses; vertical bars indicate S.E.M. The heavy horizontal line indicates chance (50%) performance. The maximum number of possible alternations is nine. (Reprinted from reference 22 with permission.)

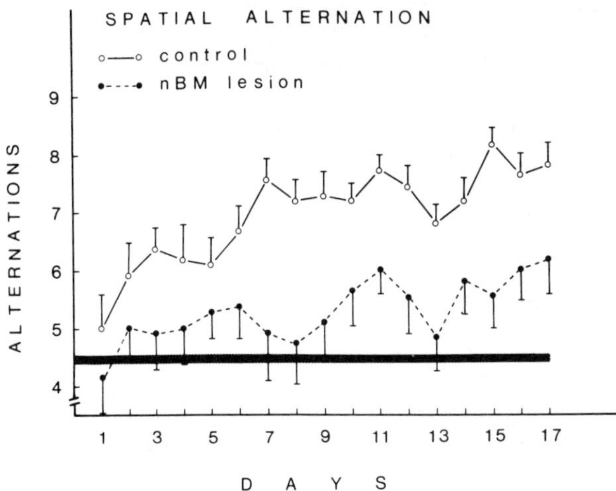

Fig. 4. Effects of ibotenate-induced lesions of the nBM on the acquisition of rewarded spatial alternation. Data are mean correct responses (alternations); vertical bars indicate S.E.M. The dark horizontal line indicates chance (50%) performance. The maximum number of possible alternations is nine. (Reprinted from reference 22 with permission.)

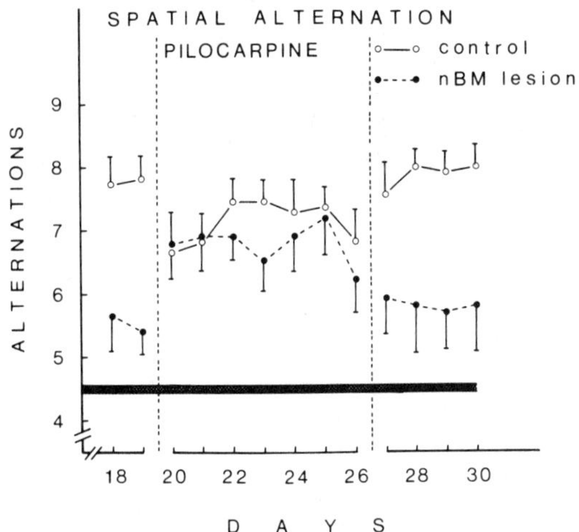

Fig. 5. Effects of pilocarpine nitrate (3 mg/kg) administered 15 min prior to each test session on spatial alternation deficits produced by lesions of the nBM. Data are mean alternated responses; vertical bars indicate S.E.M. The heavy horizontal line indicates chance (50%) performance. The maximum number of possible alternations is nine. (Reprinted from reference 22 with permission.)

5. Biochemical Neuroanatomy and Alzheimer's Disease

EDITH G. McGEER, Ph.D.
PATRICK L. McGEER, M.D., Ph.D.

Kinsmen Laboratory of Neurological Research
Department of Psychiatry University of British Columbia
2255 Wesbrook Mall Vancouver, B.C., Canada, V6T 1W5

ABSTRACT: Various neurotransmitter deficiencies have been reported in Alzheimer's disease, especially in the younger cases, but the most severe seems to be the cortical/hippocampal cholinergic defect. The cholinergic cells have been mapped in human brain using antibodies to choline acetyltransferase (CAT) and compared with structures staining for acetylcholinesterase (AChE). Counts of cholinergic cells throughout the area of the substantia innominata (basal forebrain) confirm the losses reported in Alzheimer's disease and show, moreover, age-related decreases in normal subjects and a highly significant correlation between cell counts and average cortical CAT.

γ-Glutamyl transferase (γ-GT) may be important in the transport of amino acids or peptides across the blood-brain barrier. γ-GT activities were the same in cortical samples from Alzheimer's and age-matched control brains, and there was no correlation between γ-GT and CAT or AChE levels, both of which were significantly reduced in the Alzheimer's samples. CAT and AChE activities were significantly correlated in both groups. CAT showed a negative correlation with age in the controls and a positive correlation in the Alzheimer's group.

In preliminary studies on sodium-dependent glutamate binding to cortical membranes, analysis of variance indicates the values for the Alzheimer's group are lower than those for controls but the large variability renders the data of little significance in individual cortical areas with the small numbers so far studied. Such binding may be an indicator of the integrity of glutamate nerve endings.

Introduction

The initial reports of the biochemical pathology of senile dementia of the Alzheimer's type (SDAT) came from three groups of investigators in the

United Kingdom who found sharply decreased levels of choline acetyltransferase (EC 2.3.5.6; CAT), the enzyme that synthesizes acetylcholine (ACh), in the neocortex, particularly in the hippocampus and temporal and frontal lobes (1-4). Since then, numerous groups have confirmed these findings, and much of the literature on the disease over the past 10 years has been focused on the cholinergic system because, although other types of neurons are also clearly involved, the defect in cholinergic activity seems to be the one most closely correlated with the memory losses. Much of our work in biochemical neuroanatomy has also been concentrated on the cholinergic system and aimed particularly at mapping this system, initially in the cat (5) and rat (6), but more recently in the human (7-11). In this paper, we review briefly the principal cholinergic systems identified in human and animal brains and discuss some of the problems in defining these systems in the human.

However, Alzheimer's disease (AD) clearly involves cortical pathology above and beyond degeneration of cortical cholinergic afferents. As part of a continuing study in possible pathology of SDAT, we have measured both sodium-dependent glutamate binding and γ-glutamyl transferase (EC.3.2.2; γ-GT) in cortical samples from SDAT patients and controls. The sodium-dependent glutamate binding may reflect the concentration of presynaptic glutamate uptake sites and thus the state of the glutamate nerve endings (12), whereas it has been hypothesized that γ-GT may be important in the transport of amino acids or peptides across the blood-brain barrier (13-15). Since some abnormality in the blood-brain barrier has sometimes been postulated in SDAT (16), we thought it would be worthwhile to examine this enzyme.

Cholinergic and Other Acetylcholinesterase-Positive Structures of the Human Brain

The cholinergic systems of the brain have now been described in several species using the technique of CAT immunohistochemistry. Maps of various degrees of completeness have been produced for the cat (5), rat (6-23), monkey (24-26), baboon (27) and human (7-11). There may be some species differences, but the general pattern is similar. There are relatively few major cholinergic cell groups in the brain. They can be thought of as five major systems, plus a few minor ones located mainly in the brain stem. The five major cholinergic systems are: the neostriatal-nucleus accumbens, the medial basal forebrain, the parabrachial, the reticular and the cranial motor (28). The minor systems include some nuclei associated with VIIIth nerve function such as the superior olive and some vestibular nuclei (28). Some small CAT-positive cells have been reported in the rat cortex, hippocampus and medial habenula

(18,19,21,22,29) and in the rat and cat red nucleus (5,6,24,30) but such neurons have not yet been identified in the human.

Neostriatal-Nucleus Accumbens Interneurons: It has long been known from lesions studies that internal systems of cholinergic neurons exist in the neostriatum and nucleus accumbens. Giant cells within these nuclei stain positively for CAT in all species so far studied (5,6,18,19,27) including the human (7). They constitute a surprisingly small percentage (<5%) of the total neurons in these nuclei considering the extremely high levels of ACh, CAT and acetylcholinesterase (AChE) found by biochemical measurement. Smaller cholinergic cells have also been reported in the striatum of the rat (18,31) and, although the giant cells are certainly the most prominent ones, they may not be the entire cholinergic population.

Quantitative studies in some cases of SDAT and controls of the numbers of large striatal cells stained either for CAT (7) or for AChE (32) suggest little or no pathological loss in these neurons. This is in accord with several reports indicating little loss of CAT activity in the striatum in most cases of SDAT.

The Medial Forebrain Complex: This is a more or less continuous sheet of giant cholinergic cells which starts anteriorly on the medial surface of the cortex and extends in a caudolateral direction, always maintaining its position close to the medial and ventral surfaces of the brain and terminating toward the caudal aspect of the lentiform nucleus. The names usually give to the various subregions of this complex, from rostral to caudal order, are: medial septal nucleus, nucleus of the vertical limb of the diagonal band of Broca, nucleus of the horizontal limb of the diagonal band of Broca, and the nucleus basalis of Meynert (S,V,H and M in Fig. 1) or substantia innominata. In animals, this complex has been shown to provide cholinergic innervation to the hippocampus, amygdala, interpeduncular nucleus and all neocortical areas (28,33). The horizontal portion of this complex has been mapped in the human by both CAT immunohistochemistry (7-10) (Fig. 1A) and AChE histochemistry (34). Price *et al.* (35-37) first reported loss of large cells from this area in SDAT. This finding has now been corroborated in a number of studies (7,9,10,38-46). In our own laboratory, we have been able to show that the giant cells of the medial basal forebrain are a single population of cholinergic cells (9) and, therefore, the dropout reported by Price *et al.* (35) represents a cholinergic population exclusively.

Counts of such cells in every tenth section across this region not only indicate a loss of SDAT (Fig. 1B,C,D) (7,9,10) but also a decrease with age in neurologically normal individuals (Fig. 1B) (9,10). The slope of the line of correlation is almost identical to that found for the average CAT activity in seven cortical regions as a function of age in controls (Fig. 1E);

and, in those brains where cortical samples were obtained before the brain was fixed for histological studies, there was a good correlation between the number of cholinergic neurons counted in the substantia innominata and the average cortical CAT measured (Fig. 1F). This finding provides some evidence that in the human, as in other species, much of the cortical cholinergic innervation arises from this group of cells.

Decreases in cortical CAT activity in neurologically normal individuals, such as indicated in Figure 1E, have been previously reported (47-52). It has also been reported that, as the figure also indicates, cortical CAT in SDAT increases with age, reflecting the generally more severe pathology in the younger cases.

Parabrachial System: This system is the most intense and concentrated cholinergic cell group in the brain stem. It surrounds the brachium conjunctivum commencing in the most rostral aspects of the pons and follows the direction of the brachium conjunctivum (superior cerebellar peduncles) in a caudodorsal direction. Various subnuclei are separately identified in this particular region, and the nomenclature varies somewhat from species to species. The most commonly described nucleus is the pedunculopontine tegmental nucleus in the lateral aspect at the most rostral portion of the complex (Fig. 2A and 2B). In the human, staining was also seen in the medial and lateral parabrachial nuclei. A few CAT-positive cells were also found in the human in the lateral lemniscus, and these may be related either to this parabrachial complex or to a cholinergic system associated with VIIIth nerve function.

Projections from the nuclei of this complex have been reported to the cortex, various thalamic nuclei, the hypothalamus, amygdala and substantia nigra, as well as some descending projections (28,33). Some of the ascending projections seem to be partly cholinergic, and some have been reported to contain substance P as a cotransmitter (53). However, much remains to be learned about the cholinergic tracts arising in this complex.

The Reticular System: This is composed of a scattered collection of very large cells extending throughout the gigantocellular and magnocellular tegmental fields of the reticular formation. Caudally, the gigantocellular and magnocellular CAT-containing neurons are gradually aggregated medially toward the granular layer of the raphe and ventrally to the area near the inferior olivary nucleus. Thus, these cells extend continuously from the rostral pons into the caudal medulla as a longitudinally oriented cluster. In the human, positively staining nuclei of this system include the reticularis pontis oralis and caudalis, reticularis tegmenti pontis, reticularis gigantocellularis, reticularis lateralis and the formatio reticularis centralis (medulla). Figures 3A and

3B are photomicrographs of some of the CAT-positive gigantocellular neurons in the human.

The cholinergic projections are largely unknown but probably include some to the spinal cord and cerebellum as well as ascending fibers to the thalamus and other rostral nuclei (28,33).

Motor Nuclei of the Peripheral Nerves: All motor nuclei of the cranial nerves (III-VII and IX-XII), as well as the nucleus supraspinalis, are CAT-positive in the human as well as other species. These are the counterparts of the cells in the anterior and lateral horns of the spinal cord which are also cholinergic. Figure 3C shows typical staining of cholinergic neurons in such a motor nucleus in the human.

The Vestibular System: As previously reported for the cat (5) and rat (6), minor staining of cells for CAT has been found in the human in components of the vestibular, and possibly the auditory, system. These include cells in the lateral vestibular nucleus and the superior olive (Fig. 3D) (11).

Methodology and Additional Acetylcholinesterase-Positive Structures: The cholinergic neurons of the human brain described above were mapped using a number of different antibodies to human CAT and brains which were obtained within six hours of death and fixed by perfusion. Satisfactory staining, particularly in the hindbrain, depended on the tissue being fresh and the vessels well enough preserved to permit the blood to be flushed out prior to the introduction of the fixative. Even so, the methodology is not sufficiently sensitive to provide information regarding fiber bundles and terminals, as was possible for fresh, well-fixed material in the cat (5) and rat (6). It is possible that some cholinergic structures were not stained. A possible example are the magnocellular neurons of the red nucleus which have been reported to stain positively for CAT in the cat (5) and rat (6,30) and to accumulate radioactive choline by retrograde flow from the spinal cord (54). This would suggest that the rubrospinal tract may be partially cholinergic. In the human, however, we have not seen strongly CAT-positive cells in this area, although there were strongly AChE-positive cells (11). It is not known whether this is a species difference or a relative insensitivity of the CAT immunohistochemical method in human tissue.

In the forebrain of animals, AChE histochemistry, particularly after pretreatment of the animals with diisopropyl fluorophosphate (DFP), seems to be a valuable tool for the detection of most cholinergic neurons (55). In the human, of course, pretreatment with DFP is not possible. AChE histochemistry without DFP pretreatment is useful in identifying cholinergic neurons of the medial basal forebrain complex, but the cholinergic neurons of the neostriatum and nucleus accumbens are often obscured by the dense staining of the neuropil.

In the brain stem, AChE histochemistry, even with DFP pretreatment, is not very useful in identifying cholinergic neurons because so many noncholinergic neurons are AChE-intensive. These include the catecholamine and serotonin neurons of the substantia nigra, locus coeruleus and raphe. The AChE-positive structures of human hindbrain have been mapped using a highly sensitive modification of the Karnovsky and Roots(56) procedure. The type of staining obtained is exemplified in Figures 4A and 4B. Under these conditions, all CAT-positive cells are also AChE-positive (Fig. 4A). In addition, however, as exemplified in Figures 2A and 4B, many CAT-negative neurons stain for AChE. Besides the previously mentioned catecholamine and serotonin neurons, such cells were noted in several sensory systems, including the nuclei gracilis and cuneatus, all of the sensory nuclei of the Vth nerve, the tractus solitarius and the auditory and vestibular sensory nuclei, cells and fibers in the inferior and superior colliculi, as well as the nucleus intercollicularis. Also staining for AChE were cells in the pontine gray matter and arcuate nucleus. The inferior olive and the dorsal and medial olivary nuclei showed some AChE staining (11).

The significance of the AChE-positive staining in most of these structures remains to be determined. It may be that the cells are cholinoceptive as many of them were so defined in the map of the cat brain (5). That would mean that afferent AChE-containing fibers to these structures represent terminal fields for true cholinergic neurons. Some may be cholinergic but not detectable with the relatively insensitive CAT immunohistochemical method. Future studies with more refined techniques will be necessary to define these details in the human and in other mammalian species.

The conditions necessary for AChE staining are far less exacting than those for CAT. The high sensitivity of the method of Tago *et al.* (57) for identifying AChE-positive structures, and particularly AChE-positive structures and true cholinergic cells, have been revealed by the correlative study of CAT and AChE-positive staining (11). It will be important to establish more exact connections in the future.

Sodium-Dependent Glutamate Binding

There is considerable evidence that glutamate serves as the transmitter for many cortical pyramidal cells and is important in both corticofugal and commissural pathways. Bowen and Davison (58) indicate that there is some loss of cortical pyramidal cells in SDAT. For this reason, it might be supposed that pathological changes in glutamate neurons might be important in SDAT, but a really satisfactory index of such neurons, useful in postmortem brains, does not exist. Greenamyre *et al.* (59)

reported that sodium-independent L-[^{3}H]-glutamate binding, as measured autoradiographically, was lower than normal in the cortex but normal in the caudate, putamen and claustrum in brain sections from SDAT patients. Biochemical assay of such binding in the caudate, on the other hand, was reported to show an increase in SDAT, which was thought to indicate reduced glutamate innervation with a compensating supersensitivity of receptors (60). Sodium-independent binding, in any case, presumably measures postsynaptic binding and is not a direct measure of the integrity of the glutamate neurons themselves.

Sadki *et al.* (61) report reduced levels of glutamate in cortical and subcortical areas of SDAT brains, whereas glutamate levels in the CSF have been found not to be significantly different from controls (62). Glutamate levels *per se*, however, are not a good index of glutamate neurons because of the existence of glutamate in all structures and many metabolic compartments.

Smith *et al.* (63) found normal potassium-stimulated release of glutamate from temporal lobe biopsy samples of SDAT patients despite the reduced acetylcholine synthesis seen in the same samples. This would argue against a marked effect on the glutamate systems, but further examination seems worthwhile. Studies in the caudates of normal rats and those with lesions of the corticostriatal glutamate tract suggested that sodium-dependent glutamate binding might be to presynaptic glutamate uptake sites and thus might be useful as an index of the integrity of glutamate terminals (12). Coross *et al.* (64) have similarly reported data indicating the association of sodium-dependent [^{3}H]-D-aspartate binding with high-affinity glutamate uptake sites in human brain. Preliminary studies in rats indicated the feasibility of doing such binding studies on frozen tissue.

The human brains used were all obtained between 2 and 24 hours after death. Seven cortical samples (cf Table 1), each weighing about 150-200 mg and free of pia mater, were rapidly dissected from each brain and stored at -70° C until used. Portions of these samples were used for the determination of CAT (65), AChE (66) or sodium-dependent glutamate binding. Preparation of the membranes and the binding assay procedure were essentially as previously reported (12) except that concentrations in the range of 0.125-1 μM [^{3}H]-L-glutamate were used for total binding, and specific binding was defined as that displaced by 5 mM L-glutamate. In each case, kinetic data were obtained on one or two of the cortical samples and the binding of the other samples determined at 0.51 μM of [^{3}H]-ligand. The brains were coded so that the nature of the case was not known to the person doing the assays.

The sodium-dependent glutamate binding tended to be similar in the various cortical samples from a single brain but showed a great deal of variability from brain to brain. In the small group studied, no relation could be seen with sex or age. There seemed to be a tendency toward lower values with greater the postmortem delay, but the correlation did not reach significance in this small group. There was no significant difference in the average postmortem delay, age or distribution of sexes between the SDAT and control groups.

The binding affinities determined by Scatchard plot also showed considerable variation from brain to brain, but there was no significant difference between the means for the SDAT (0.70 ± 0.58 μM) and control (0.82 ± 0.32 μM) groups. Overall, analysis of variance showed that the binding site density at 0.51 μM (Table 1) in the SDAT tissue was significantly lower than in control specimens ($F = 10.25$, $df = 94$). Very similar statistics were found when the B^{max} data calculated on the individually determined affinity constants were used (data not shown). The variability was such, however, that t-tests indicated no significant difference between the mean values obtained in any of the seven individual cortices, although the CAT data on these same cortices all revealed a significant difference between control and SDAT groups at the $p<0.01$ level (Table 1). There was no overall linear correlation between the individual CAT and glutamate binding data. In the control group, the calculated coefficients of correlation tended to be low and negative, whereas in the SDAT group they were all positive, and some (particularly in the temporal tip and frontal pole) almost reached significance. The K_d(s) found are in the same range as those reported by Cross *et al.* (64) for human cerebellar cortex; the densities of binding sietes are higher than those found by Cross *et al.* (64) but that would be expected since we were working with cortex whereas they were working with cerebellum. In our hands, sodium-independent binding in rat cerebellum is only about 45% of that found in cortex, and this is in accord with the much lower glutamate uptake in the former tissue (65). The data on sodium-dependent glutamate binding are in accord with the hypothesis of some pathology in cortical glutamate neurons in SDAT but might be taken to mean that the degeneration of cortical glutamate nerve endings may be less than the degeneration of cholinergic afferents. Lesion experiments in animals, however, suggest that the percentage loss in glutamate uptake sites is considerably less than the percentage loss in presumed glutamate nerve terminals, suggesting the presence of uptake sites on other structures, glia being a likely possibility. The small percentage loss in sodium-dependent glutamate binding may, therefore, reflect a larger loss in glutamate nerve endings. More data are clearly needed, particularly in view of the large variability encountered.

γ-Glutamyl Transferase

γ-Glutamyl transferase catalyzes the transfer of the γ-glutamyl group of various γ-glutamyl compounds to amino acids or peptides and is believed to function in the transport of amino acids and peptides across biological membranes (13,15). It has been isolated from brain microvessels and may play a role in transport across the blood-brain barrier (14,15). Recently Vesely and Cernoch (67) showed that microvessels from mouse, rat and bovine brains retained their γ-GT activity for at least four days postmortem and that reasonable activities could be measured in postmortem human brain. Since some abnormality of the blood-brain barrier has been frequently postulated in SDAT (16), it seemed worthwhile to measure γ-GT activities in SDAT as compared to control brains. Brain samples for this study were obtained and stored as described in the preceding section. The diagnosis of SDAT was based on histological determination of the numbers of plaques and tangles in cortical and hippocampal areas.

γ-GT was determined essentially by the method of Pajari (68). Initial experiments with portions of rat brain confirmed reports (67,68) that the amount of tissue and time of reaction were in the range giving linear results. The activities found for various rat brain regions were in good accord with those reported by others, and the activity of the homogenates prepared from fresh rat brain samples was similar to those found in homogenates of rat brain tissue stored for several days at -70° C before homogenization, indicating that frozen human samples probably could be used.

Nineteen brains from persons suffering from SDAT and 12 from neurologically normal controls were examined in this series. The SDAT cases ranged in age from 54 to 88 years (mean ± S.E. = 76.28 ± 1.43) and the controls from 51 to 98 years (78.75 ± 3.23). All patients were of western European extraction. There was no significant difference in mean delay between death and autopsy or in mean storage time at -70° C between the two groups, and no significant correlation of either of these variables or of sex with the enzyme data.

The mean γ-GT activities showed no significant difference between SDAT and control groups in any of the seven cortical regions examined (data not shown) or in the average cortical activity (Table 2).

As expected, the mean CAT activities in the SDAT cases were significantly lower than in the control cases in all the cortical regions examined (data not shown), as well as in the average for the individual brains (Table 2). AChE levels also were significantly lower in all cortical regions in the SDAT as compared to the control cases, and the correlation between the average individual CAT and AChE activities was highly significant in both groups (r = 0.577 for controls and r = 0.615 for SDAT cases). Neither CAT nor AChE activities were significantly correlated with γ-GT activities in either group.

The almost identical values obtained overall for γ-GT between the SDAT and control groups, as well as the lack of any correlation between CAT or AChE and γ-GT data, indicate that there probably is no gross abnormality in γ-GT in the cortex in SDAT such as is found in the enzymes related to the cholinergic system. These data therefore confirm the report of Bowen *et al.* (69) that the activity of an enzyme they called Y-glutamyl transpeptidase, but which is presumably γ-GT, is not abnormal in the prefrontal cortex in SDAT. Since the present data on γ-GT were obtained only at one, relatively low, concentration of the substrate, γ-glutamyl-p-nitroanilide, they do not rule out possible changes in γ-GT kinetics in SDAT, nor do they rule out possible shifts in the proportion of the various isoenzymes, assuming that such isoenzymes exist in human as in rat brain (70). In particular, since we used serine-borate buffer to produce individual assay "blanks," we would not have detected any difference that might exist between SDAT and controls in the isoenzyme not inhibited by this combination. However, these "blanks" were a very small fraction of total activity and seemed not to vary consistently with brain type.

Further work is clearly required to clarify these points but, insofar as the present data are negative and a role for the enzyme in transport across the blood-brain barrier can be assumed, these data are consistent with previous reports that the blood-brain barrier is not markedly affected in SDAT (71). It must be emphasized, however, that the relation of γ-GT to the blood-brain barrier is hypothetical; Bowen *et al.* (69) regarded the activity as an index of capillary density (58).

Acknowledgments

This research was supported by grants from the Medical Research Council of Canada, the Mr. and Mrs. P.A. Woodward's Foundation, the B.C. Medical Services Foundation and the Alzheimer's Support Association of B.C. We thank the Departments of Pathology in hospitals in the greater Vancouver area for their assistance with autopsies. The work reviewed includes that of many colleagues, in particular Drs. H. Kimura, K. Mizukawa, T. Nagai and H. Tago. We would also like to thank Joane Suzuki, Kim Singh, Ann Bui and Ron Walker for technical assistance.

References

1. Bowen, D.M., Smith, C.B., White, P. & Davison, A.N. (1976) *Brain* **99**, 459-495.
2. Davies, P. & Maloney, A.J.F. (1976) *Lancet* **2**, 1403.
3. Perry, E.K., Gibson, P.H., Blessed, G. & Tomlinson, B.E. (1977) *J. Neurol. Sci.* **34**, 247-265.
4. Perry, E.K., Perry, R.H., Blessed, G. & Tomlinson, B.E. (1977) *Lancet* **1**, 189.
5. Kimura, H., McGeer, P.L., Peng J.H. & McGeer. E.G. (1981) *J. Comp. Neurol.* **200**, 151-201.
6. Kimura, H., McGeer, P.L. & Peng, J.H. (1984) In: *Handbook of Chemical Neuroanatomy*, eds. Bjorklund, A. & Hokfelt, T. (Elsevier, Amsterdam) pp. 51-67.
7. Nagai, T., McGeer, P.L., Peng, J.H., McGeer, E.G. & Dolman, C.E. (1983) *Neurosci. Lett.* **36**, 195-199.
8. Nagai, T., Pearson, T., Peng, J.H., McGeer, E.G. & McGeer, P.L. (1983) *Brain Res.* **265**, 300-306.
9. McGeer, P.L., McGeer, E.G., Suzuki, J., Dolman, C.E. & Nagai, T. (1984) *Neurology* **34**, 741-745.
10. McGeer, P.L. (1984) *Can. J. Physiol. Pharmacol.* **62**, 741-754.
11. Mizukawa, K., McGeer, P.L., Tago, H., Peng, J.H., McGeer, E.G. & Kimura, H. (1986) *Brain Res.* (in press)
12. Vincent, S.R. & McGeer, E.G. (1980) *Brain Res.* **104**, 99-108.
13. Meister, A. (1973) *Science* **180**, 33-39.
14. Orlowski, M. & Meister, A. (1970) *Proc. Natl. Acad. Sci. USA* **67**, 1248-1255.
15. Orlowski, M., Sessa, G. & Green, J.P. (1974) *Science* **184**, 66-68.
16. Wisniewski, H.M. & Kozlowski, P.B. (1982) *Ann. NY Acad. Sci.* **396**, 119-129.
17. Eckenstein, F. & Sofroniew, M.V. (1983) *J. Neurosci.* **3**, 2286-2292.
18. Armstrong, D.M., Saper, C.B., Levey, A.I., Wainer B.H. & Terry, R.D. (1983) *J. Comp. Neurol.* **216**, 53-68.
19. Houser, C.R., Crawford, G.D., Barber, R.P., Salvaterra, P.M. & Vaughn, J.E. (1983) *Brain Res.* **266**, 97-119.
20. Levey, A.I., Wainer, B.H., Mufson, E.J. & Mesulam, M.M. (1983) *Neuroscience* **9**, 9-22.
21. Sofroniew, M.V., Eckenstein, F., Thoenen, H. & Cuello, A.C. (1982) *Neurosci. Lett.* **33**, 7-12.
22. Houser, C.R., Crawford, G.D., Salvaterra, P.M. & Vaughn, J.E. (1985) *J. Comp. Neurol.* **234**, 17-34.
23. Satoh, K. Armstrong, D.M. & Fibiger, H.C. (1983) *Brain. Res. Bull.* **11**, 693-720.

24. Hedreen, J.C., Bacon, S.J., Cork, L.C., Kitt, C.A., Crawford, G.D., Salvaterra, G.D. & Price, D.L. (1983) *Neurosci. Lett.* **43**, 173.
25. Mesulam, M.M., Mufson, E.J., Levey, A.I. & Wainer, B.H. (1983) *J. Comp. Neurol.* **214**, 170-197.
26. Mesulam, M.M., Mufson, E.J., Levey, A.I. & Wainer, B.H. (1984) *Neuroscience* **12**, 669-686.
27. Satoh, K. & Fibiger, H.C. (1985) *J. Comp. Neurol.* **236**, 197-214.
28. McGeer, P.L., McGeer, E.G. & Peng, J.H. (1984) *Life Sci.* **34**, 2319-2338.
29. Matthews, D.A., Salvaterra, P.M., Crawford, G.D., Houser, C.R. & Vaughn J.E. (1983) *Soc. Neurosci. Abstr.* **9**, 79.
30. Sofroniew, M.V., Eckstein, F., Thoenen, H. & Cuello, A.C. (1982) *Soc. Neurosci. Abstr.* **8**, 516.
31. Hattori, T., McGeer, E.G., Singh, V.K. & McGeer, P.L. (1977) *Exp. Neurol.* **55**, 666-679.
32. Parent, A., Csonka, C. & Etienne, P. (1984) *Brain Res.* **291**, 154-158.
33. McGeer, P. L. & McGeer, E.G. (1984) In: *Handbook of Neurochemistry*, 2nd edition. Vol. 6. ed. Lajtha, A. (Plenum Press, New York) pp. 379-410.
34. Hedreen, J.C., Struble, R.G., Whitehouse, P.J. & Price, D.L. (1984) *J. Neuropathol. Exp. Neurol.* **43**, 1-21.
35. Price, D.L., Whitehouse, P.J., Struble, R.G., Clark, A.W., Coyle, J.T., DeLong, M.D. & Hedreen, J.C. (1982) *Neurosci. Comm.* **1**, 84-92.
36. Whitehouse, P.J., Price, D.L., Clark, A.W., Coyle, J.T. & DeLong, M.R. (1981) *Ann. Neurol.* **10**, 122-126.
37. Whitehouse, P.J., Hedreen, J.C., White, C.L. & Price, D.L. (1983) *Ann. Neurol.* **13**, 243-248.
38. Mann, D.M.A., Yates, P.O. & Marcyniuk, B. (1984) *Mech. Aging Dev.* **25**, 189-204.
39. Mann, D.M.A., Yates, P.O. & Marcyniuk, B. (1986) *J. Neurol. Neurosurg. Psychiatr.* **49**, 310-312.
40. Perry, R.H., Candy, J.M., Perry, E.K., Irving, D., Blessed, G., Fairbairn, A.F. & Tomlinson, B.E. (1982) *Neurosci. Lett.* **33**, 311-331.
41. Rogers, J.D., Brogan, D. & Mira, S.S. (1985) *Ann. Neurol.* **17**, 163-170.
42. Saper, C.B., German, D.C. & White, C.L. III (1985) *Neurology* **35**, 1089-1095.
43. Tagliavini, F., Pilleri, G., Bouras, C. & Constantinidis, J. (1984) *Neurosci. Lett.* **44**, 37-42.
44. Tagliavini, F. & Pilleri, G. (1983) *Lancet* **1**, 469-470.

45. Wilcock, G.K., Esiri, M.M., Bowen, D.M. & Smith, C.C. (1983) *Neuropathol. Appl. Neurobiol.* **9**, 175-179.
46. Candy, J.M., Perry, R.H., Perry, E.K., Irving, D., Blessed, G., Fairbairn, A.F. & Tomlinson, B.E. (1983) *J. Neurol. Sci.* **59**, 277-289.
47. McGeer, E.G. & McGeer, P.L. (1975) In: *Neurobiology of Aging*, eds. Ordy, J.M. & Brizzee, K.R. (Plenum Press, New York & London) pp. 287-305.
48. Perry, E.K., Perry, R.H., Gibson, P.H., Blessed, G. & Tomlinson, B.E. (1977) *Neurosci. Lett.* **6**, 85-89.
49. Perry, E.K., Tomlinson, B.E., Blessed, G., Bergman, K., Gibson, P.H. & Perry, R.H. (1978) *Br. Med. J.* **2**, 1457-1459.
50. Davies, P. (1979) *Brain Res.* **171**, 319-327.
51. Rossor, M.J., Fahrenkrug., Emson, P.C., Mountjoy, C.Q., Iversen, L.L. & Roth, M. (1980) *Brain Res.* **201**, 249-253.
52. Allen, S.J., Benton, J.S., Goodhardt M.J., Haan E.A., Sims N.R., Smith, C.T., Spillane, J.A., Bowen D.M. & Davison, A.N. (1983) *J. Neurochem.* **41**, 256-265.
53. Vincent, S.R., Satoh, K., Armstrong, D.M. & Fibiger, H.C. (1983) *Nature* **306**, 688-690.
54. Pare, M.F., Jones, B.E. & Beaudet, A. (1982) *Soc. Neurosci. Abstr.* **8**, 517.
55. Lehmann, J. & Fibiger, H.C. (1979) *Life Sci.* **25**, 1939.
56. Karnovsky, M.J. & Roots, L. (1964) *J. Histochem. Cytochem.* **12**, 219-221.
57. Tago, H., Kimura, H. & Maeda, T. (1986) *J. Histochem. Cytochem.* (in press)
58. Bowen, D.M. & Davison, A.N. (1986) *Br. Med. Bull.* **42**, 75-80.
59. Greenamyre, J.T., Penney, J.B., Young, A.B., D'Amato, C.J., Hicks, S.P. & Shoulson, I. (1985) *Science* **227**, 1496-1499.
60. Pearce, B.R., Palmer, A.M., Bowen, D.M., Wilcock, G.K., Esiri, M.M. & Davison, A.N. (1984) *Neurochem. Pathol.* **2**, 221-232.
61. Sasaki, H., Muramoto, O., Kanazawa, I., Arai, H., Kosaka, K. & Iisuki, R. (1986) *Ann. Neurol.* **19**, 263-269.
62. Smith, C.C.T., Bowen, D.M., Francis, P.T., Snowden, J.S. & Neary, D. (1985) *J. Neurol. Neurosurg. Psychiatr.* **48**, 469-471.
63. Smith, C.C.T., Bowen, D.M., Sims, N.R., Neary, D. & Davison, A.N. (1983) *Brain Res.* **264**, 138-141.
64. Cross, A.J., Skan, W.J. & Slater, P. (1986) *Neurosci. Lett.* **63**, 121-124.
65. McGeer, E.G., Singh, E.A. & McGeer, P.L. (1986) *Alzheimer Disease and Associated Disorders Int. J.* (in press).
66. Sung, S.C. & Ruff, B.A. (1983) *Neurochem. Res.* **8**, 303-311.

67. Vesely, J. & Cernoch, M. (1984) *Neurochem. Res.* **9**, 917-923.
68. Pajari, M. (1984) *Int. J. Dev. Neurosci.* **2**, 197-202.
69. Bowen, D.M., Smith, C.B., White, P. & Davison, A.N. (1976) *Brain* **99**, 459-496.
70. Reyes, E. & Barela, T.D. (1980) *Neurochem. Res.* **5**, 159-170.
71. Dean, R.L. (1984) *Neurobiol. Aging* **5**, 357-359.

TABLE 1. Specific sodium-dependent binding at 0.51 μM [^{3}H]-L-glutamate and choline acetyltransferase in cortical tissue from some cases of Alzheimer's disease and neurologically normal controls*

Cortical Area	*Glutamate binding (pm/mg protein)*			*Choline acetyltransferase μm/h-100 mg protein*		
	SDAT	*Controls*	*SDAT/ Controls*	*SDAT*	*Controls*	*SDAT/ Controls*
Temporal tip	19.1±12.6	24.4±13.1	78%	0.22±0.11	0.88±0.49	27%
Mid temporal	12.9± 6.9	29.5±29.1	44%	0.18±0.14	0.68±0.15	27%
Postcentral	12.8± 7.6	15.2± 3.3	84%	0.24±0.20	0.74±0.40	32%
Occipital	14.4±10.2	25.2±23.1	57%	0.16±0.13	0.46±0.18	35%
Frontal pole	20.4± 8.4	24.5±13.5	82%	0.29±0.20	0.72±0.37	40%
Broca's area	16.8±13.6	27.7±13.6	60%	0.25±0.15	0.60±0.24	42%
Precentral	13.7± 7.3	19.8± 8.1	69%	0.34±0.23	0.77±0.31	44%
Average	15.6± 9.7	24.1±16.3	65%	0.24±0.18	0.65±0.29	37%

**Data are given in terms of mean* ± S.D. There were 6 controls aged 79 ± 2.5 yr and 10 SDAT cases, aged 77 ± 5.8 yr. The average of the activities in the seven cortical areas for each individual is plotted in Figures 1E and 1F and used for the calculation of the group mean averages shown above.

TABLE 2. Average activity in seven cortical areas of γ-glutamate transferase (γ-GT) choline acetyltransferase (CAT) and acetylcholinesterase (AChE)*

	γ-GT	*CAT*	*AChE*
SDAT cases (19)	31.89 ± 1.74	0.21 ± 0.004†	29.44 ± 2.32†
Controls (12)	31.95 ± 2.78	0.77 ± 0.07	51.84 ± 3.17

*All data are in μm/hr - 100 mg protein and given as mean ± S.E. More detailed data will be published (65). † Significantly different from control value at $p<0.001$.

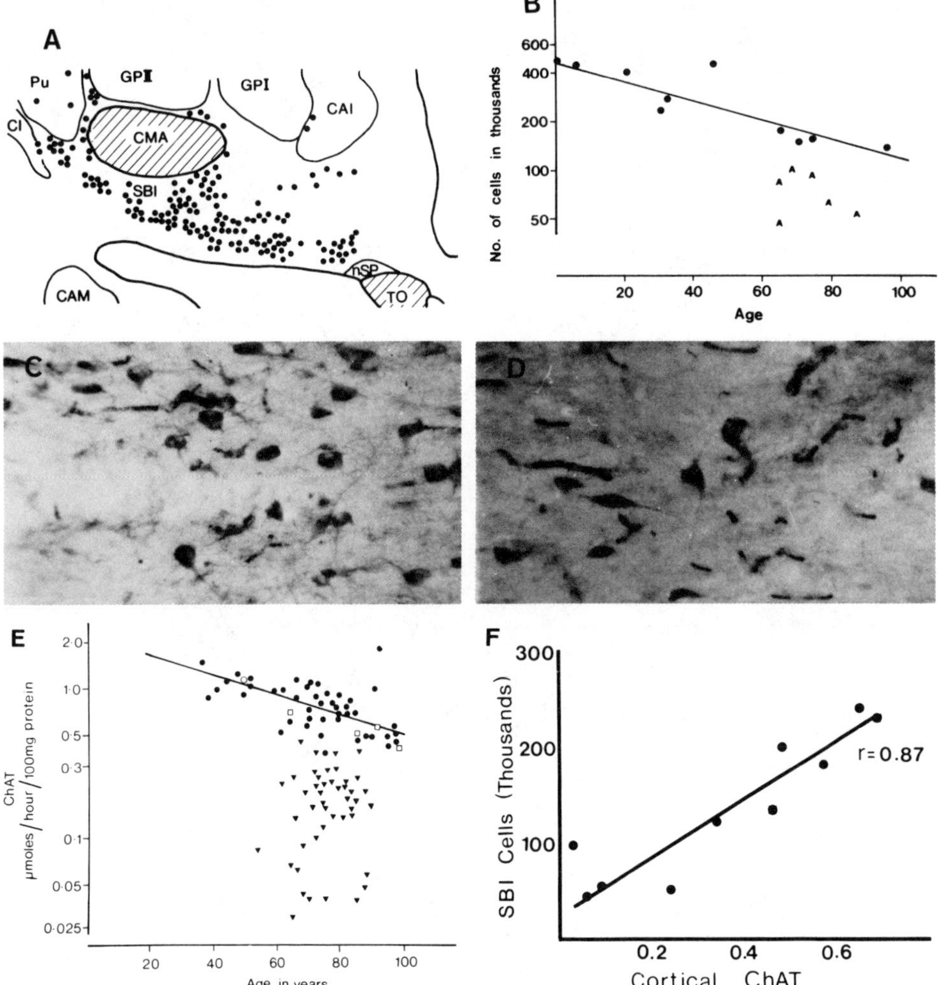

Fig. 1. (*A*) Coronal diagram of human brain showing location of cholinergic neurons at midsagittal level of substantia innominata (SBI). Other abbreviations: Pu = putamen; CMA = anterior commissure; Cl = claustrum; CAM = amygdala; GPpl = globus pallidus pars lateralis; GPpm = globus pallidus pars medialis; CA1 = internal capsule; nSP = supraoptic nucleus; TO = optic tract. (*B*) Semilogarithmic plot of age against the number of cells in the substantia innominata in Alzheimer's cases (*A*) and the neurologically normal controls (●). The correlation of the control data with age is highly significant (r = -0.87). (*C, D*) Examples of CAT-positive staining seen in the substantia innominata in a typical normal (*C*) and SDAT case (*D*). Bar = 100 μm. (*E*) Semi-log plot of age against average CAT activity in seven cortical regions (see Table 1) for controls (●), Alzheimer's cases (▼), and demented individuals without Alzheimer's pathology (□). The (○) is the CAT activity in a biopsy of temporal cortex from an epileptic patient. Correlation of the control data with age is highly significant (r = -0.73). (*F*) Plot of number of cholinergic cells in the SBI in individual brains against the average CAT activity measured in seven cortical areas.

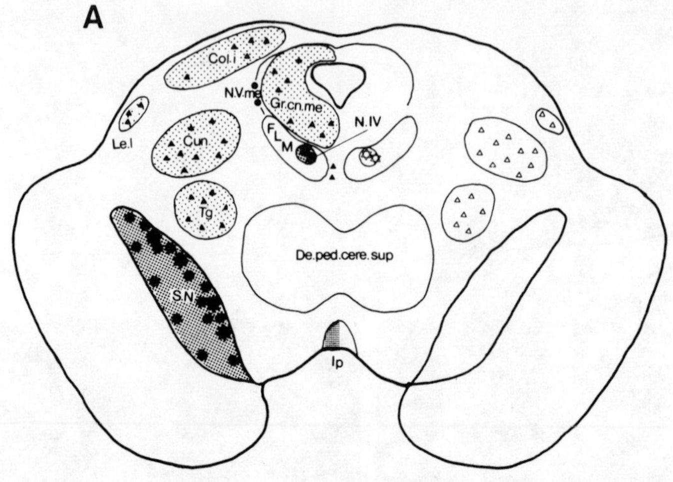

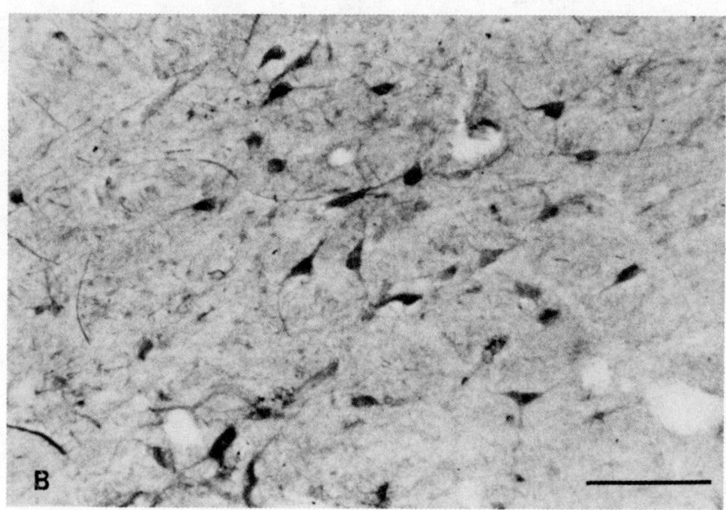

Fig. 2. (*A*) One of eight cross-sectional maps of human brain stem from Mizukawa *et al.* (32) indicating AChE-containing structures (left side) and CAT-containing structures (right side). Abbreviations are: CGM = corpus geniculatum medialis; CS = superior colliculus: EW =n. accessorius nervi oculomotorii; FLM = fasciculus longitudinalis medialis; IP = n. interpeduncularis; LM = medial lemniscus; MRF = mesencephalic reticular formation; NCF = n. cuneiformis; NR = n. ruber; NTM = n. mesencephalicus nervi trigemini; SGC = substantia grisea centralis; SN = substantia nigra; TTC = tractus tegmentalis centralis; III = n. nervi oculomotorii. Symbols: ✸ or ✧ large, intensely AChE- or CAT-positive cells with prominent processes; ▼ or ▽ small or medium-size, AChE- or CAT-positive cells with less prominent processes; ⁘⁘⁘ intense AChE fiber staining; ⁛⁛⁛ moderate AChE fiber staining; ∴∴ light AChE fiber staining. (*B*) CAT staining of the nucleus tegmentalis pedunculopontinus showing medium-size, multipolar cells with some prominent processes. Bar = 50 μm.

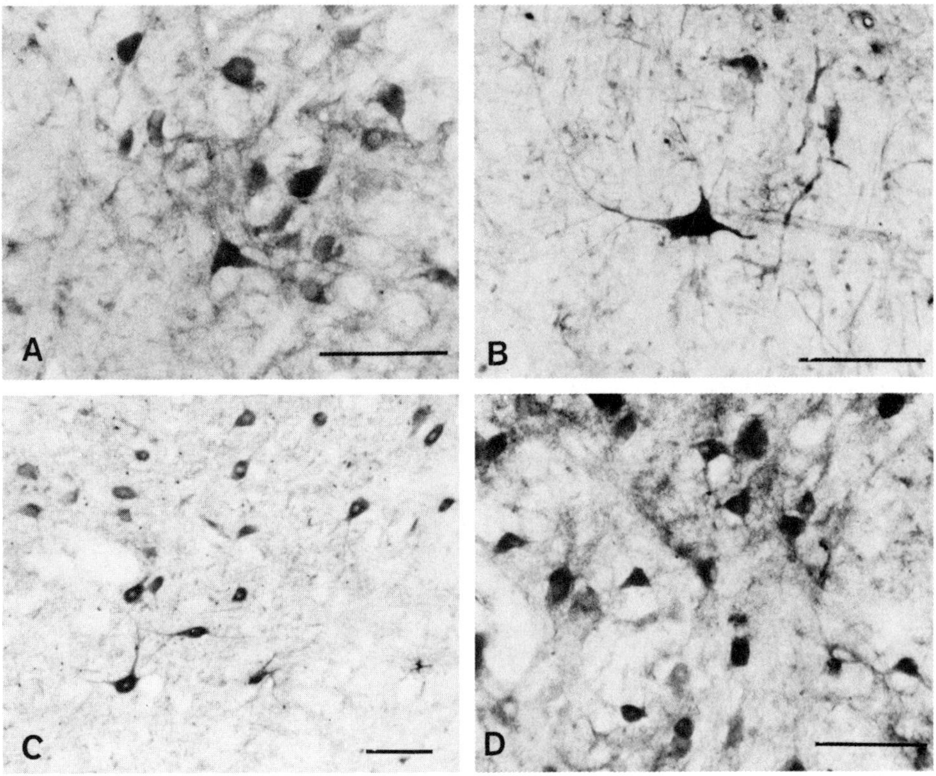

Fig. 3. (*A*) CAT-positive cells in the nucleus gigantocellularis, demonstrating few processes. These tend to occur in clusters. (*B*) Isolated cells in the same nucleus with prominent processes. (*C*) CAT-positive staining of cells of nucleus motorius nervi trigemini. (*D*) CAT-positive staining of nucleus vestibularis. The cells are relatively weakly stained and do not demonstrate prominent processes. Bars = 50 μm.

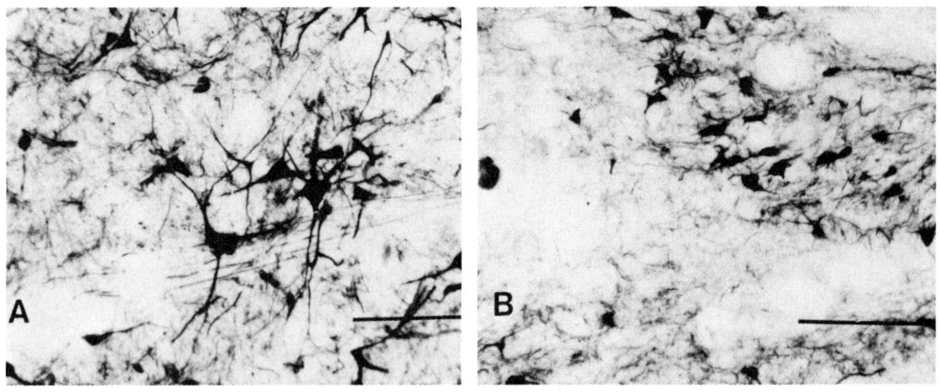

Fig. 4. (*A*) AChE-positive staining of cells of the nucleus gigantocellularis (compare with Figures 3A, 3B). (*B*)AChE-positive staining of cells of the mucleus gracilis. Bars = 50μm.

6. Catecholamines in Association Cortex and Age-Related Decline in Representational Memory: Neurobiological Studies in Nonhuman Primates

PATRICIA S. GOLDMAN-RAKIC, Ph.D.

Department of Neuroanatomy Yale School of Medicine
New Haven, CT 06510

ABSTRACT: Studies of the functions, neurochemistry and circuitry of central nervous system structures in nonhuman primates have provided important insights into the processes of memory in normal and aged subjects and have suggested promising therapeutic approaches to memory decline in the aged and demented human. This chapter focuses on studies of the prefrontal cortex, which is particularly relevant to aging and dementia because of its involvement in short-term (working) memory and which is the site of high concentrations of senile plaques in patients with Alzheimer's disease (AD). Our results demonstrate the important role of catecholamine deficiency in memory deficits of aged primates. We have shown that the performance of these animals on delayed-response tests of visuospatial memory can be restored with alpha-2-adrenergic agonists, possibly via a mechanism of postsynaptic supersensitivity.

Introduction

Age-related decline in memory and information-processing capacity is well known to the average person and scientist alike. It is a subject of intensifying interest and increasing urgency as the number of persons surviving to old age increases rapidly and a proportion of these aged succumb to the dementing diseases of old age. It would seem logical that an understanding of the age-related pathology of memory be based on knowledge of the mechanisms that mediate memory and cognition in the young healthy adult brain. Although our knowledge of the neural systems crucial for cognitive functions still lags behind our appreciation of the neural systems that mediate central sensory and motor processes, some significant advances have been achieved in this field. Studies of nonhuman primates have played an important role in these advances because of the close phyletic relationship of these animals to humans and their similar brain organization.

In this chapter, I briefly review some of the findings from my own laboratory on the functions, neurochemistry and circuitry of central nervous system structures underlying cognitive and mnemonic functions in nonhuman primates. Such studies have contributed important insights about the aging process and suggested promising therapeutic approaches to memory decline in the aged and demented human (*e.g.*, 1-4). My focus here is on the prefrontal cortex, which is located in the anterior half of the frontal lobe (Fig. 1) and is particularly relevant to aging and dementia because of its involvement in short-term or working memory (reviewed in 5-9). The prefrontal cortex has also been implicated in selective attention, loss of initiative and fluency, "self-ordering" functions involving sequences of actions, affective responses and, in man, abstract reasoning (reviewed in 5,7, and 10). Alterations in these functions are frequent in senile dementia; indeed, the vegetative state toward which the most seriously ill are driven in this disease is not unlike that associated with the global effects of frontal lobotomy.

Delayed-Response Task

Visuospatial memory is well developed in rhesus monkeys, and thus this type of memory has served in my laboratory as a model system for studies of the anatomical, neurochemical and physiological basis of working memory. The task that has proved most useful for this purpose is the delayed response. In the classical version of this test, the subject is shown the location of a food morsel that is then hidden from view by an opaque screen (Fig. 2). Following a delay of several seconds, the subject chooses the correct location from two or more options. In this situation, the subject must remember where the bait had been placed a few seconds earlier. In a variation of this task, spatial delayed alternation, the subject is required to alternate between left and right food wells on successive trials that are separated by delays. Since, in the latter task, the animal is not permitted to observe the experimenter baiting the food wells in the delay periods, to be correct on any given trial requires keeping track of which response was made last. The essence of the delayed-response test is that it indexes an animal's ability to use short-term representational memory; *e.g.*, of the spatial location of an object, to guide behavior in the absence of informative external cues. A key difference between the delayed-response tasks and many other tasks is that in the former, *no information is provided to the animal by external stimuli at the time of response*; instead, the response is guided by an internalized representation. Prefrontal lesions do not disturb performance on a wide variety of associative memory tasks in which two different stimuli are presented simultaneously and responses to one are consistently reinforced. It seems that prefrontal cortex is necessary precisely when behavior must be regulated by memories of stimuli rather than by the stimuli themselves (7,9,11). In this context, it is interesting to note that, according to Craik, age differences in human memory "appear to be slightest when mental processes are 'driven' rather directly by the stimulus or are strongly determined or supported by the environment..." and are "greatest, on the other hand, when the task requires 'going beyond' the information given — where processes are self-initiated..and/or where a different 'set' must be established from the person's habitual set or the set induced by the environment" (p. 7, ref. 12).

Anatomical Connections: Information-Processing Circuitry

The prefrontal cortex in primates has a number of cytoarchitectonic and functional subdivisions, each of which has multiple afferent and efferent connections with the posterior sensory association cortices, the limbic cortices and the basal ganglia that are in a "chain of command" for the processes of perception, information storage and execution or inhibition of motor responses. By virtue of these connections, each of the subdivisions of the prefrontal cortex may be considered a type of executive center for integrating events in space and time and utilizing stored representations of the outside world to guide behavior. This section briefly describes the major connections of the principal sulcus. This is the subarea of prefrontal cortex that is most relevant to short-term spatial memory, in that the capacity to perform delayed-response tasks depends on the bilateral integrity of this cortex and on that of no other cortical area (reviewed in 7). Moreover, during the past decade, its circuitry has been worked out to the point that relations between specific connections and specific processes can be analyzed in detail.

As revealed by its role in delayed-response performance, the principal sulcus cortex in monkeys is specialized for guiding response choice on the basis of spatial information and thus should have access to a visuospatial coordinate system. In harmony with this role, it receives its major corticocortical input from the posterior parietal cortex (Fig. 3B; 13-16), where spatial information about the outside world is perceived and processed (17,18).

The principal sulcus is also prominently connected with hippocampally related cortical areas and with the presubicular portion of the hippocampus proper (19). These recently described multiple direct and indirect connections of the principal sulcus with the hippocampus presumably allow the principal sulcus to access stored representations via hippocampal retrieval mechanisms (Fig. 3C; 19). Indeed, the metabolic activity of the dentate gyrus and pyramidal-cell layers of the hippocampus is elevated when monkeys perform the spatial delayed-response tasks, indicating that hippocampal mechanisms are engaged in delayed response, presumably through the circuitry that has been outlined (20).

The anatomy of motor control by which principal-sulcus neurons participate in the selection or inhibition of responses has been worked out in outline (Fig. 3D). This anatomy includes projections from the principal sulcus to the caudate nucleus (*e.g.*, 21,22), connections with the motor thalamus (*e.g.*, 8) and with the deep "motor" layers of the superior colliculus (23,24). The ability to initiate behavior or to inhibit inappropriate response must somehow require these pathways.

The conclusion from these studies is that all circuitry exists for regulation of behavior by representational memory: visuospatial input (parietal-prefrontal connections), storage/recall mechanisms (prefrontal-hippocampal circuits) and, importantly, motor commands (prefrontal connections with motor structures). However, details of synaptic organization are less well defined. A starting point for future dissection of intracortical circuit diagrams is the knowledge that prefrontal cortex, like all other neocortical areas, has a distinct laminar plan. For example, pyramidal neurons in Layer III project primarily to other cortical areas, both within the same (associational neurons) and opposite (callosal neurons) hemispheres (Fig. 4). Whereas >80% of corticocortical neurons originate in layer III, layer V is the principal source of projections to the caudate nucleus and putamen, to the colliculus and to other subcortical structures; neurons in layer VI project selectively to the thalamus. Knowing these facts, one can begin to appreciate the synaptic architecture and wiring diagrams underlying a specific cortical function. It is of interest that neuropathological changes associated with Alzheimer's disease (AD), namely senile plaques, are present in high concentration in prefrontal cortex (3); and layer III, from which the corticocortical neurons originate, has a particularly high density of neuritic plaques in cortical association areas (25).

Anatomical Connections: The Ascending and Descending Monoaminergic Systems

As in other species, the prefrontal cortex of the monkey contains significant levels of dopamine (DA), norepinephrine (NE) and serotonin (26). Nuclei labeled following injections of horseradish peroxidase (HRP) into the principal sulcus and various other subdivisions of the prefrontal and cingulate cortex include the locus coeruleus, the central superior nucleus and caudal portion of the dorsal raphe nucleus as well as cells in the ventral tegmental area, the medial one-third of the substantia nigra, pars compacta and the retrorubral nucleus (Fig. 5; also ref. 27). Most of the neurons labeled in the brain stem after injections of HRP into the prefrontal cortex correspond in location and morphology to those identified as monoamine-containing and are therefore the main source of the DA, NE and serotonin found in the prefrontal and anterior cingulate areas.

Histofluorescence and immunohistochemical methods have confirmed the presence of catecholamine-containing fibers in prefrontal cortex and have offered important new details about the topographic and laminar distribution of these axons within the cortical layers (28,29). An important observation is that the catecholaminergic (CA) fiber systems within the cortex are distributed in particular layers. Most areas of cortex examined possess a bilaminar pattern, with one concentration of CA-containing exons present in a supragranular layer and the other deep to layer IV. In the principal sulcus, for example, CA-containing exons are concentrated in upper layer III and in the deep layers V and VI and are more sparse in other layers (28). This layer-specific innervation suggests that monoamine-containing afferents modulate specific classes of projection neurons that reside in these layers (see below).

Finally, the prefrontal cortex not only receives a substantial CA projection from the locus coeruleus and ventral tegmental areas, but also it is one of the few areas to issue a reciprocal descending projection to the region of the locus coeruleus, as well as to the raphe nuclei and the ventral tegmental areas directly (Fig. 6; also ref. 1). These studies indicate that the prefrontal cortex may have a direct or indirect (through interneurons) descending influence on its own activation and very possibly on that of other cortical regions. The baseline firing rate of locus coeruleus neurons has been related to the behavioral relevance and significance of sensory stimuli (*e.g.*, 30). Perhaps the prefrontal cortex can convey highly processed information to the locus coeruleus by the corticofugal pathway described, informing locus coeruleus neurons when and how much to alert the rest of the central nervous system for an impending event or demand.

Concentration and Synthesis of Catecholamines in Primate Prefrontal Cortex

Biochemical studies of primate prefrontal cortex in the mid-1970's revealed marked regional differences in the endogenous concentrations and turnover rates of DA, NE and serotonin in different cytoarchitectonic areas of the cerebral cortex (31). Dopamine and NE are found in highest concentrations in the prefrontal and anterior temporal cortex; with a few exceptions, these neurotransmitter substances decrease along the fronto-occipital axis and are present in considerably lower concentration in the primary visual cortex (26). Rates of catecholamine synthesis generally parallel the concentration data and are especially high in various areas of the association cortex, including prefrontal cortex, and lowest in the primary visual cortex (26). In agreement with these biochemical studies, recent immunohistochemical studies of DA-beta-hydroxylase (DBH) in the parietal and occipital lobe have revealed that DBH is almost absent from the lateral geniculate nucleus of the thalamus and sparse in the primary visual cortex. This study also revealed a qualitative difference in the concentration of DBH-positive fibers in the pulvinar–lateral posterior complex of the thalamus and in the posterior parietal cortex relative to the primary visual system (32). These findings collectively suggest that noradrenergic fibers innervate a large number of structures involved in visuospatial analysis more densely than those involved in visual feature extraction and pattern analysis (32). This idea is consistent with the failure of catecholamine agonists to affect visual-discrimination performance in behavioral studies (see below).

Neurochemical Deficits of Aging

The prefrontal cortex appears to be especially sensitive to catecholamine loss with aging (33). In our regional biochemical studies of aged (10- to 18-year-old) rhesus monkeys, we found large (50%) decreases in DA in prefrontal cortex but not in premotor or motor areas of the frontal lobe. Catecholamine synthesis was compromised throughout the cerebral cortex and was reduced by >60% in prefrontal cortex, whereas neither serotonin levels nor 5-hydroxytryptamine (5-HT) accumulation was changed (33). Our biochemical study was carried out in relatively "young" aged monkeys (≤18 years); we expect that adrenergic loss would be even more severe in older animals. The CA deficits observed in prefrontal cortex of aged monkeys raised the possibility that such deficits account in part for the delayed-response deficits that had been described in aged monkeys (2) and, indeed, we now have good evidence that this is the case (see below).

Deficits in catecholamine content have also been reported for prefrontal cortex in aged and senile humans and may play a role in their memory loss. Attention in the study of aging has focused on two diffuse ascending systems: the cholinergic basal forebrain system and the adrenergic projections of the locus coeruleus. Degeneration of the cholinergic neurons of the basal forebrain in patients with AD is well documented (*e.g.*, 4). However, it is now clear that neurons of the locus coeruleus also degenerate in this disease and, indeed, a loss of $\leq$80% of the neurons in this nucleus can occur in the most severely demented patients (34). In line with the loss of adrenergic cells, there is a significant reduction in NE in the prefrontal cortex of senile demented patients (35), as well as marked reduction in the DBH content of the cerebral cortices of patients dying with senile dementia of the Alzheimer type (SDAT) (36). However, the available evidence indicates that both alpha-1-and alpha-2-adrenergic receptor density in Alzheimer patients does not fall below the level in normal aged brain (37), encouraging the belief that agonists acting at these receptors might have palliative effects (see below).

Replacement Therapy for Working-Memory Deficits in Young Adult Monkeys

It is widely believe that catecholamines play a modulatory role in synaptic function. For example, iontophoretic application of NE in rat somatosensory cortex enhances response to excitatory or inhibitory synaptic inputs produced either by natural stimulation of the contralateral forepaw or by microiontophoresis of excitatory or inhibitory neurotransmitters (38). Recent studies (described below) indicate that a similar modulatory action of DA and NE could occur in primate principal sulcus and contribute to the regulation of its cognitive functions, possibly through activation of alpha-adrenergic receptors.

In the first of two studies relevant to the issue of neuromodulation, young adult rhesus monkeys were first trained on the delayed-alternation task as well as on a visual-pattern discrimination task that does not require prefrontal cortex. After the animals completed training, catecholamines were depleted in the principal sulcus by intracerebral microinjections of the catecholamine toxin 6-hydroxydopamine (6-OHDA) alone or in combination with desmethylimipramine (DMI) (39). Control groups were injected with 5,6-dihydroxytamine to deplete serotonin or with vehicle alone to assess the effect of nonspecific damage from the injections. In an additional group, the cortex in the principal sulcus was surgically removed. Postmortem biochemical analysis at the end of the experiment revealed that the experimental group given 6-OHDA plus DMI had the largest depletion of catecholamines in principal sulcus (an 87% depletion of DA and a 76% depletion of NE) and were the only group to show a large postoperative impairment on the delayed-alternation task. Importantly, this group maintained normal performance on the visual-discrimination task.

Dose-response curves for a variety of drugs obtained in these monkeys both preoperatively and postoperatively revealed that certain catecholamine agonists reversed the delayed-alternation impairments expressed in the most-affected group: L-dopa, apomorphine and clonidine each improved performance in one or more animals. These results provided the first direct evidence that loss of a cognitive function could be caused by catecholamine deficiency in the cortex, in this case, in the principal sulcal cortex, and further indicated that such loss could be treated successfully by "replacement" therapy (31).

Cognitive Decline and Replacement Therapy in Aged Rhesus Monkeys

Given that experimentally induced catecholamine loss could produce a deficit in one of the family of delayed-response tasks, it seemed reasonable to hypothesize that the endogenous loss in cortical catecholamines that we had shown occurs in aging monkeys (33) could also account for their reported delayed-response impairments (2). In order to assess the contribution of cortical catecholamine deficiency to the age-related spatial-memory deficits, Arnsten and Goldman-Rakic recently examined the effects of catecholamine agonists on the delayed-alternation performance of aged monkeys (1). A number of drugs were tried; the alpha-2-adrenergic agonist clonidine consistently improved spatial delayed-response performance in a dose-dependent manner in all monkeys tested: to date, 13 of 13 (1; Arnsten and Goldman-Rakic, unpublished observations). Furthermore, the effects are pharmacologically, behaviorally and site specific. The beneficial effects of clonidine can be blocked in a dose-dependent manner by the alpha-2-antagonist yohimbine, which, given alone, intensifies the behavioral impairment of the aged animals. The effects of clonidine and yohimbine are specific to the delayed-response test and have no effect on visual-pattern discrimination performance. This profile of behavioral impairment in the aged monkey implicates the principal sulcus as the site of clonidine's beneficial effects on delayed-response performance. Supporting this conclusion, monkeys in whom the principal sulcal region had been surgically ablated show no improvement with clonidine, whereas young adult monkeys with experimental depletion of catecholamines in the principal sulcus are improved by clonidine in a manner consistent with receptor supersensitivity (1). Additionally, as discussed in greater detail below, [^{3}H]-clonidine binding sites are found in high concentration in just those layers of the principal sulcus that are most consistent with a role in enhancing information processing.

Location of the Alpha-2 Receptor in Prefrontal Cortex

Quantitative autoradiography of receptor [^{3}H]-clonidine binding in the cerebral cortex reveals that the alpha-2-adrenergic receptor is concentrated in layers I and III of prefrontal cortex including the principal sulcus (Goldman-Rakic and Gallagher, unpublished observations) (Fig. 7). As layer III in this region is the principal origin of callosal and associational (corticocortical) neurons and layer I a major target of incoming corticocortical axons, this finding provides strong evidence of a link between CA afferents and the information-processing machinery of the prefrontal cortex.

The binding of [^{3}H]-clonidine is characterized by high affinity, saturability and the pharmacology associated with alpha-2-adrenergic receptors (oxymetazoline NE phenylephrine, and alpha-1-adrenergic agonist). Scatchard analysis of saturation experiments generated from data on autoradiograms shows K_d values for binding in cortical layers in the dorsal principal sulcus in reasonable agreement with data from whole-brain sections. However, B_{max} values for autoradiographic data obtained in specific anatomically defined layers show laminar-specific labeling, as described above.

An important issue that cannot be resolved at present is whether the alpha-adrenergic receptors described here are presynaptic or postsynapic or, possibly, both. Although considerable pharmacologic evidence indicates that noradrenergic nerve terminals possess autoreceptors, such autoreceptors have not been conclusively demonstrated in cortex. It is relevant that kinetic and saturation experiment with [^{3}H]-clonidine in rat brain reveal the highest concentrations of high- and low-affinity binding sites in frontal cortex (40). Furthermore, in almost all regions examined in rodent brain, including frontal cortex, neither high- nor low-affinity [^{3}H]-clonidine binding was decreased by 6-OHDA lesions of noradrenergic terminals. Rather, both the low-affinity and, especially, the high-affinity binding sites actually increased in frontal cortex after chemical deafferentation, suggesting that [^{3}H]-clonidine binding in cortex is partly or largely postsynaptic. This conclusion is consistent with our pharmacological findings, discussed above, that clonidine induces marked improvements in performance of aged rhesus monkeys on a cognitive task mediated by the principal sulcal cortex. The ameliorative effects of clonidine are blocked by the alpha-2-receptor blocker yohimbine, and the cognitive performance of young monkeys with large experimentally induced depletion of NE in the prefrontal cortex is improved by lower doses of clonidine than are needed in monkeys with smaller NE deficits, who generally require higher doses before exhibiting improvements (1). As we have shown that old monkeys exhibit large endogeneous losses of CA in prefrontal cortex (31) and also respond to lower doses of clonidine than do "younger" aged animals (1), these various findings suggest that clonidine may improve memory by enhancing cortical function at supersensitive postsynaptic alpha-2-receptor sites. This model is currently being tested in our laboratory (Arnsten and Goldman-Rakic, unpublished observations).

Circuit Basis for Neuromodulation in Principal Sulcus

The relatively rapid reversal of deficits by drugs fits well with the idea that the catecholamines play a modulatory role in cognitive processing. The rapid restoration of behavior on a dose-dependent basis implies that the aged animal has adequate access to the sensory information, as well as to the working memory and motor-control mechanisms necessary for performing the task under appropriate conditions. However, the circuit basis for CA effects on cognition is not known: we do not know whether the receptor lies on the cell bodies or proximal dendrites of cortical neurons, on interneurons or on incoming afferents. Our working hypothesis is that brain-stem catecholamine-containing afferents target specific columns of projection neurons either directly or through interneurons and could thereby influence the computational processes carried out by corticocortical networks. For example, alpha-2 receptors may in fact be associated with layer III projection neurons that are mainly of the corticocortical type. Therefore, catecholamine-containing axons might directly facilitate communication between interconnected areas of prefrontal, parietal and limbic cortex. This idea is supported by the correspondence of the location of ^{3}H binding sites within the principal sulcus with the cell bodies, dendrites and terminals of corticocortical projection systems. Additionally, layer III contains the highest concentration of NE-sensitive cells in rhesus prefrontal cortex (41). Finally, as mentioned previously, in patients with AD, layer III contains particularly high concentrations of neurofibrillary tangles and neuritic plaques (25). Alpha-2 receptors are also present in the outer part of layer I, where their concentration is higher than in any other layer; layer 1 receives a high density of callosal and associational terminals (Fig. 4; 16,39).

Conclusions

More than 80% of the human cerebral cortex is devoted to so-called associative functions, neither strictly sensory nor strictly motor but rather integrative. It is these association areas that are most involved in diseases affecting mental capacity. It is important to realize that these areas are anatomically interconnected. For example, the prefrontal and parietal cortices are connected with the subiculum and entorhinal cortex that recent studies have shown are also affected in AD (42). Thus, a "lesion" in one part of the system can be expected to affect activity in other parts. Only part of the complex circuitry of association cortex has been reviewed here; for a more extensive review, see reference 7. Nonetheless, we can conclude that the prefrontal cortex is part of a widespread neural system of association areas that work together and are crucial for the regulation of cognitive behavior; *i.e.*, that behavior which is regulated by representational knowledge. An important feature of the prefrontal role in this network is that it appears to be crucial for translating knowledge into action.

Knowledge of the anatomical, neurochemical and functional properties of prefrontal cortex in nonhuman primates has led to an animal model of cognitive function in young and aged humans. Our studies demonstrate the important role of catecholamine deficiency in the memory deficits of aged primates without excluding the contribution of other lesions. We have shown that the performance of aged monkeys on delayed-response tasks can be restored with an alpha-2-adrenergic agonist and that the mechanism of action may be through postsynaptic supersensitivity. Support for this model comes from the similar nature of catecholamine loss in aged-human cortex and the correspondence of the pathological changes in the brains of patients with AD with the findings in aged rhesus monkeys. Efforts are now underway to examine the therapeutic efficacy of alpha-2-adrenergic compounds in the treatment of human age-related memory decline. Whatever the outcome of these studies, the present program of research has identified a particular receptor in cerebral cortex that may be relevant to cognitive processes, opening up study of cortical function at a molecular level.

References

1. Arsten, A.F.T. & Goldman-Rakic, P.S. (1985) *Science* **230**, 1273-1276.
2. Artus, R.T., Fleming, D. & Johnson, H.R. (1978) *J. Gerontol.* **33**, 858-871.
3. Kitt, C.A., Struble, R.G., Cork, L.C., Mobley, W.C., Walker, L.C., Joh, T.H. & Price, D.L. (1985) *Neuroscience* **16**, 691-699.
4. Price, D.L., Whitehouse, P.J., Struble, R.G., Price, D.L., Jr., Cork, L.C., Hedreen, J.C. & Kitt, C.A. (1983) *Banbury Rep.* **15**, 65-77.
5. Fuster, J.M. (1985) *The Prefrontal Cortex.* (Raven Press, New York).

6. Fuster, J.M. (1985) In: *Cerebral Cortex,* ed. Jones, E.G. & Peters, A. (Plenum Press, New York) pp. 151-177.
7. Goldman-Rakic, P.S. In: *Handbook of Physiology,* ed. Plum, F. & Mountcastle, V. (American Physiological Society, Bethesda) (in press).
8. Ilinsky, I., Jouandet, M.L. & Goldman-Rakic, P.S. (1985) *J. Comp. Neurol.* **236**, 315-330.
9. Passingham, R.E. (1985) *Behav. Neurosci.* **99**, 3-21.
10. Stuss, D.T. & Benson, D.F. (1984) *Psychol. Bull.* **95**, 3-28.
11. Jacobsen, C.F. (1936) *Comp. Psychol. Monogr.* **13**, 1-68.
12. Craik, F.I.M. (1984) In: *Neuropsychology of Memory,* ed. Squire, L. & Butters, N. (The Guilford Press, New York) pp. 3-12.
13. Cavada, C. & Goldman-Rakic, P.S. (1985) *Soc. Neurosci. Abstr.* **11**, 323.
14. Goldman-Rakic, P.S. & Schwartz, M.L. (1982) *Science* **216**, 755-757.
15. Petrides, M. & Pandya, D.N. (1985) *J. Comp. Neurol.* **228**, 105-116.
16. Schwartz, M.L. & Goldman-Rakic, P.S. (1984) *J. Comp. Neurol.* **226**, 403-420.
17. Lynch, J.C., Mountcastle, V.B., Talbot, W.H. & Yin, T.C.T. (1977) *J. Neurophysiol.* **40**, 362-389.
18. Mountcastle, V.B., Motter, B.C., Steinmetz, M.A. & Duffy, C.J. (1984) In: *Dynamic Aspects of Neocortical Function,* ed. Edelman, G.M., Gall, W.E. & Cowan, W.M. (John Wiley & Sons, New York) pp. 159-193.
19. Goldman-Rakic, P.S., Selemon, L.D. & Schwartz, M.L. (1984) *Neuroscience* **12**, 719-743.
20. Friedman, H. & Goldman-Rakic, P.S. (1985) *Soc. Neurosci. Abstr.* **11**, 460.
21. Selemon, L. & Goldman-Rakic, P.S. (1985) *J. Neurosci.* **5**, 776-794.
22. Yeterian, E.H. & Van Hoesen, G.W. (1978) *Brain Res.* **139**, 43-63.
23. Fries, W. (1984) *J. Comp. Neurol.* **230**, 55-76.
24. Goldman-Rakic, P.S. & Nauta, W.J.H. (1976) *Brain Res.* **116**, 145-149.
25. Pearson, R.C.A., Esiri, M.M., Hjorns, R.W., Wilcock, G.K. & Powell, T.P.S. (1985) *Proc. Natl. Acad. Sci. USA* **82**, 4531-4534.
26. Brown, R.M., Crane, A.M. & Goldman, P.S. (1977) *Brain Res.* **124**, 576-580.
27. Porrino, L. & Goldman-Rakic, P.S. (1982) *J. Comp. Neurol.* **205**, 63-76.
28. Levitt, P., Rakic, P. & Goldman-Rakic, P.S. (1984) *J. Comp. Neurol.* **225**, 1-14.
29. Morrison, J.H. & Foote, S.L. (1986) *J. Comp. Neurol.* **243**, 717-738.
30. Aston-Jones, G. & Bloom, F.E. (1981) *J. Neurocytol.* **1**, 887-900.

31. Brozoski, T., Brown, R.M., Rosvold, H.E. & Goldman, P.S. (1979) *Science* **205**, 929-931.
32. Morrison, J.H., Foote, S.L., O'Connor, D. & Bloom, F.E. (1982) *Brain Res. Bull.* **9**, 309-319.
33. Goldman-Rakic, P.S. & Brown, R.M. (1981) *Neuroscience* **6**, 177-187.
34. Bondareff, W., Mountjoy, Q. & Roth, M. (1982) *Neurology* **32**, 164-168.
35. Adolfsson, R., Gottfries, C.G., Roos, B.E. & Windblad, B. (1979) *Br. J. Psychiatr.* **135**, 216-223.
36. Cross, A.J., Crow, T.J., Perry, E.K., Perry, R.H., Blessed, G. & Tomlinson, B.E. (1981) *Br. Med. J.* **282**, 93-94.
37. Cross, A.J., Crow, T.J., Johnson, J.A., Perry, E.K., Perry, R.H., Blessed, G. & Tomlinson, B.D. (1984) *J. Neurol. Sci.* **64**, 109-117.
38. Waterhouse, B.D. & Woodward, D.J. (1980) *Exp. Neurol.* **67**, 11-34.
39. Bugbee, N.M. & Goldman-Rakic, P.S. (1984) *J. Comp. Neurol.* **220**, 355-364.
40. U'Prichard, D.C., Bechtel, W.D., Rouot, B.M. & Snyder, S.H. (1979) *Mol. Pharmacol.* **16**, 47-60.
41. Sawaguchi, T. & Matsumura, M. (1985) *Neurosci. Res.* **2**, 255-273.
42. Hyman, B.T., Van Hoesen, G.W., Damasio, A.R. & Barnes, C.L. (1984) *Science* **225**, 1168-1170.

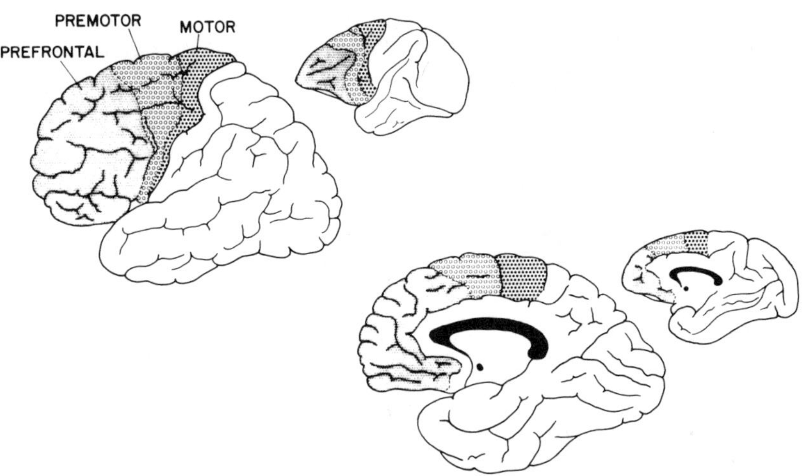

Fig. 1. Lateral and medial views of human and monkey cerebral cortex showing position and relative size of prefrontal, premotor and motor territories of frontal lobe.

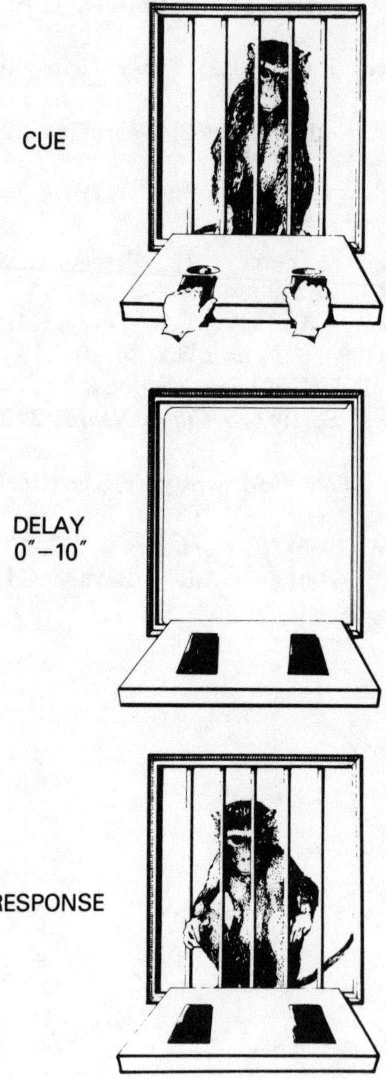

Fig. 2. Components of spatial delayed-response trial. In the cue period (top panel), monkey watches as experimenter baits one well with morsel of food and then both wells are covered with cardboard plaques. During the delay phase (middle panel), opaque screen is lowered for $\geq$1 sec; this effectively prevents animal from responding immediately. In the response phase (lower panel), screen is raised and monkey is allowed to select which of two identically marked wells contains the reward. (Reprinted with permission from reference 19.)

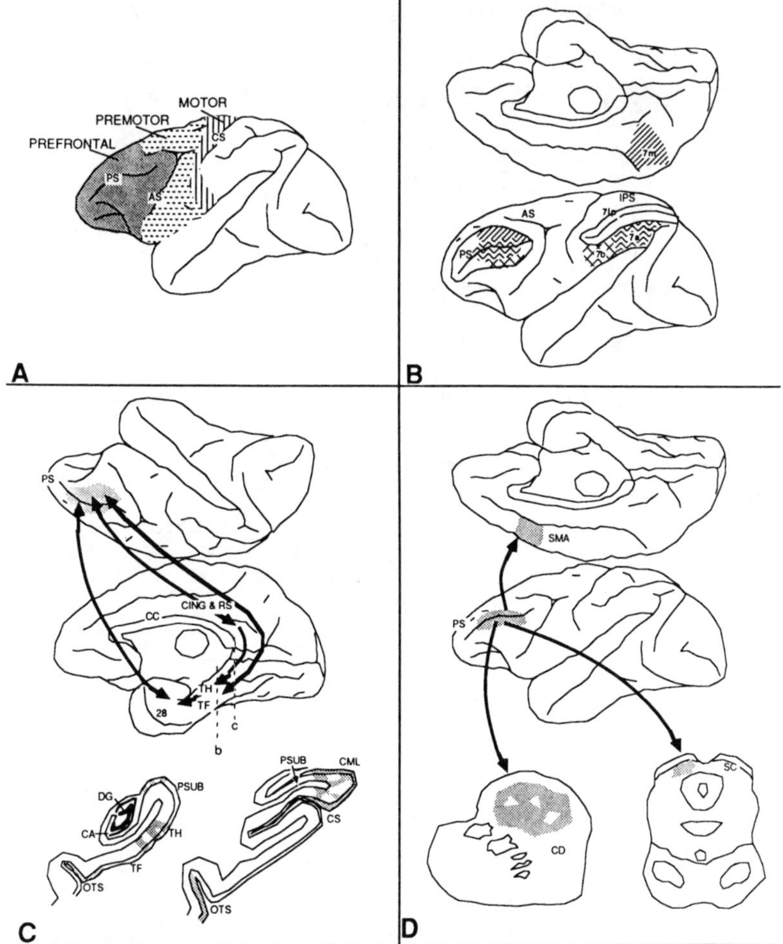

Fig. 3. A. View of cerebral cortex. B. Summary of areas in posterior parietal cortex that process visuospatial (7a, 7m, and 7ip) and somatic-related information (7b) and the distribution of their projections in principal sulcus as revealed by correspondence in zip-a-tone pattern. Area 7m is interconnected with dorsal bank and rim of caudal principal sulcus; 7a is interconnected with fundus and lower portion of each bank and 7b with upper portion and rim of ventral bank of principal sulcus; area 7ip in caudal bank of intraparietal sulcus (IpS) is connected with anterior bank of arcuate sulcus (ArcS). C. Summary of direct and indirect circuits linking principal sulcus with structures involved in memory: the hippocampal formation. D. Summary of major projections from principal sulcus to areas of brain involved in motor control. Other abbreviations: IS = intraparietal sulcus; CA = Ammon's horn of the hippocampus; CC = corpus callosum; CD = caudate nucleus; Cing and RS = cingulate and retrosplenial cortices; CML = caudomedial lobule; CS = collateral sulcus; DG = dentate gyrus; PSUB = presubiculum; TH, TF and 28 = parahippocampal areas; OTS = occipitotemporal sulcus; SC = superior colliculus; and SMA = supplementary motor cortex. (Reprinted with permission from reference 7.)

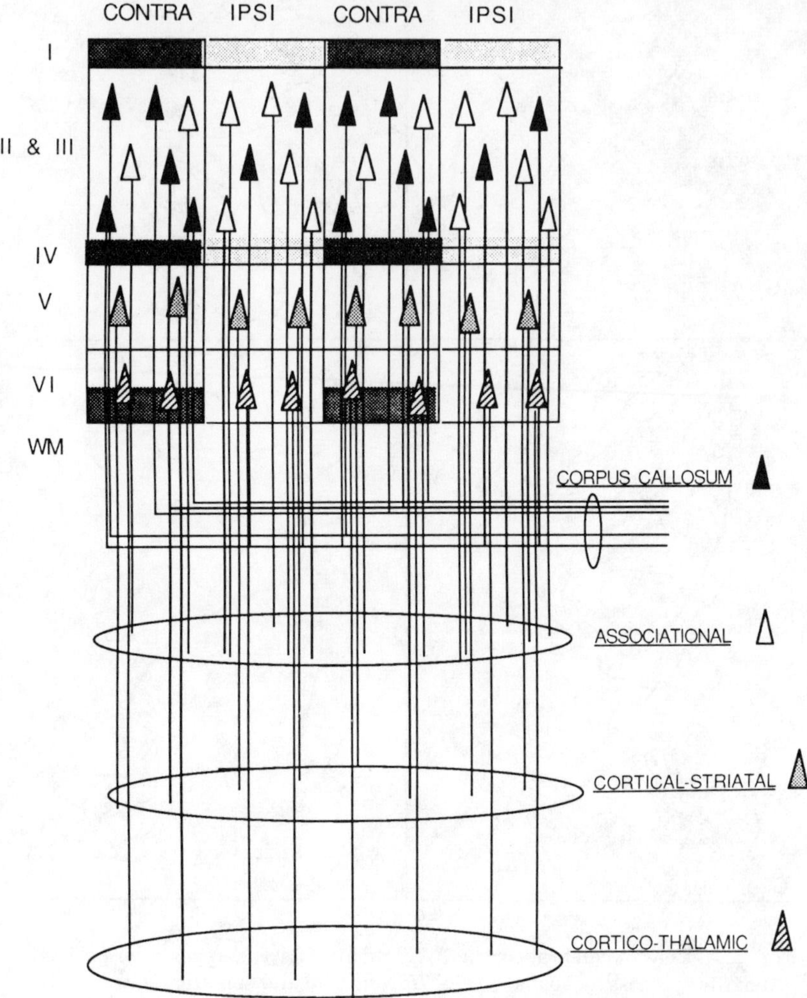

Fig. 4. Simplified circuit diagram illustrating terminal fields of parietal associational fibers (light stipple) and callosal fibers (dark stipple) in layers I, IV and VI of adjacent columns in principal sulcus. Also shown are callosal (dark triangles) and associational (light triangles) projection neurons that send axons to contralateral prefrontal cortex and to ipsilateral parietal cortex, respectivey. Note that callosal neurons are more concentrated in columns defined by callosal afferents and associational neurons are more concentrated in columns receiving dense associational fiber input. As described in reference 16, layer III contains around 80% of callosal and associational projection neurons; the remaining 20% are distributed in layers V and VI. Precise organization of the inputs and output neurons in principal sulcus encourages belief that its circuitry can be known at the cellular and synaptic level. (Reprinted with permission from reference 16.)

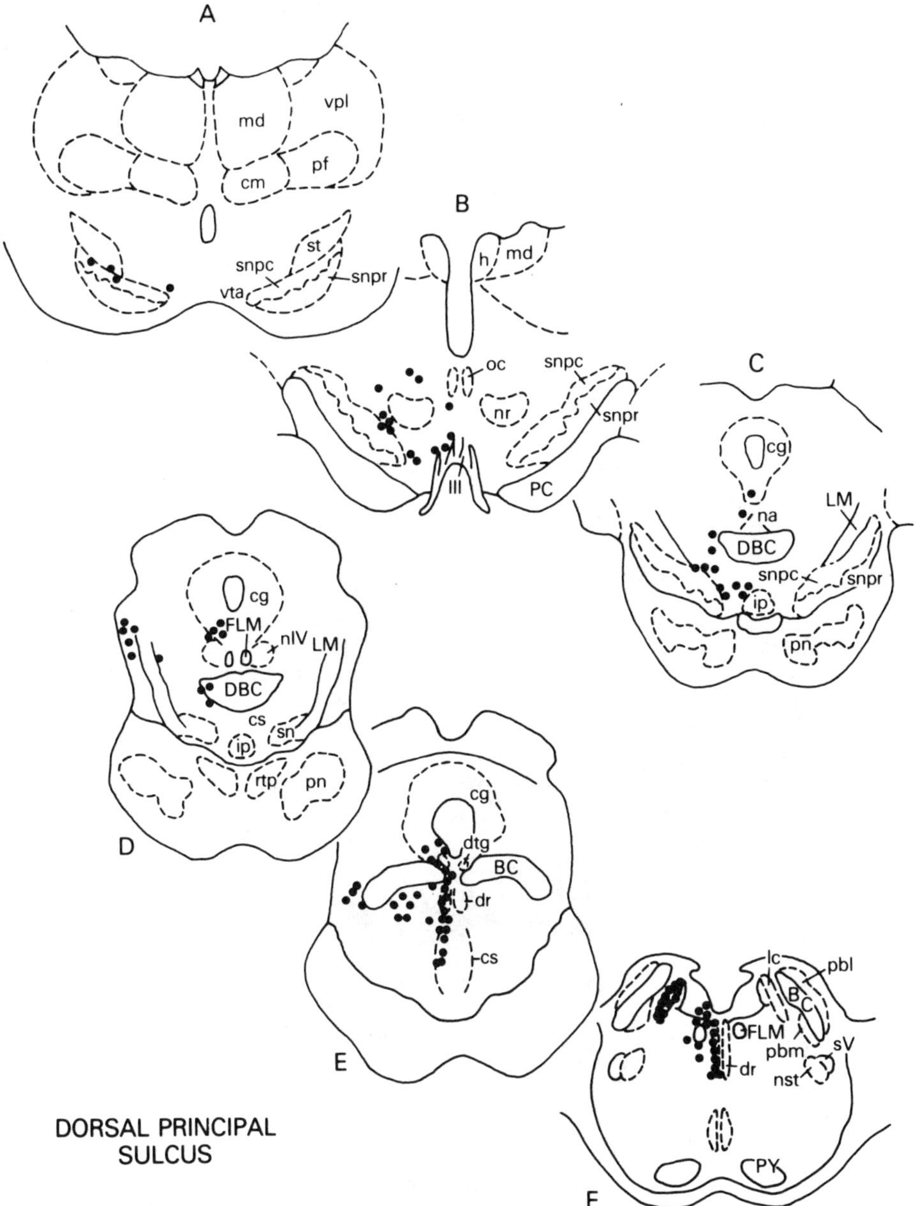

Fig. 5. Location of retrogradely labeled neurons (black dots) in brain-stem monoamine nuclei of monkey injected with free HRP into dorsal bank of principal sulcus. Selected abbreviations: bc = brachium conjunctivum; dr = dorsal raphe; cs = central superior nucleus; lc = locus coeruleus; nST = nucleus of the solitary tract; py = pyramids; snpc = substantia nigra, pars compacta; snpr = substantia nigra, pars reticulata. (Reprinted with permission from reference 27.)

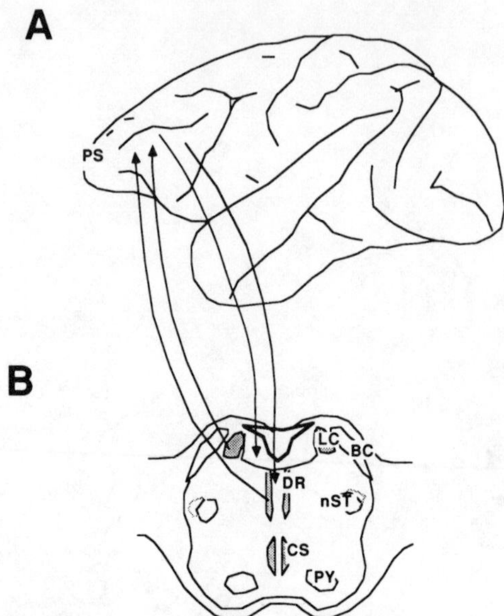

Fig. 6. Summary of prefrontal interconnections with several of brain-stem monoaminergic cell groups thought to be involved in activational processes (based on data from 1 and 27). PS = principal sulcus; other abbreviations as in Figure 5. (Reprinted with permission from reference 7).

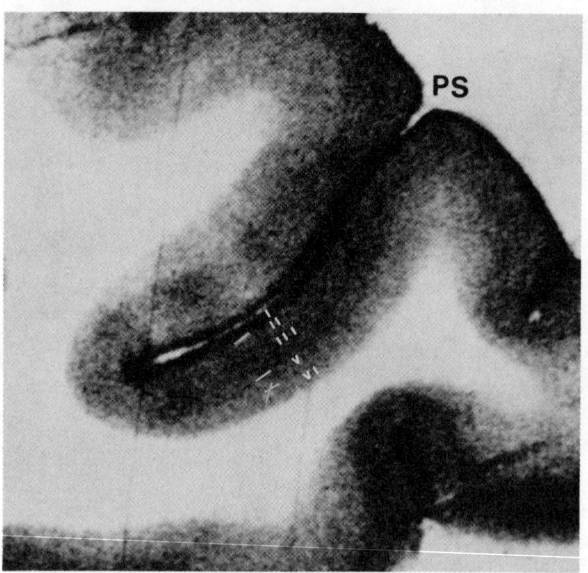

Fig. 7. Diagram illustrating distribution of [^{3}H]-clonidine binding (alpha-2 receptor) in principal sulcus. Density of ^{3}H binding is greatest in layers I (particularly in outer part) and III. (Goldman-Rakic and Gallagher, unpublished observations).

7. Synaptic Plasticity, Aging and Alzheimer's Disease

CARL W. COTMAN, Ph.D.

Department of Psychobiology University of California, Irvine
Irvine, CA 92717

ABSTRACT: Synapse replacement in response to cell death may be a powerful compensatory mechanism in aging and disease-related neuronal loss within defined neuronal populations. Axon sprouting, similar to that observed in rodents after creation of entorhinal lesions, occurs in the dentate gyrus of patients with Alzheimer's disease. It appears that septal fibers sprout as well as those of intrinsic CA4 fibers. Septal stimulation *in vivo* facilitates entorhinal synaptic transmission. Accordingly, the additional input from the sprouting fibers is probably similarly efficacious and a natural compensatory mechanism. Sprouting of the CA4 input also may help preserve function. Thus, replacement of new synapses after partial denervation may participate in functional restoration, even though the original afferents are not exclusively replaced. In doing so, however, the hippocampus may paradoxically become more susceptible to excitotoxic-mediated cellular damage. Enhanced plasticity may thus be gained at the price of increased vulnerability.

Introduction

Alzheimer's disease (AD) is a neurodegenerative disorder characterized neuropathologically by the presence of neurofibrillary tangles, neuritic plaques and severe neuronal cell losses in specific cortical and subcortical areas. The disease runs its course over several years, resulting in serious cognitive loss as the brain deteriorates. Research over the past many years has focused largely on characterizing the degenerative process and finding the causes of these pathological changes. It is commonly believed that the brain has little if any natural defense against the loss of its circuits and thus no defense against its own degenerative changes.

One of the hallmark changes of AD is the loss of neuronal populations, which occurs throughout the course of the disease. In addition to a profound loss of cholinergic neurons, there is a loss of particular cortical associational neurons. Studies on brain tissues obtained postmortem from patients with AD have demonstrated severe loss in select areas of the limbic system. Hyman and colleagues reported that AD is accompanied by a selective loss of layer II and III stellate cells of the entorhinal cortex and pyramidal neurons of the subiculum (1). These entorhinal neurons are the primary source of cortical input to the hippocampus, so the loss of the entorhinal input plus the subiculum functionally isolates the hippocampus and may account for the loss of cognitive functions which are dependent on the hippocampus. Thus, any particular compensatory mechanisms which can preserve and/or rebuild this vital entorhinal pathway would be critical early in the course of the disease.

In this article, we show that the brain of a patient with AD has the capacity to regenerate some of its lost circuitries after entorhinal cell death through axon sprouting and the formation of new connections. In the first section, we describe animal models relevant to entorhinal neuron loss and the induction of axon sprouting. In the second section, we describe parallel experiments carried out in the brains of AD patients obtained postmortem, which illustrate similar effects. We suggest that these changes can help maintain circuit function early in the course of this disease.

Organization and Function of Entorhinal and Dentate Gyrus Circuitry

The entorhinal cortex receives input from numerous cortical areas representing visual, somatosensory, auditory and olfactory sensory systems (Fig. 1). Additionally, the entorhinal cortex receives a major input from the amygdala, which further links the entorhinal area with limbic functions. This cortex thus is a highly specialized associational area, and it is, therefore, not surprising that damage to these cells would have serious consequences for hippocampal function.

Layer II and III stellate cells in the entorhinal area project by way of the perforant path to the outermost portion of the granule cell dendrites, providing a powerful excitatory drive to these cells. In the rodent brain, approximately 80% of the fibers to the outer portion are entorhinal. Recent evidence indicates that the entorhinal input to the dentate gyrus granule cells uses an excitatory amino acid as the neurotransmitter (2).

Activation of layer II-III stellate cells excites the granule cells in the dentate gyrus. When activated, these cells in turn drive CA3 and CA4 pyramidal neurons. The CA4 pyramidal neurons, in turn, project back onto the granule cells, synapsing on the inner one-third of the granule cell dendritic field immediately proximal to the zone of entorhinal termination. Thus, the entorhinal dentate CA4 loop comprises a reverberating circuit so that a train of entorhinal inputs is bilaterally directed and enchanced by the output of the CA4 neurons.

The dendritic field of the granule cells also receives inputs from various brain stem nuclei, including the locus ceruleus, raphe nuclei and a prominant projection from the septal area and diagonal band. Activation of the medial septum appears to enhance excitatory input to the hippocampus. The septal input acts as a type of conditional input, facilitating ongoing excitation.

Upon clearing the dentate gyrus, information is fed through the primary hippocampal circuit, starting with granule cell input to CA3 cells. The CA3 cells, in turn, project by way of the Schaeffer collateral system to CA1 pyramidal cells. CA3 neurons also project to the lateral septum, whereas the CA1 cells project to the subiculum, which distributes information to areas such as the limbic cortex, amygdala, hypothalamus and thalamus.

In AD, not only is there a loss of entorhinal and subicular cells, but in addition some of the intrinsic neurons within the hippocampus are compromised (3). It is well known that the hippocampus is the primary location of neuritic plaques and tangles. Thus, the potential loss of hippocampal functions is severe, and the burden on healthy cells to maintain function increases.

Axon Sprouting in the Hippocampus of the Rodent

Research carried out over the past several years in animal models has shown that the remaining healthy neurons can sprout new connections after the loss of input from the entorhinal cortex to the dentate gyrus (4,5). In response to the loss of entorhinal cells, the remaining undamaged neurons are capable of sprouting new connections and forming new functional synapses to replace those lost. This, temporarily at least, may offset the precipitous loss of neurons and could, in principle, stabilize circuitries. The nature of the reactive growth is predictable and has been well defined in animal models.

In animals, unilateral ablation of the entorhinal cortex causes a widespread loss of connections, which are gradually replaced such that virtually the entire population of the synapses is eventually restored. New synapses begin to innervate their targets 2 to 4 days after the lesion is created and continue to appear until prelesion levels are restored after several weeks (6,7).

Several inputs contribute to the restored circuitries (Fig. 2). In animals in which the contralateral entorhinal cortex is spared, the small crossed entorhinal pathway sprouts and increases the innervation of this zone.

This increased input is physiologically potent enough to excite the partially denervated granule cells (8). Thus, the system is capable of restoring bilateral cortical input. It has been postulated that sprouting of this input is a significant factor in the recovery of function after unilateral entorhinal ablation (9,10).

Cholinergic projections from the septal nuclei also sprout after creation of entorhinal lesions (11,12). These cholinergic afferents can be monitored easily with a histochemical stain for the enzyme acetylcholinesterase (AChE). In a normal brain, the molecular layer is only mildly innervated, as evidenced by light, even staining in the outer zone. This is in marked contrast to an animal that has had entorhinal damage, in which there is dark, intense staining in the outer molecular layer indicative of the proliferation of the septal hippocampal projections.

Commissural/associational afferents from CA4 neurons that innervate the inner one-third of the molecular layer also sprout in response to an entorhinal lesion. These fibers expand their terminal fields and sprout part way into the denervated zone. This expansion which can be observed by silver staining, autoradiographic or HRP methods, rapidly and completely repopulates the area of expansion (13-15). Recently, it has been shown that the commissural/associational axons appear to use an excitatory amino acid as neurotransmitter, and receptors for kainic acid, a glutamate analog, appear to be concentrated in the inner zone (16,17). Corresponding to the expansion of the fiber plexus, the kainic acid-binding sites also appear to increase in number in the zone where the fibers have sprouted (18). This suggests that the appropriate receptors are available to subserve synaptic transmission. These new synapses appear capable of enhancing the drive of the dentate granule cells (19). Since these fibers form a recurrent excitatory loop, such sprouting may serve to amplify signals passing through this relay.

Axon sprouting may have its most important functional significance in the aged brain, where neuronal death can occur across the lifespan and in which neurodegenerative diseases are more common. It is clear that the brain of aged rodents is capable of axon sprouting and synaptogenesis throughout the lifespan. Aged animals, as well as adult and young animals, mobilize a robust regenerative reaction which is qualitatively extremely similar to that in younger animals. The principal difference appears to be a reduction in the initial rate of onset rather than in the extent of regrowth (20,21).

In the hippocampal circuitry, virtually every lesion-induced response has been extensively characterized and evaluated with respect to the resultant circuitry. The hippocampal formation of the rodent demonstrates a remarkable degree of plasticity, regardless of the age of the animal. In general, the following conclusions can be drawn:

1. Reinnervation proceeds until a normal or near-normal synaptic density is achieved in all major regions of the hippocampal formation.
2. Aged animals also support lesion-induced neuronal growth, although the onset of reinnervation is delayed.
3. New synaptic connections are formed in response to a loss of synaptic input, and in most instances, a different circuitry is created when compared with the intact system. However, only those inputs already present on denervated neurons increase in abundance.
4. Homotypic inputs appear to be preferred in replacing lost synapses in severe cases; *e.g.*, associational inputs selectively replace commissural input in the dentate gyrus and in area CA1. Homosynaptic reinnervation may compensate for lost synaptic terminals by an expansion of the remaining inputs. In these cases, circuit function *per se* may not be altered except that redundancy is decreased.
5. In the dentate gyrus, sprouting after creation of entorhinal lesions is both homotypic and heterotypic. In this case, heterotypic reinnervation may also be compensatory, since the sprouted heterosynaptic input (C/A and septal inputs) can augment the residual (contralateral and/or ipsilateral entorhinal) pathways.

Hippocampal Plasticity in Alzheimer's Disease

On the basis of this information gained from rodent models, it would be predicted that sprouting might occur in the brain of patients with AD. However, there are at least two reasons why such sprouting might not occur. First, it may be that the degenerative state of the brain is incapable of or incompatible with regenerative growth responses. In other words, the system is in a pure state of catabolism, such that anabolic reactions are unsuccessful: the system degrades more rapidly than it can possibly rebuild. Second, it is not known whether the gradual and partial loss of cells from a population is in itself capable of triggering a regrowth. In animal models, lesions that cause a *rapid* loss of input are used to trigger growth. In contrast, in AD, there is a slow, gradual loss of cells, which may not be sufficient to incite regrowth.

As noted in the introduction, Hyman and colleagues (1) reported that AD is accompanied by a selective loss of layer II and III stellate cells of the entorhinal cortex. Thus, does the loss of entorhinal cells in AD trigger sprouting and reactive synaptogenesis, as in animals with traumatic lesions? Do the commissural/associational fibers sprout in AD brains? Since it is not possible to study these fibers directly in man, it is necessary to use an indirect approach such as the distribution of excitatory amino acid receptors used by the C/A system. The kainic acid-binding pattern in the hippocampus of control patients is similar to that observed in the normal brain. A region of high density of kainic acid sites exists in the inner third of the molecular layer, the innervation zone of the C/A fibers.

In rodents with entorhinal lesions, these kainate binding sites expand so that they occupy one half or more the molecular layer (Fig. 3). In the brains of patients with AD, the kainic acid-binding sites also expand into the outer molecular layer so that they are present in more than half of the zone. This expansion is similar to that which occurs in rodents with entorhinal lesions. These results suggest that C/A fibers in the human brain sprout in response to pathologically induced neuronal loss.

In rodents, entorhinal lesions also trigger growth of the cholinergic septal input to the dentate gyrus. In many cases of AD, there is a selective and profound loss of the basal forebrain cholinergic neurons (22). However, in some cases, neuronal loss in the entorhinal hippocampal subicular complex has been described without a corresponding loss of the forebrain cholinergic neurons.

In those patients in whom significant cholinergic input is present, intensification of AChE activity is found in the outer half of the dentate molecular layer (18; Fig. 4). This finding indicates that these neurons are capable of sprouting in the course of AD. This reaction is qualitatively similar to that described in the rodent brain after entorhinal cell loss.

Thus it appears that the neuronal loss in the entorhinal cortex of AD patients may act as a stimulus much as does a lesion in the rat brain. The loss removes the perforant path input to the hippocampus and dentate gyrus, inducing a compensatory response from adjacent C/A system afferents and from septal afferents, if present. The observed expansion of a receptor field and the increase in the activity of a transmitter-metabolizing enzyme are in marked contrast to the numerous reports of reductions in transmitter-related substances in this disease. Compensatory growth in the course of a degenerative disease indicates that the resultant circuitry cannot simply be considered as a loss of neural elements.

In the dentate gyrus, NMDA receptors are present which appear to mediate long-term potentiation, a synaptic analog of memory. These receptors seem to be well preserved in AD, showing at most only small losses (23), in contrast to previous reports indicating significant neuronal loss of these receptor types (24). Thus, many of the systems necessary to maintain function through a dentate gyrus integration center are preserved or are rebuilt in the course of neuronal loss.

Senile Plaques as Aberrant Sprout-Stimulating Structures

In several cases of AD, we observed that there are numerous AChE-positive plaques in the denervated dentate molecular layer, precisely corresponding to the enhanced sprouting response in this region (18). Their disposition corresponds to the density and distribution of plaques, as revealed by silver stain procedures. From evidence obtained to date, it seems to us that septal sprouting precedes plaque formation. For example, Fig. 5 illustrates a case in which sprouting coexists with plaques within the molecular layer, whereas in an adjacent area of the dentate one can see no sprouting and no plaques. This picture is consistent with the hypothesis that in an early phase of plaque formation, there may be an aberrant process of greatly increased sprouting. The growth of septal fibers may become overstimulated, thereby contributing to an overabundance of reactivity within the plaque. It could be that sprouting is caused by localized degeneration which causes an increase in trophic factors (4). Reactive astrocytes, and possibly neurite-stimulating cells in the area, may cause enhanced sprouting in clusters in the developing plaque. For example, recent studies indicate that astrocytes, and possibly macrophages, produce growth factors, as well as cell-surface molecules such as laminin, which can stimulate sprouting of central neurons. Finally, septal cells appear to degenerate and lose their input to the dentate gyrus. Lacking their proper target, the cells finally lack proper trophic signals, as if they had been axotomized, and this loss contributes to their ultimate demise. Although the mechanisms and details of plaque formation are unknown, this information on sprouting and plaque formation as predecessors to cell degeneration provides an alternative to pure degenerative processes in the sequel of plaque formation.

Discussion

It is our hypothesis that axon sprouting, while plaque formation is minimal, may serve as a natural compensatory reaction to maintain functions that would otherwise decline more rapidly in patients with AD. For example, septal stimulation has been shown to facilitate entorhinal to hippocampal synaptic transmission (25). Thus, additional cholinergic input may be beneficial with regard to hippocampal function, much as increased cholinergic function created by agonists or other pharmacological manipulations can facilitate the function of key relays. CA4 sprouting in the hippocampus provides another example of a possible beneficial reaction. These fibers comprise one of the several feedback loops, part of reverberating circuits within the hippocampus.

After the loss of entorhinal input, the growth of these fibers may act to enhance and build up entorhinal signals which would otherwise be too weak. The CA4 sprouting, then, increases the strength of incoming cortical signals, which can then be relayed to subsequent integrative centers along the pathway. In Alzheimer's patients, it is possible that residual entorhinal inputs may also sprout, thus sustaining input in the wake of partial neuronal loss. However, unlike in animal models, this has not been demonstrated in the brains of patients with AD.

Thus, as the cells are lost, either new connections made by the healthy cells from within the population can assume parallel functions or the fibers from converging pathways can, as illustrated, boost weakened signals and maintain functional stability in the wake of cell loss. Reactive growth can, in principle, help maintain function if a portion of the relay is still intact. The clinical threshold, where functions may disappear, at least is postponed so that the nervous system can counteract the loss of its circuits. Once the system decays to the point where the circuits break, however, we predict a rapid functional decline. Reactive sprouting may be a natural mechanism in aging but also may function in the course of some degenerative disorders. Perhaps, by elucidating the process, it will be possible to develop therapies along these natural lines of defense so that it will be possible to improve the outcome of such central nervous system disorders. Research in this area may also provide new clues on the fundamental issue: what leads to cell loss in the first place? Reactive regrowth of neural circuitries certainly indicates that the brain can mobilize its resources and that the system is sufficiently viable to respond to various interventions.

References

1. Hyman, B.T., Van Hoesen, G.W., Damasio, A.R. & Barnes, C.L. (1984) *Science* **225**, 1168-1170.
2. Cotman, C.W. & Nadler, J.V. (1981) In: *Glutamate: Transmitter in the Central Nervous System*, eds. Roberts, P.J., Storm-Mathisen, J. & Johnston, G.A.R. (John Wiley and Sons, Ltd., London) pp. 117-154.
3. Ball, M.J., Hachinski, V., Fox, A., et al. (1985) *Lancet* **1**, 14-16.
4. Cotman, C.W. & Nieto-Sampedro, M. (1984) *Science* **225**, 1287-1294.
5. Cotman, C.W. & Anderson, K.J. (1986) In: *Physiologic Basis for Functional Recovery in Neurological Disease,* ed. Waxman, S. (Raven Press, New York) in press.
6. Matthews, D.A., Cotman, C.W. & Lynch, G. (1976) *Brain Res.* **115**, 1-21.

7. Matthews, D.A., Cotman, C.W. & Lynch, G. (1976) *Brain Res.* **115**, 23-41.
8. Steward, O., Cotman, C.W. & Lynch, G.S. (1973) *Exp. Brain Res.* **18**, 396-414.
9. Scheff, S.W. & Cotman, C.W. (1977) *Behav. Biol.* **21**, 286-293.
10. Loesche, J. and Steward, O. (1977) *Brain Res. Bull.* **2**, 31-39.
11. Cotman, C.W., Matthews, D.A., Taylor, D. & Lynch, G. (1973) *Proc. Natl. Acad. Sci. USA* **70**, 3473-3477.
12. Lynch, G.S., Matthews, D.A., Mosko, S., Parks, T. & Cotman, C.W. (1972) *Brain Res.* **42**, 311-318.
13. Lynch, G., Gall, C. & Cotman, C.W. (1977) *Exp. Neurol.* **54**, 179-183.
14. Zimmer, J. (1973) *Brain Res.* **64**, 293-311.
15. Scheff, S.W., Benardo, L.S. & Cotman, C.W. (1980) *Brain Res.* **199**, 21-38.
16. Monaghan, D.T. & Cotman, C.W. (1982) *Brain Res.* **252**, 91-100.
17. Monaghan, D.T., Holets, V., Toy, D. & Cotman, C.W. (1983) *Nature* **306**, 176-179.
18. Geddes, J.W., Monaghan, D.T., Cotman, C.W., Lott, I.T., Kim, R.C. & Chui, H.C. (1985) *Science* **230**, 1179-1181.
19. West, J., Deadwyler, S., Cotman, C.W. & Lynch, G. (1975) *Brain Res.* **97**, 215-233.
20. Hoff, S.F., Scheff, S.W., Benardo, L.S. & Cotman, C.W. (1982) *J. Comp. Neurol.* **205**, 246-252.
21. Hoff, S.F., Scheff, S.W., Benardo, L.S. & Cotman, C.W. (1982) *J. Comp. Neurol.* **205**, 253-259.
22. Coyle, J.T., Price, D.L. & DeLong, M.R. (1983) *Science* **219**, 1184-1190.
23. Geddes, J.W. & Cotman, C.W. (1986) *Neurosci. Res.* in press.
24. Greenamyre, J.T., Penney, J.B., Young, A.B., D'Amato, C.J., Hicks, S.P. & Shoulson, I. (1985) *Science* **227**, 1496-1499.
25. Fantie, B.D. & Goddard, G.V. (1982) *Brain Res.* **252**, 227-237.

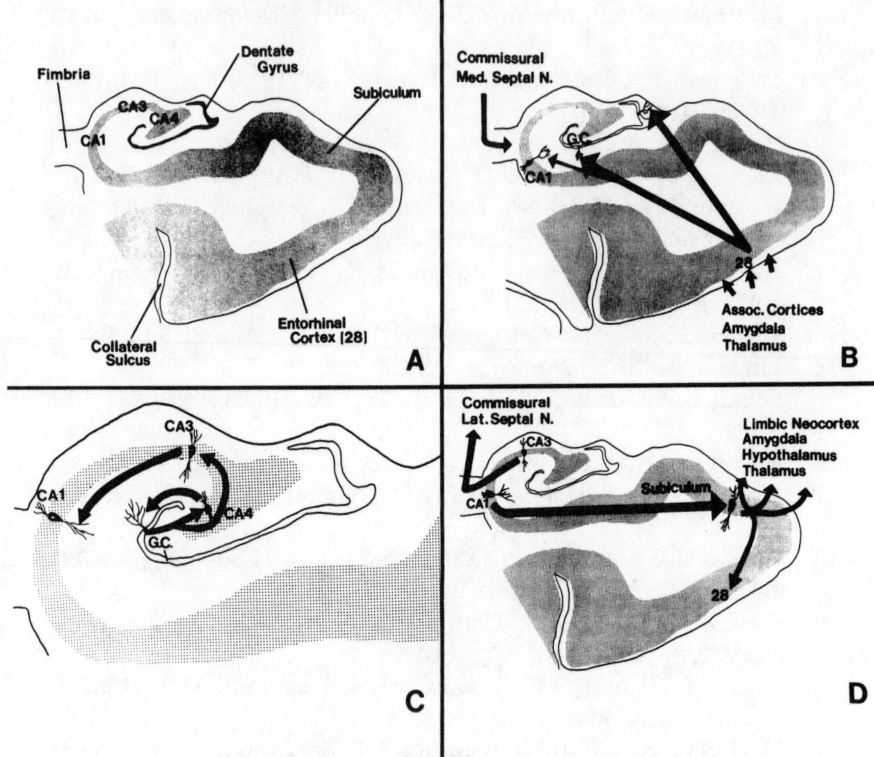

Fig. 1. Summary of the major connections of the hippocampal formation. *A.* Coronal section through human hippocampal formation and overlying parahippocampal gyrus; major cell populations are indicated by shading and include the entorhinal cortex (Brodmann's area 28), subiculum, subdivisions of Ammon's horn (areas CA1-CA4) and the dentate gyrus. *B.* Major inputs to the entorhinal cortex (28). The entorhinal cortex projects primarily to the dentate gyrus granule neurons (large arrows). *C.* Dentate granule cells (G.C.) project to both CA3 and CA4 pyramidal neurons. CA4 pyramidal neurons send a bilateral fiber projection back onto inner dendrites of dentate granule cells (commissural/associational afferents). CA3 neurons project bilaterally to dendrites of CA1 pyramidal neurons. *D.* Outflow of transmission from hippocampal formation. CA1 neurons project heavily to the subiculum which, in turn, projects to limbic neocortex, amygdala, hypothalamic nuclei and thalamus. Additional outputs from hippocampal formation arise from CA3 neurons, giving rise to commissural and septal projections.

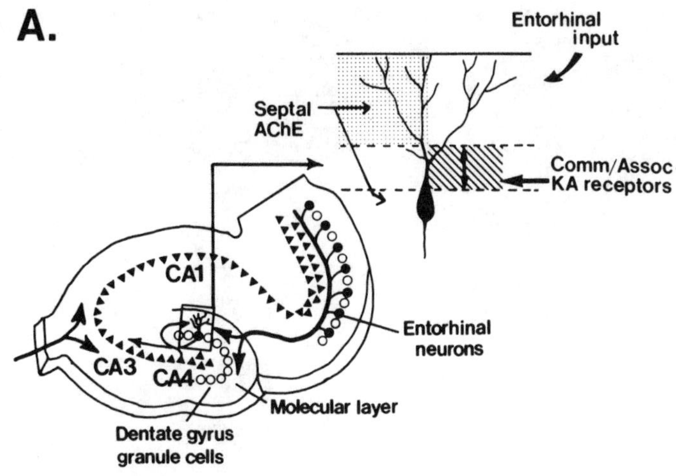

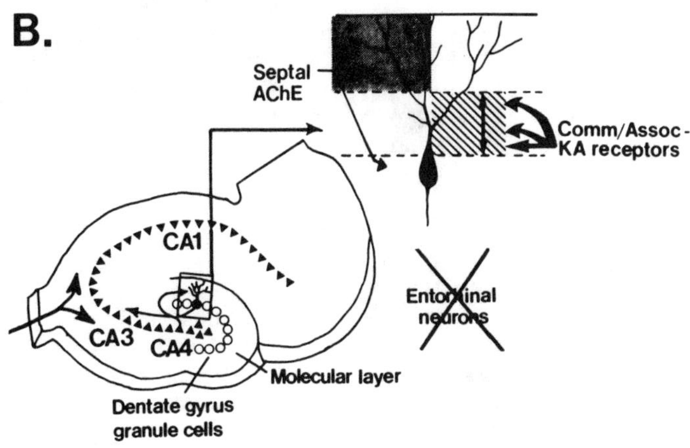

Fig. 2. Changes in dentate gyrus molecular layer following creation of unilateral entorhinal lesion. *A*. Normal distribution of entorhinal input to outer two-thirds of molecular layer, commissural/associational inputs (Comm/Assoc) and kainic acid (KA) receptors in the inner one-third of the molecular layer. Septal inputs occupy outer molecular layer as well as a thin band of fibers in supragranular zone. *B*. After entorhinal ablation, septal afferents as well as commissural and associational afferents sprout.

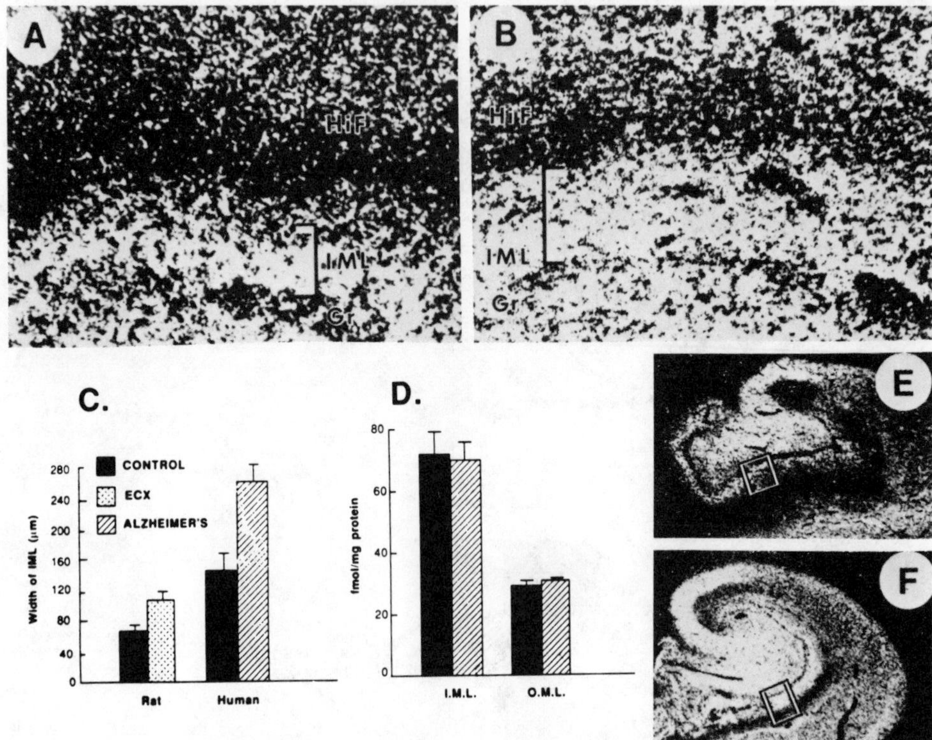

Fig. 3. [^{3}H]-kainic acid (KA) binding in the human hippocampal dentate gyrus. *A.* Autoradiographic distribution of [^{3}H]-KA binding from control subject. Receptors are concentrated in inner molecular layer (IML) immediately subjacent to granule cell layer (Gr). The outer boundary of the dentate gyrus is the hippocampal fissure (HiF). *B.* [^{3}H]-KA binding in Alzheimer's brain. Note that receptor distribution has expanded to occupy more than half of the molecular layer. *C.* Averaged widths of the [^{3}H]-KA binding in inner molecular layer compared in rats that have received an entorhinal cortical lesion (ECX) and controls and in Alzheimer's and control brains. *D.* Total [^{3}H]-KA binding in Alzheimer's brains and controls in the inner (IML) and outer (OML) molecular layers; no significant difference in total binding in the groups. *E.* Low-power autoradiograph of [^{3}H]-KA binding in entire hippocampal formation from control brain (E) and Alzheimer's brain (F). Boxes indicate areas similar to the higher magnifications shown in *A* and *B*.

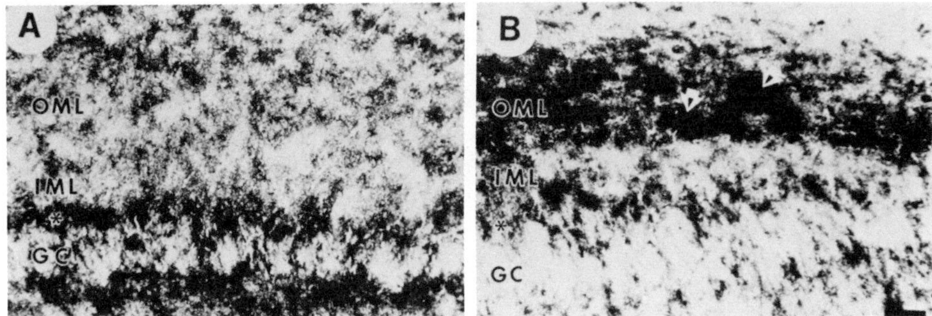

Fig. 4. AChE staining in human hippocampal dentate gyrus. *A*. Control subject; most AChE activity is seen in regions adjacent to granule cell layer (G.C.); *e.g.*, supragranular zone (asterisk). Less-intense staining is seen in the outer (OML) and inner (IML) molecular layers. *B*. Alzheimer's brain; note intensification of activity in outer molecular layer and presence of AChE-positive plaques (arrowheads). Calibration bar = 25 μm.

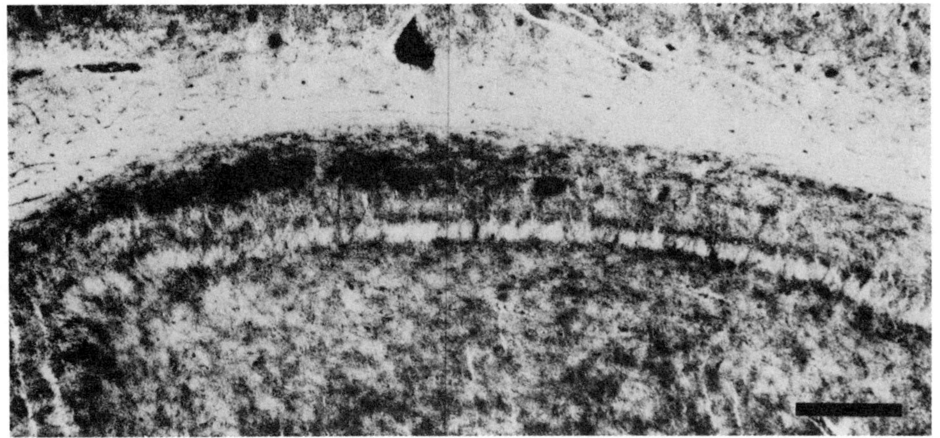

Fig. 5. AChE staining in hippocampal dentate gyrus from Alzheimer's brain; note AChE-positive plaques and intensification in left portion of dentate molecular layer. Right portion appears comparatively normal. Calibration bar = 500 μm.

8. Central Nervous System Degeneration Caused by Prions

MICHAEL R. D. SCOTT, M.D.

Department of Neurology University of California
San Francisco, CA 94143

DAVID WESTAWAY, Ph.D,* STEPHEN J. DeARMOND, M.D.,‡ MICHAEL P. McKINLEY, Ph.D.,* STANLEY B. PRUSINER, M.D.*†

ABSTRACT: Prions cause degenerative neurological diseases: scrapie in animals and Creutzfeldt-Jakob disease in humans. Progress in purification of the scrapie agent, or prion, over the last decade has led to an explosion of new information about slow infections causing brain degeneration. The novel properties and structure of the prion distinguish it from viruses. Besides demonstrating that prions are unique biological particles, our studies have shown that cerebral amyloids may not be inert waste products, as most investigators have assumed for nearly a century. Indeed, scrapie prions fulfill all of the criteria required for their classification as a form of cerebral amyloid. The significance of prion research for understanding nontransmissible degenerative disorders such as Alzheimer's disease (AD) is as yet unknown.

Introduction

Scrapie is rapidly becoming one of the best understood degenerative neurological diseases. Progress in purification of the scrapie agent, or prion, over the last decade has led to an explosion of new information about slow infections causing brain degeneration. Perhaps the most unexpected discovery has been the identification of the cellular isoform of the scrapie prion protein (1). Although the function of this protein in normal cells is unknown, the presence of related PrP genes in virtually all eukaryotes ranging from yeast to humans suggests that cellular prion proteins play an important role in the metabolism of healthy cells.

Departments of *Neurology, †Biochemistry and Biophysics, and ‡Pathology, University of California, San Francisco, CA.

As recently as two years ago, all knowledge about the scrapie agent was derived from bioassays requiring from 2 to 4 months. Now, PrP monoclonal antibodies (2), as well as cloned PrP genes and cDNAs (1), are being used to study the genetic origin and mode of replication of prions as well as the pathogenetic mechanisms of prion diseases.

The significance of prion research for understanding non-transmissible degenerative disorders such as Alzheimer's disease (AD) is unknown. Certainly, many additional studies are necessary to decipher whether knowledge from studies of prions will be helpful in investigating AD, as seems likely.

Scrapie Prions Contain a Sialoglycoprotein

Purification led to the first identification of a putative macromolecule within the scrapie prion (3-7). This molecule (PrP 27-30) is a sialoglycoprotein with an apparent M_r of 27,000 to 30,000 (Table 1) (8). The development of a large-scale purification protocol has allowed determination of the N-terminal sequence of PrP 27-30 and production of antibodies against the protein (6,9,10). Other investigators, using purification steps similar to those we developed, likewise seem to have demonstrated the presence of this protein in their preparations (11,12).

That PrP 27-30, which is derived from PrP 33-35^{Sc}, is a component of the infectious scrapie prion is supported by four principal lines of evidence: (a) PrP 27-30 and scrapie prions copurify (13); PrP 27-30 is the most abundant macromolecule in purified preparations of prions (3); (b) PrP 27-30 concentration is proportional to prion titer (4,5); (c) procedures that denature, hydrolyze or selectively modify PrP 27-30 also diminish prion titer (5,7); and (d) the PrP gene (*Prn-p*) in mice is linked to a gene controlling scrapie incubation times (*Prn-i*) (14). To date, all attempts to separate the scrapie isoform of the prion protein (PrP 33-35^{Sc}) from infectivity have been unsuccessful.

Some investigators have suggested that the scrapie prion protein (PrP 27-30 or PrP 33-35^{Sc}) is unrelated to scrapie infectivity (15-17). They seem not to have considered the differences between the cellular and scrapie isoforms of the prion protein (Table 2). Furthermore, no macromolecule other than PrP 27-30 has been associated with scrapie infectivity.

Considerable evidence suggests that the infectious particles or prions causing scrapie and Creutzfeldt-Jakob disease (CJD) are composed largely if not entirely of protein, although the unlikely possibility that prions contain a small nucleic acid molecule cannot be excluded by available experimental data. How prions multiply is unknown, for they do not contain a gene encoding the prion protein: that gene is found in the host-cellular DNA.

The product of the PrP gene in healthy cells is a protein designated PrP 33-35^C (1,18,19). This protein has an M_r of 33,000 to 35,000, is sensitive to proteases and does not polymerize (1,19). The counterpart of this protein, found only in scrapie-infected animals and called PrP 33-35^{Sc}, is resistant to proteases and does polymerize into amyloid rods and filaments (Table 2). Since PrP 33-35^{Sc} is the only known component of the scrapie infectious particle or prion, learning how PrP 33-35^{Sc} differs chemically from its cellular isoform, PrP 33-35^C, is crucial.

Immunologic Studies of Prion Proteins

One of the most perplexing questions in scrapie and CJD research is now beginning to yield: the lack of an immune response to a lethal "slow infection" has posed a biological puzzle which is unprecedented. Our discovery of PrP 33-35^C may explain why animals and humans do not mount an immune response to PrP 33-35^{Sc} during scrapie or CJD infection (1). This tolerance induced by PrP 33-35^C may also explain why antibodies to PrP 33-35^{Sc} were so difficult to raise (9,20). Nonetheless, we recently succeeded in producing monoclonal antibodies (MAb) to PrP 27-30 (PrP Mab) (2) that recognize both PrP 33-35^C and PrP 33-35^{Sc}. Besides unequivocally establishing the relation between PrP 33-35^C and PrP 33-35^{Sc}, PrP MAb should be of great value in virtually all future phases of scrapie and CJD research.

In homogenates of scrapie-infected hamster brain, two proteins, PrP 33-35^C and PrP 33-35^{Sc}, of M_r 33,000 to 35,000 were recognized by antisera raised against PrP 27-30 (Table 2). After treatment of the homogenates with proteinase K under conditions which do not alter scrapie infectivity, the M_r of PrP 33-35^{Sc} was reduced to 27,000 to 30,000. In homogenates from normal brain, PrP 33-35^C of M_r 33,000 to 35,000 was also found by Western blotting; however, exposure to proteinase K resulted in extensive digestion. The same results were obtained with antisera purified by affinity chromatography using a PrP 27-30 column or with antisera raised against a 13-amino-acid synthetic peptide (PrP-P1) corresponding to the N-terminus of PrP 27-30 (2). Thus, uninfected brain contains a protein of M_r 33,000 to 35,000 which shares antigenic determinants with PrP 27-30 but which is not protease-resistant and does not polymerize into amyloid rods and filaments (Table 2).

Prion Proteins Are Integral Membrane Proteins

Analysis of the PrP cDNA sequence showed that the protein is translated with a 22-amino-acid signal peptide at the N-terminus. Two hydrophobic helices are found within the interior of the protein, and they are of sufficient length to span the membrane (1).

On the basis of these results, subcellular fractionation of scrapie-infected and normal hamster brains was undertaken (19). Both PrP 33-35^{C} and PrP 33-35^{Sc} were found to be membrane-bound (Table 2). Whereas PrP 33-35^{Sc} is absent from normal brain, it increases progressively during scrapie infection. In contrast, the PrP 33-35^{C} concentration remains constant. Detergent extraction of brain microsomes from scrapie-infected hamsters disrupts the membrane and produces prion rods; extraction of normal microsomes does not produce rod-shaped particles (Table 2). These experiments emphasize the differences in physical properties between PrP 33-35^{C} and PrP 33-35^{Sc}.

Cell-free-translation studies with brain mRNA and RNA transcribed from the PrP cDNA produced transmembrane prion proteins (B. Hay, R.A. Barry, I. Lieberburg and S.B. Prusiner, submitted for publication). Using proteolytic digestion of the translation products coupled with antisera produced against a PrP synthetic peptide and lectin-affinity chromatography, the transmembrane orientation of the prion protein was established. The prion protein crosses the membrane bilayer at least twice. To date, we have been unable to produce a protease-resistant form of the prion protein.

Structure of the Prion Protein Deduced from PrP cDNA Sequence

Recent studies (21) have shown that initiation of translation at an ATG codon begins 42 nucleotides upstream from the ATG near the 5′ end of the cDNA clone initially reported (1). The initiation Met is the first of 22 amino acid residues which comprise a signal peptide (Fig. 1). The signal peptide is cleaved by cellular proteases as the native prion protein is synthesized. The first 67 amino acids of PrP 33-35 are not found in PrP 27-30; these amino acids are hydrolyzed during purification which utilizes proteinase K digestion. Western blot analysis shows that homogenates of scrapie-infected brain contain two immunoreactive proteins of apparent M_r 33,000 to 35,000 (19). One protein, PrP 33-35^{C}, is degraded upon digestion with proteinase K, whereas the other, PrP 33-35^{Sc}, is converted to PrP 27-30 during proteinase K digestion (Table 2). The region of the protein which is proteolytically digested contains an interesting set of repeated sequences. Two small repeats of GG(N/S)RYP are followed by a longer set of five repeats of P(H/Q)GGG(/T)WGQ. Although these repeats possess a high degree of beta structure, they are unnecessary for the amyloid properties exhibited by PrP polymers (3). The significance of these repeats is unknown, but it is of interest that they are highly conserved in the hamster, mouse and human proteins (1,15,22). Since these repeats are hydrolyzed when PrP 27-30 is generated and there is no loss of scrapie infectivity, we surmise that they may be important for the cellular function of the prion protein.

As noted above, the deduced prion protein cDNA sequence shows that it has a hydrophobic C-terminus and a hydrophobic domain near the N-terminus (1). The sequence between the hydrophobic regions presumably exhibits considerable beta structure, and there is a segment which probably folds into an amphipathic helix (23). The hydrophobic domains, as well as the amphipathic helix, are probably buried within cellular membranes, since recent studies have shown that the prion protein is an integral membrane protein which spans the membrane bilayer at least twice (B. Hay, R.A. Barry, I. Liebergur, S.B. Prusiner, and V.R. Lingappa, submitted for publication). The finding of multiple forms of scrapie prions has been attributed to their hydrophobicity (24), and numerous studies have documented the association of scrapie infectivity with membranes (25).

The difference between the predicted ($\approx$19 or less) and observed (27 to 30) molecular weights of PrP 27-30 appears to be due to glycosylation (8). Chemical deglycosylation of PrP 27-30 with hydrogen fluoride or trifluoromethane sulfonic acid followed by SDS polyacrylamide gel electrophoresis has yielded a protein of about M_r 20,000 (T. Haraguchi, R.A. Barry and S.B. Prusiner, in preparation). There are two potential N-glycoslylation sites of the type Asn-X-Thr at codons 181 to 183 and 197 to 199. (1,21).

Attempts to find meaningful sequence homologies for the PrP cDNA or its translated protein sequence with other macromolecules in computerized data bases (26,27) have been unsuccessful to date. The amino acid and cDNA sequences of the prion protein were also compared with that of known amyloids, and no homology was found. Thus, the prion protein appears to be unique amongst known macromolecules.

The Hamster PrP Gene

Once correspondence between the cDNA and the amino acid sequence was established, the cDNA was used to probe the genome of the hamster. Both normal and scrapie-infected animals exhibit the same restriction nuclease patterns on Southern blot analysis. A single restriction fragment of 2.6 kb was observed after Eco RI digestion (28), suggesting that the gene for the prion protein might be compact. More recent studies show that the entire open reading frame is contained within a single exon (Fig. 2) (21). The 5′ end of the PrP gene contains multiple initiation sites located between 82 and 50 nucleotides upstream of a splice donor site. These start sites have been defined by S_1 nuclease and primer extension analysis of brain RNA and also by *in vitro* transcription of cloned DNA. (Due to a cloning artifact, the 33 terminal nucleotides of the cDNA clone HaPrPcDNA-s11 are an inverted version of the genomic sequences.) The transcription start sites are preceded by a G+C-rich region which contains three direct repeats of the nonanucleotide GCCCCGCCC. This tandem array strikingly resembles the consensus binding site of the Spl protein (29-31) and the GC motifs found in several viral and cellular promoters (32-35). This promoter structure, which lacks a "TATA" box, is reminiscent of several housekeeping genes. A 10-kb intron follows the splice donor site. A splice acceptor precedes an uninterrupted block of coding sequences which define the remainder of the PrP mRNA. An ATG codon possessing the features of an initiation site (36,37) is located 11 nucleotides downstream of this splice site. This corresponds to the ATG at nucleotide positions 91 to 93 of the HaPrPcDNA-s11 sequence (21).

Hamster chromosomal DNA was cleaved with individual restriction enzymes, electrophoresed through an agarose gel and analyzed by Southern blotting (28) using the radiolabeled PrP gene probes. We have constructed three probes corresponding to (a) the first exon, (b) the intron (21) and (c) the second exon (1); both normal and scrapie-infected animals (75 days after inoculation) gave the same restriction patterns with these probes. From these results, we concluded that PrP 27-30 is encoded by a cellular gene and that rearrangements of this gene are unlikely to figure in the pathogenesis of scrapie. These and other experimental results demonstrate that the PrP gene is single copy.

The degree of sequence conservation between hamster and human PrP is consistent with filter hybridization experiments which revealed that mouse, rat, sheep, goat, nematode, Drosophila and, possibly, yeast harbor candidate PrP gene sequences (38). It is therefore likely that all mammals susceptible to scrapie contain PrP genes. Our results suggest that all mammals may have PrP-related sequences and raise the question of how many other prion diseases exist.

Human PrP cDNA and Creutzfeldt-Jakob Disease Prions

Hybridization (1) and immunochemical (40) studies on CJD prion proteins have implied that the human genome contains a PrP gene. A single RNA species of $\approx$2.5 kb was observed in human polyadenylated RNA samples on a Northern transfer (22).

A human retinal cDNA library was screened using a hamster PrP cDNA probe under conditions of reduced stringency (1), and nine positive clones were identified and selected. Using the established hamster PrP cDNA sequence as a guide for computer arrangement (41) of the human cDNA fragments, a PrP-related open reading frame was established in the human cDNA (22). The predicted amino acid sequence of this human PrP protein has been aligned with the hamster PrP sequence in Figure 3 (1,21). These protein sequences differ in length by one amino acid (253 *vs.* 254). Twenty-seven amino acid residues differ between the hamster and human sequences; this sequence divergency (10.67%) is paralleled by the 96/759 (12.65%) variation in the nucleotide sequences.

The N-terminus of the human PrP protein displays a segment of 22 residues typical of signal peptides (42). These characteristics include a hydrophobic core (MLVLFV) and a small uncharged residue (C) at the putative signal-sequence cleavage site; we predict that the mature protein commences at the Lys residue 23 and that prior to post-translational modification, human PrP has an M_r of 25,239 daltons. Seven of 22 of the putative signal-peptide residues differ from the hamster PrP sequence (Fig. 3). Such signal-peptide sequence variation is well documented (43,44).

Biochemical similarities have been established between the prions causing scrapie and those causing CJD in that antibodies raised against hamster scrapie PrP 27-30 or PrP synthetic peptides cross-react with human CJD prion proteins (40) as well as amyloid plaques from patients with CJD or Gerstmann-Straussler syndrome (GSS) (45). Subsequently, other investigators also demonstrated cross-reactivity between rodent and human prion proteins (46-49). Molecular cloning studies demonstrate that this cross-immunoreactivity results from the highly conserved sequences amongst PrP molecules (1,22). Furthermore, like scrapie prion proteins, CJD prion proteins polymerize into amyloid rods and exhibit green birefringence after staining with Congo red.

Human and Mouse PrP Gene Chromosomal Localization

Studies with somatic-cell hybrids have localized the human PrP gene (PRNP) to chromosome 20 and the mouse PrP gene (*Prn-p*) to chromosome 2 (50). These assignments of the genes to the homologous chromosomes of these organisms provide additional evidence for the hypothesis that a common ancestor of man and mouse possessed a PrP gene. *In situ* hybridization studies have localized PRNP to band 20p12 ⟶ pter. Linkage analysis of the mouse *Prn-p* has located it within 10 cM of the agouti locus on chromosome 2 (51). Additional studies, described below, have shown that *Prn-p* is tightly linked to a gene controlling the scrapie incubation time (*Prn-i*) (14). *Prn-p* and *Prn-i* have been designated the prion gene complex (*Prn*).

Scrapie and Creutzfeldt-Jakob Disease Incubation-Time Genes

A facinating question concerns the mechanism controlling the long incubation periods in prion diseases. For example, in CJD and kuru, incubation times of 30 years appear to be common (52). Early studies with sheep showed that the genetic background of the host could influence both incubation times and susceptibility to scrapie (53). Dickinson and coworkers, using specific inbred strains of mice and "strains" of scrapie prions, defined a genetic locus in mice which they labeled *Sinc* (54,55). They were unable to link *Sinc* to any known genetic markers or to determine its chromosomal location. Neither the strains of mice nor the prions have been made available to other investigators, and little progress in understanding *Sinc* has been made (56).

Two genes which influence prion incubation periods in mice have been identified and their chromosomal assignments determined. *Pid-1* is located on chromosome 17 within the D-subregion of the H-2 (major histocompatibility) complex (57). This gene modulates the incubation period of experimental CJD in congenic mice. Of greater influence in both experimental scrapie and CJD is the *Prn-i* gene, the dominant allele of which codes for longer incubation times (14). Using a restriction-fragment-length polymorphism, *Prn-i* has been shown to be linked to the gene encoding the prion protein (*Prn-p*) (14). Indeed, *Prn-p* and *Prn-i* may be one and the same. If no recombinants are found, then the identity of these two genes can be tested directly using transgenic and chimeric mice.

Defining the precise nucleotide sequences responsible for short and long incubation times will be of paramount importance. Such studies should, for the first time, begin to elucidate the molecular mechanisms controlling incubation times in prion diseases and may help us understand why many degenerative diseases manifest themselves late in life. It is tempting to speculate that the prion clock gene (*Prn-i*) has a more general influence, perhaps even playing a role in the timing of senescence.

Expression of PrP mRNA

Polyadenylated RNA prepared from brains of normal and scrapie-infected hamsters at different times after inoculation with prions was analyzed by Northern blotting (58) using a PrP cDNA (1). There was no significant difference between the samples obtained from infected and control animals. Using a mouse PrP cDNA probe, Chesebro *et al.* (15) obtained similar results.

In situ hybridization of normal and scrapie-infected hamster brains showed that neurons contain the highest levels of PrP mRNA (equivalent to 50 copies per cell). In contrast, glial cells contain <3 mRNA copies per cell (59). These findings are in accord with the well-established observation that central nervous system (CNS) neurons are probably the only cell type which undergoes degeneration in prion diseases (60).

Although PrP mRNA levels were unchanged throughout the course of scrapie infection, we have found that the expression of the PrP gene is developmentally regulated (61). During the first 20 days after birth, PrP mRNA increases in the neonatal hamster brain, as measured by Northern blot analysis of polyadenylated RNA and cell-free translation of total brain RNA (61). By 20 days of age, PrP mRNA levels reach a maximum. Apparently, the levels of PrP mRNA remain constant throughout the adult life of the hamster.

Recent studies have shown that PrP mRNA levels in the septal nucleus of the developing hamster brain can be modulated by nerve growth factor (NGF). Newborn hamsters injected intraventricularly with NGF 2, 5 and 7 days after birth showed a 15- to 20-fold increase in their septal PrP mRNA levels (W. Mobley, M.P. McKinley and S.B. Prusiner, in preparation).

Search for a Prion Genome

The size of the smallest infectious unit causing scrapie remains controversial, principally because of the extreme heterogeneity and apparent hydrophobicity of the prion. Early studies by Alper and her colleagues suggested an M_r of 60,000 to 150,000 based on ionizing-radiation particle-size estimates (62,63). Although an alternate interpretation of the data has been proposed (12), there is no firm evidence that Alper's M_r calculations are incorrect. In fact, in recent studies, purified preparations of prions exhibited the same resistance to inactivation by ionizing radiation observed by Alper for the scrapie agent in brain homogenates nearly 20 years earlier. In addition, sucrose-gradient sedimentation, molecular-sieve chromatography and membrane-filtration studies all suggest that a significant portion of the infectious particles are considerably smaller than the smallest known viruses (64). However, the propensity of the scrapie agent to aggregate makes M_r determinations by each of these methods subject to artifact.

To date, no experimental data have indicated that scrapie infectivity depends on nucleic acid within the particle. Attempts to inactivate scrapie prions with nucleases, ultraviolet radiation (254 nm), zinc-catalyzed hydrolysis, psoralen photoadduct formation and chemical modification by hydroxylamine have all yielded negative results, even in preparations that contain one major protein as determined by amino acid sequencing (39,64,65). Although these negative results cannot prove the absence of a nucleic acid genome within the prion, they make such absence likely. Moreover, the many attempts to identify a prion-specific, subgenomic nucleic acid of 10 to 2,000 bases using silver staining and [^{32}P]-5′-end labeling have been unsuccessful to date.

Purified preparations of prions obtained by detergent extraction, differential centrifugation and sucrose-gradient sedimentation were disrupted by phenol extraction and blotted on nitrocellulose. Under conditions optimal for hybridization of the cDNA with either RNA or DNA, no annealing of the radiolabeled PrP cDNA with the phenol extracts of the purified prions was observed. Less than 0.004 nucleic acid molecules per ID_{50} unit were found, demonstrating that prions do not carry a genomic nucleic acid encoding the prion protein (1).

These observations of DNA encoding PrP 27-30 within the hamster genome but not within the infectious prion particles show that prions are not typical viruses. The presence of a genomic nucleic acid within the DNA of the host which encodes PrP 27-30 is reminiscent of the integrated genomes of retrovirus proteins; however, unlike retroviruses, infectious prion particles contain no RNA or DNA molecules encoding their protein. This observation forces us to reject the hypothesis that the scrapie prion is an elusive but typical virus, as typical viruses contain either an RNA or a DNA genome which encodes at least one protein of their coat or capsid. However, it is conceivable that a novel defective virus might derive its capsid protein from sequences encoded by the host instead of by a helper virus. In the case of the prion, only one protein has been found associated with the infectivity, and this protein is clearly encoded within the host genome.

Several hypothetical structures and replication mechanisms for the prion can now be eliminated (66,67). For example, our results exclude the need for an unprecedented process such as reverse translation or protein-directed protein synthesis to explain the multiplication of PrP 27-30 molecules during scrapie infection. It is still possible that prions are novel defective viruses. In other words, prions might contain a small nucleic acid which has not been detected and derive their protective capsid from host-encoded proteins which are modified into a protease-resistant form during infection. However, there is no evidence for such a nucleic acid.

Ultrastructural Studies of Scrapie and Creutzfeldt-Jakob Disease Prions

Many investigators have used the electron microscope to search for a scrapie-specific particle. Spheres, rods, fibrils and tubules have been described in scrapie-, kuru- and CJD-infected brain tissue (68-75). Notable amongst the early studies are reports of filamentous virus-like particles 15 nm in diameter in human CJD brain (73) and rod-shaped particles measuring 15 to 26 nm in brains of sheep, rats and mice with scrapie (74,75). Studies with ruthenium red and lanthanum nitrate suggest that the rod-shaped particles possess surface polysaccharides; these findings are of special interest since PrP 27-30 is a sialoglycoprotein (8).

In purified fractions prepared from scrapie-infected brains, rod-shaped particles measuring 10 to 20 nm in diameter and 100 to 200 nm in length were found (3,13). Although no unit morphologic structure could be identified, most of the rods exhibited a relatively uniform diameter and appeared as flattened cylinders. Some of the rods had a twisted structure, suggesting that they might be composed of protofilaments. In the fractions containing rods, one major protein (PrP 27-30) and $\approx 10^{9.5}$ ID_{50} units of prions per milliliter were found. The high degree of purity of our preparations, demonstrated by radiolabeling and SDS polyacrylamide gel electrophoresis, allowed us to establish that the rods are composed of PrP 27-30 molecules. Since PrP 27-30 had already been shown to be required for and inseparable from infectivity (5), we concluded that the rods must be a form of the prion (76). Immunoelectron microscopic studies using antibodies raised against PrP 27-30 have confirmed that the rods are composed of PrP 27-30 molecules (77).

Recent studies have shown that the rod-shaped particles in purified preparations of prions are created upon detergent extraction of membranes containing PrP $33\text{-}35^{Sc}$ (Fig. 4A and B) (19). Detergent extraction of membranes containing only PrP $33\text{-}35^{C}$ did not produce rods (Table 2). These observations support our hypothesis that the rods are aggregates of prions (3,13).

Sonication of the prion rods reduced their mean length to 60 nm and generated many spherical particles without altering infectivity titers (Fig. 4C) (61). In contrast, fragmentation of the M-13 filamentous bacteriophage by brief sonication reduced infectivity significantly. These studies demonstrate that the scrapie agent is not a filamentous animal virus, as some investigators have suggested (78).

Scrapie and Creutzfeldt-Jakob Disease Prion Proteins Form Amyloids

The ultrastructure of the prion rods is indistinguishable from that of many purified amyloids (3). Histochemical studies with Congo red have extended this analogy to purified preparations of prions (3) as well as to scrapie-infected brain, where amyloid plaques stain with antibodies to PrP 27-30 (9). In addition, Prp 27-30 stains with periodic acid-Schiff reagent (8); amyloid plaques in tissue sections likewise readily bind this reagent.

Recent immunocytochemical studies with antibodies to PrP 27-30 have shown that filaments measuring approximately 16 nm in diameter and up to 1500 nm in length within amyloid plaques of scrapie-infected hamster brain are composed of prion proteins (79). The antibodies to PrP 27-30 did not react with neurofilaments, glial filaments, microtubules or microfilaments in brain tissue. The prion filaments have relatively uniform diameter, rarely showing narrowings, and possess all the morphologic features of amyloid. Except for their length, the prion filaments appear to be identical ultrastructurally to the rods found in purified fractions of prions.

In extracts of scrapie-infected rodent brains, abnormal structures were found by electron microscopy and labeled scrapie-associated fibrils (80). These abnormal fibrils were distinguished from other filamentous structures including amyloids by their characteristic and well-defined morphology (78,80,81). Some investigators have equated these fibrils with the prion rods (82) even though the rods are both ultrastructurally and histochemically identical to many amyloids (3). Whereas the rods are composed largely if not entirely of scrapie or CJD prion proteins, the composition of the fibrils remains to be established.

Alzheimer's Disease and Prions

Besides demonstrating that prions are unique biological particles and fundamentally different from viruses, our studies have shown that cerebral amyloids may not be inert waste products, as most investigators have assumed for nearly a century (3,9,82). Indeed, scrapie prions fulfill all the criteria required for their classification as a form of cerebral amyloid. This discovery has intensified interest in the possible etiologic role of amyloids in AD (82). For nearly a century, the accumulation of amyloid filaments with senile plaques and neurofibrillary tangles (NFT) was appreciated, but their significance in the causation of AD has been a subject of continuing controversy (83).

Recent studies have shown that the major protein of vascular amyloid in AD and probably in AD senile plaques is unrelated to the prion protein; this conclusion is based on both amino acid sequencing (84-88) and immunostaining studies (45,89; G.W. Roberts, R. Lofthouse, R. Brown, T.J. Crow, R.A. Barry and S.B. Prusiner, submitted for publication). The proteins comprising paired helical filaments (PHF) of the NFT are less well characterized (90-97). Interestingly, some antisera raised against partially purified PHF from AD brains do stain amyloid plaques in CJD, GSS and kuru; the molecular basis for this cross-reactivity remains to be established (98).

The lack of AD transmissibility to experimental animals was the first evidence that the etiologic molecules in AD were not CJD prions even though the two diseases share many clinical and pathologic features (99). On the other hand, learning about the molecular changes which differentiate the cellular prion protein from its CJD isoform may be informative in understanding the pathogenesis of AD. Of interest are familial pedigrees which contain multiple cases of both AD and CJD (100). Whether these pedigrees demonstrate a significant relation between these two dementing degenerative CNS disorders or whether AD is simply an incidental finding in familial CJD is unknown.

It will be important to define the human prion gene complex and learn whether any gene within or near the complex plays any role in the pathogenesis of AD. Presumably, a human prion incubation-time gene controls the timing of CJD, GSS and kuru. Perhaps this same clock gene regulates the age-dependent degenerative CNS diseases such as AD, Parkinson's disease and amyotrophic lateral sclerosis.

Clearly, the approaches developed first for the investigation of experimental scrapie in rodents have proved to be directly applicable to the study of CNS degeneration in humans caused by CJD prions. Perhaps most important, the current study of prions may represent a point of departure for future investigations of other degenerative diseases. Many disorders may eventually be shown to be caused by prion-like macromolecules. The genetic origin of prions and the slow amplification mechanisms which account for their replication make these unique macromolecules interesting candidates for involvement in many diseases that occur later in life.

Acknowledgments

Portions of this chapter were adapted from an article to be published in *Annual Reviews of Medicine.* Important contributions from Drs. R. Barry, C. Bellinger-Kawahara, J. Bockman, K. Gilles and R. Mayer are gratefully acknowledged. Collaborative studies with Drs. G. Carlson, J. Cleaver, T. Diener, W. Hadlow, L. Hood, S. Kent, D. Kingsbury, B. Oesch, D. Riesner and C. Weissmann have been important to the progress of these studies and are greatly appreciated. The authors thank K. Bowman, D. Groth, M. Vincent and M. Walchli for technical assistance as well as L. Gallagher and S. Coleman for editorial and administrative assistance. This work was supported by research grants from the National Institutes of Health (AGO2132 and NS14069) as well as by gifts from R.J. Reynolds Industries, Inc. and the Sherman Fairchild Foundation.

References

1. Oesch, R., Westaway, D., Walchli, M., McKinley, M.P., Kent, S.B., Aebersold, R., Barry, R.A., Tempst, P., Teplow, D.B., Hood, L.E., Prusiner, S.B. & Weissmann, C. (1985) *Cell* **40**, 735-746.
2. Barry, R.A. & Prusiner, S.B. (1986) *J. Infect. Dis.* (in press).
3. Prusiner, S.B., McKinley, M.P., Bowman, K.A., Bolton, D.C., Bendheim, P.E., Groth, D.F. & Glenner, G.G. (1983) *Cell* **35**, 349-358.
4. Bolton, D.C., McKinley, M.P. & Prusiner, S.B. (1982) *Science* **218**, 1309-1311.
5. McKinley, M.P., Bolton, D.C. & Prusiner, S.B. (1983) *Cell* **35**, 57-62.
6. Prusiner, S.B., Groth, D.F., Bolton, D.C., Kent, S.B. & Hood, L.E. (1984) *Cell* **38**, 127-134.
7. Bolton, D.C., McKinley, M.P. & Prusiner, S.B. (1984) *Biochemistry* **23**, 5898-5905.
8. Bolton, D.C., Meyer, R.K. & Prusiner, S.B. (1985) *J. Virol.* **53**, 596-606.
9. Bendheim, P.E., Barry, R.A., DeArmond, S.J., Stites, D.P. & Prusiner, S.B. (1984) *Nature* **310**, 418-421.
10. Bendheim, P.E., Bockman, J.M., McKinley, M.P., Kingsbury, D.T. & Prusiner, S.B. (1985) *Proc. Natl. Acad. Sci. USA* **82**, 997-1001.
11. Diringer, H., Gelderblom, H., Hilmert, H., Ozel, M., Edelbluth, C. & Kimberlin, R.H. (1983) *Nature* **306**, 476-478.
12. Hilmert, H. & Diringer, H. (1984) *Biosci. Rep.* **4**, 165-170.
13. Prusiner, S.B., Bolton, D.C., Groth, D.F., Bowman, K.A., Cochran, S.P. & McKinley, M.P. (1982) *Biochemistry* **21**, 6942-6950.
14. Carlson, G.A., Kingsbury, D.T., Goodman, P., Coleman, S., Marshall, S.T., DeArmond, S.J., Westaway, D. & Prusiner, S.B. (1986) *Cell* **46**, 503-511.
15. Chesebro, B., Race, R., Wehrly, K., Nishio, J., Bloom, M., Lechner, D., Bergstrom, S., Robbins, K., Mayer, L., Keith, J.M., Garon, C. & Haase, A. (1985) *Nature* **315**, 331-333.
16. Weitgrefe, S., Zupancic, M., Haase, A., Chesebro, B., Race, R., Frey, W. II, Rustan, T. & Friedman, R.L. (1985) *Science* **230**, 1177-1181.
17. Braig, H.R. & Diringer, H. (1985) *EMBO J.* **4**, 2309-2312.
18. Barry, R.A., Kent, S.B., McKinley, M.P., Meyer, R.K., DeArmond, S.J., Hood, L.E. & Prusiner, S.B. (1986) *J. Infect. Dis.* **153**, 848-854.
19. Meyer, R.K., McKinley, M.P., Bowman, K.A., Barry, R.A. & Prusiner, S.B. (1986) *Proc. Natl. Acad. Sci. USA* **83**, 2310-2314.

20. Kasper, K.C., Bowman, K., Stites, D.P. & Prusiner, S.B. (1981) In: *Hamster Immune Responses in Infectious and Oncologic Diseases*, ed. Streilein, J.W., Hart, D.A., Stein-Streilein, J., Duncan, W.R. & Billingham, R.E. (Plenum Press, New York) pp. 401-413.
21. Basler, K., Oesch, B., Scott, M., Westaway, D., Walchli, M., Groth, D.F., McKinley, M.P., Prusiner S.B. & Weissmann, C. (1986) *Cell* **46**, 417-428.
22. Kretzschmar, H.A., Stowring, L.E., Westaway, D., Stubblebine, W.H., Prusiner, S.B. & DeArmond, S.J. (1986) *DNA* **5**, 315-324.
23. Finer-Moore, J. & Stroud, R.M. (1984) *Proc. Natl. Acad. Sci. USA* **81**, 155-159.
24. Prusiner, S.B., Hadlow, W.J., Garfin, D.E., Cochran, S.P., Baringer, J.R., Race, R.E. & Eklund, C.M. (1978) *Biochemistry* **17**, 4993-4997.
25. Hunter, G.D. (1979) In: *Slow Transmissible Diseases of the Nervous System*, ed. Prusiner, S.B. & Hadlow, W.J. (Academic Press, New York) Vol. 2, pp. 365-385.
26. Genetic Sequence Data Bank. 1 August 1984. Genbank (R) Release 23.0. 4088 Loci, 3220532 Bases, from 5198 Repeated Sequences.
27. Protein Sequence Database of the Protein Identification Resource (PIR), Supported by the Division of Research Resources of the National Institutes of Health, Release 2.1. August 13, 1984. Barker, W.C., Hart, L.T., Orcutt, B.C., George, D.G., Yeh, L.S., Chen, H.R., Blomquist, M.C., Johnson, G.C., Seibel-Ross, E.I., Ledley, R.S. National Biomedical Research Foundation, Washington, D.C.
28. Southern, E.M. (1975) *J. Mol. Biol.* **98**, 503-517.
29. Dynan, W.S. & Tijian, R. (1983) *Cell* **32**, 669-680.
30. Dynan, W.S., Sazer, S., Tijian, R. & Schimke, R.T. (1986) *Nature* **319**, 246-248.
31. Kadonaga, J.R., Jones, K.A. & Tijian, R. (1986) *Trends Biochem. Sci.* **11**, 20-23.
32. Fromm, M. & Berg, P. (1982) *J. Mol. Appl. Genet.* **1**, 457-481.
33. McKnight, S.L. & Kingsbury, R. (1982) *Science* **217**, 316-325.
34. Reynolds, G.A., Basu, S.K., Osborne, T.F., Chin, D.J., Gil, G., Brown, M.S., Goldstein, J.L. & Luskey, K.L. (1984) *Cell* **38**, 275-285.
35. Valerio, D., Duyvesteyn, M.G., Dekker, B.M., Weeda, G., Berkvens, T.M., van der Voorn, L., van Ormondt, H. & van der Eb, A.J. (1985) *EMBO J.* **4**, 437-443.
36. Kozak, M. (1984) *Nucleic Acids Res.* **12**, 857-872.
37. Kozak, M. (1984) *Nature* **308**, 241-246.
38. Westaway, D. & Prusiner, S.B. (1986) *Nucleic Acids Res.* **14**, 2035-2044.

39. McKinley, M.P., Masiarz, F.R., Isaacs, S.T., Hearst, J.E. & Prusiner, S.B. (1983) *Photochem. Photobiol.* **37**, 539-545.
40. Bockman, J.M., Kingsbury, D.T., McKinley, M.P., Bendheim, P.E. & Prusiner, S.B. (1985) *N. Engl. J. Med.* **312**, 73-78.
41. Conrad, B. & Mount, D.W. (1982) *Nucleic Acids Res.* **10**, 31-38.
42. von Heijne, G. (1985) *J. Mol. Biol.* **184**, 99-105.
43. Sabatini, D.D., Kreibich, G., Morimoto, T. & Adesnik, M. (1982) *J. Cell Biol.* **92**, 1-22.
44. von Heijne, G. (1983) *Eur. J. Biochem.* **133**, 17-21.
45. Kitamoto, T., Tateishi, J., Tashima, I., Takeshita, I., Barry, R.A., DeArmond, S.J. & Prusiner, S.B. (1986) *Ann. Neurol.* (in press).
46. Gibbs, C.J. Jr., Joy, A., Heffner, R., Franko, M., Miyazaki, M., Asher, D.M., Parisi, J.E., Brown, P.W., Gajdusek, D.C. (1985) *N. Engl. J. Med.* **313**, 734-738.
47. Bode, L., Pocchiari, M., Gelderblom, H. & Diringer, H. (1985) *J. Gen. Virol.* **66**, 2471-2478.
48. Brown, P., Gajdusek, D.C., Gibbs, C.J. Jr. & Asher, D.M. (1985) *N. Engl. J. Med.* **313**, 728-731.
49. Manuelidis, L., Valley, S. & Manuelidis, E.E. (1985) *Proc. Natl. Acad. Sci. USA* **82**, 263-267.
50. Sparkes, R.S., Simon, M., Cohn, V.H., Fournier, R.E., Lem, J., Klisak, I., Heinzmann, C., Blatt, C., Lucero, M., Mohandas, T., DeArmond, S.J., Westaway, D., Prusiner, S.B. & Weiner, L.P. (1986) *Proc. Natl. Acad. Sci. USA* (in press).
51. Carlson, G.A., Lovett, M., Epstein, C.J., Westaway, D., Goodman, P.A., Marshall, S.T. & Prusiner, S.B. (1986) *Molecular and Biochemical Genetics Workshop* (Abstr.)
52. Gajdusek, D.C. (1977) *Science* **197**, 943-960.
53. Parry, H.B., ed. (1983) In: *Scrapie Disease in Sheep* (Academic Press, New York).
54. Dickinson, A.G. & Meikle, V.M. (1971) *Mol. Gen. Genet.* **112**, 73-79.
55. Dickinson, A.G., Bruce, M.E., Outram, G.W. & Kimberlin, R.H. (1984) In: *Proceedings of Workshop on Slow Transmissible Diseases,* Tokyo, pp. 105-118.
56. Kimberlin, R.H. (1986) *Neuropathol. Appl. Neurobiol.* **12**, 131-147.
57. Kingsbury, D.T., Kasper, K.C., Stites, D.P., Watson, J.C., Hogan, R.N. & Prusiner, S.B. (1983) *J. Immunol.* **131**, 491-496.
58. Thomas, P.S. (1980) *Proc. Natl. Acad. Sci. USA* **77**, 5201-5205.
59. Kretzschmar, H.A., Prusiner, S.B., Stowring, L.E. & DeArmond, S.J. (1986) *Am. J. Pathol.* **122**, 1-5.
60. Zlotnik, I. (1962) *Acta Neuropathol. (Berlin)* **1 (suppl.)**, 61-70.
61. McKinley, M.P., Braunfeld, M.B., Bellinger, C.G. & Prusiner, S.B. (1986) *J. Infect. Dis.* **154**, 110-120.

62. Alper, T., Haig, D.A. & Clarke, M.C. (1966) *Biochem. Biophys. Res. Commun.* **22**, 278-284.
63. Latarjet, R. (1979) In: *Slow Transmissible Diseases of the Nervous System*, ed. Prusiner, S.B. & Hadlow, W.J. (Academic Press, New York) Vol. 2, pp. 387-408.
64. Prusiner, S.B. (1982) *Science* **216**, 136-144.
65. Diener, T.O., McKinley, M.P. & Prusiner, S.B. (1982) *Proc. Natl. Acad. Sci. USA* **79**, 5220-5224.
66. Prusiner, S.B., Cochran, S.P., Groth, D.F., Downey, D.E., Bowman, K.A. & Martinez, H.M. (1982) *Ann. Neurol.* **11**, 353-358.
67. Prusiner, S.B. (1984) *Sci. Am.* **251**, 50-59.
68. David-Ferreira, J.F., David-Ferreira, K.L., Gibbs, C.J. Jr. & Morris, J.A. (1968) *Proc. Soc. Exp. Biol. Med.* **127**, 313-320.
69. Bignami, A. & Parry, H.B. (1971) *Science* **171**, 389-399.
70. Lampert, P.W., Gajdusek, D.C. & Gibbs, C.J. Jr. (1971) *J. Neuropathol. Exp. Neurol.* **30**, 20-32.
71. Baringer, J.R. & Prusiner, S.B. (1978) *Ann. Neurol.* **4**, 205-211.
72. Field, E.J., Mathews, J.D. & Raine, C.S. (1969) *J. Neurol. Sci.* **8**, 209-224.
73. Vernon, M.L., Horta-Barbosa, L., Fuccillo, D.A., Sever, J. L., Baringer, J.R. & Birnbaum, G. (1970) *Lancet* **1**, 964-966.
74. Field, E.J. & Narang, H.K. (1972) *J. Neurol. Sci.* **17**, 347-364.
75. Narang, H.K. (1974) *Acta Neuropathol. (Berlin)* **28**, 317-329.
76. Rasool, C.G. & Selkoe, D.J. (1985) *N. Engl. J. Med.* **312**, 700-705.
77. Barry, R.A., McKinley, M.P., Bendheim, P.E., Lewis, G.K., DeArmond, S.J. & Prusiner, S.B. (1985) *J. Immunol.* **135**, 603-613.
78. Merz, P.A., Rohwer, R.G., Kascsak, R., Wisniewski, H.M., Somerville, R.A., Gibbs, C.J. Jr. & Gajdusek, D.C. (1984) *Science* **225**, 437-440.
79. DeArmond, S.J., McKinley, M.P., Barry, R.A., Braunfeld, M.B., McColloch, J.R. & Prusiner, S.B. (1985) *Cell* **41**, 221-235.
80. Merz, P.A., Somerville, R.A., Wisniewski, H.M. & Iqbal, K. (1981) *Acta Neuropathol. (Berlin)* **54**, 63-74.
81. Merz, P.A., Wisniewski, H.M., Somerville, R.A., Bobin, S.A., Masters, C.L. & Iqbal, K. (1983) *Acta Neuropathol. (Berlin)* **60**, 113-124.
82. Diringer, H., Gelderblom, H., Hilmert, H., Ozel, M., Edelbluth, C. & Kimberlin, R.H. (1983) *Nature* **306**, 476-478.
83. Katzman, R. (1986) *N. Engl. J. Med.* **314**, 964-973.
84. Wong, C.W., Quaranta, V. & Glenner, G.G. (1985) *Proc. Natl. Acad. Sci. USA* **82**, 8729-8732.
85. Glenner, G.G. & Wong, C.W. (1984) *Biochem. Biophys. Res. Commun.* **122**, 1131-1135.

86. Glenner, G.G. & Wong, C.W. (1984) *Biochem. Biophys. Res. Commun.* **120**, 885-890.
87. Masters, C.L., Simms, G., Weinman, N.A., Multhaup, G., McDonald, B.L. & Beyreuther, K. (1985) *Proc. Natl. Acad. Sci. USA* **82**, 4245-4249.
88. Roher, A., Wolfe, D., Paultke, M. & Kukuruga, D. (1986) *Proc. Natl. Acad. Sci. USA* **83**, 2662-2666.
89. Brown, P., Coker-Vann, M., Pomeroy, K., Franko, M., Asher, D.M., Gibbs, C.J. Jr. & Gajdusek, D.C. (1986) *N. Engl. J. Med.* **314**, 547-551.
90. Kosik, K.S., Joachim, C.L. & Selkoe, D.J. (1986) *Proc. Natl. Acad. Sci. USA* **83**, 4044-4048.
91. Wood, J.G., Mirra, S.S., Pollock, N.J. & Binder, L.I. (1986) *Proc. Natl. Acad. Sci. USA* **83**, 4040-4043.
92. Grundke-Iqbal, I., Iqbal, K., Tung, Y., Quinlan, M., Wisniewski, H.M. & Binder, L.I. (1986) *Proc. Natl. Acad. Sci. USA* **83**, 4913-4917.
93. Sternberger, N.H., Sternberger, L.A. & Ulrich, J. (1985) *Proc. Natl. Acad. Sci. USA* **82**, 4274-4276.
94. Masters, C.L., Multhaup, G., Simms, G., Pottgiesser, J., Martins, R.N. & Beyreuther, K. (1985) *EMBO J.* **4**, 2757-2763.
95. Crowther, R.A & Wischik, C.M. (1985) *EMBO J.* **4**, 3661-3665.
96. Miller, C.C.J., Brion, J.-P., Calvert, R., Chin, T.K., Eagles, P.A.M., Downes, M.J., Flament-Durand, J., Haugh, M., Kahn, J., Probst, A., Ulrich, J. & Anderton, B.H. (1986) *EMBO J.* **5**, 269-276.
97. Perry, G., Rizzuto, N., Autilio-Gambetti, A. & Gambetti, P. (1985) *Proc. Natl. Acad. Sci. USA* **82**, 3916-3920.
98. Kates, J., DeArmond, S.J., Borcich, J., Barry, R.A. & Prusiner, S.B. (1986) *Neurology* **36 (Suppl. 1)**:224 (Abstr.)
99. Goudsmit, J., Morrow, C.H., Asher, D.M., Yanagihara, R.T., Masters, C.L., Gibbs, C.J. Jr. & Gajdusek, D.C. (1980) *Neurology* **30**, 945-950.
100. Masters, C.L., Gajdusek, D.C. & Gibbs, C.J. Jr. (1981) *Brain* **104**, 535-558.

TABLE 1. Glossary of prion terminology

Prion	Small *pro*teinacous *in*fectious particle which resists inactivation by procedures that modify nucleic acids. It causes scrapie and Creutzfeldt-Jakob disease (CJD). "Scrapie agent" is a synonym.
PrP 27-30	This protein is the only identifiable macromolecule in purified preparations of hamster scrapie prions. Digestion of PrP 33-35^{Sc} with proteinase K generates PrP 27-30.
PrP 33-35^{Sc} or PrP^{Sc}	Scrapie isoform of the prion protein (PrP).
PrP 33-35^{C} or PrP^{C}	Cellular isoform of the prion protein (PrP).
Prn-p	Prp gene in mice; located on chromosome 2.
PRNP	Prp gene in humans; located on chromosome 20.
Pid-1	Gene in mice on chromosome 17 controlling scrapie incubation times.
Prn-i	Gene in mice on chromosome 2 controlling scrapie incubation times. *Prn-i* and *Prn-p* form the prion gene complex.
Sinc	Genetic locus in mice controlling scrapie incubation times; location unknown.
Prion rod	An aggregate of prions composed largely, if not entirely, of PrP^{Sc} or PrP 27-30 molecules. Created by detergent extraction of membranes. Morphologically and histochemically indistinguishable from many amyloids.

TABLE 2. Cellular and scrapie prion protein isoforms in hamsters

Properties	*PrP 33-35^{C}*	*PrP 33-35^{Sc}*
Uninfected brain	Present	Absent
Scrapie brain	Level unchanged	Accumulates
Concentration*	<1 μg/g	≈10μg/g
Purified prions	Absent	10^4 molecules/ID_{50}
Genetic origin	One cellular gene	One cellular gene
mRNA	2.1 kb	2.1 kb
Location:		
Intracellular	Membrane-bound	Membrane-bound
Extracellular	None	Amyloid filaments with plaques
Detergent extraction	Soluble	Amyloid rods formed
Protease digestion	Degraded	Converted to PrP 27-30†

*Expressed as micrograms of prion protein per gram of brain tissue; † PrP 27-30 is derived from PrP 33-35^{Sc} during proteinase K digestion in the absence or presence of detergent.

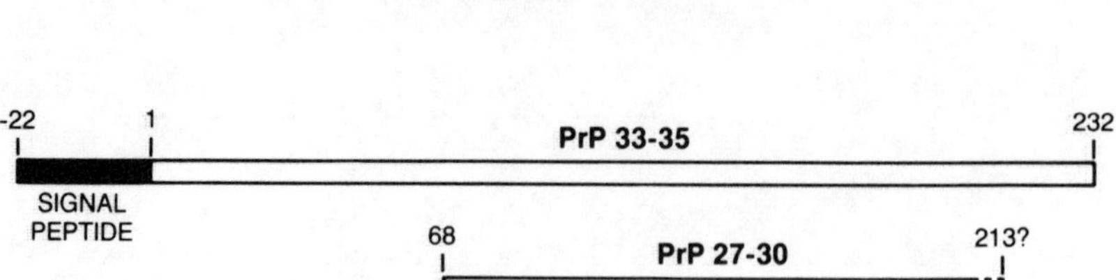

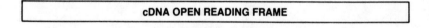

Fig. 1. Structure of the hamster prion protein (PrP). The open reading frame encodes a protein of 254 amino acids. The first 22 amino acids comprise a signal peptide which is cleaved during synthesis of PrP 33-35. Digestion of the scrapie isoform of PrP 33-35^{Sc} with proteinase K generates a smaller protease-resistant polypeptide designated PrP 27-30.

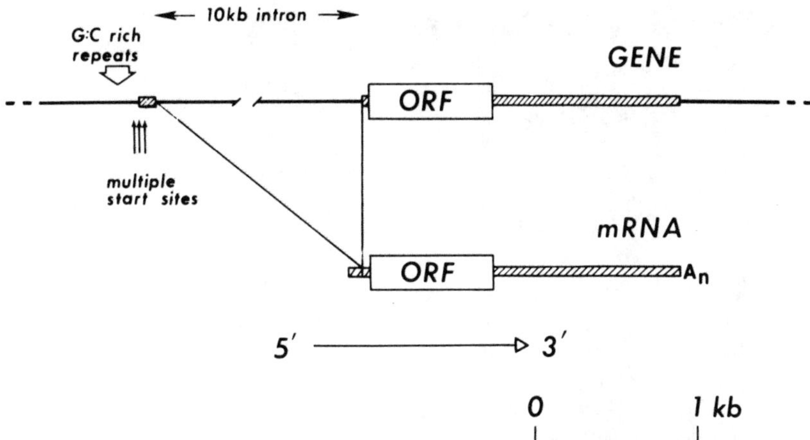

Fig. 2. Structure of the hamster PrP gene and mRNA. The features were deduced from the nucleotide sequences of PrP genomic and cDNA clones. Untranslated regions of the mRNA are represented by hatched boxes; open reading frame is represented by an open box. A splicing event which joins the 5′ leader sequences to the remainder of the coding sequences is shown by a vertical and a diagonal line.

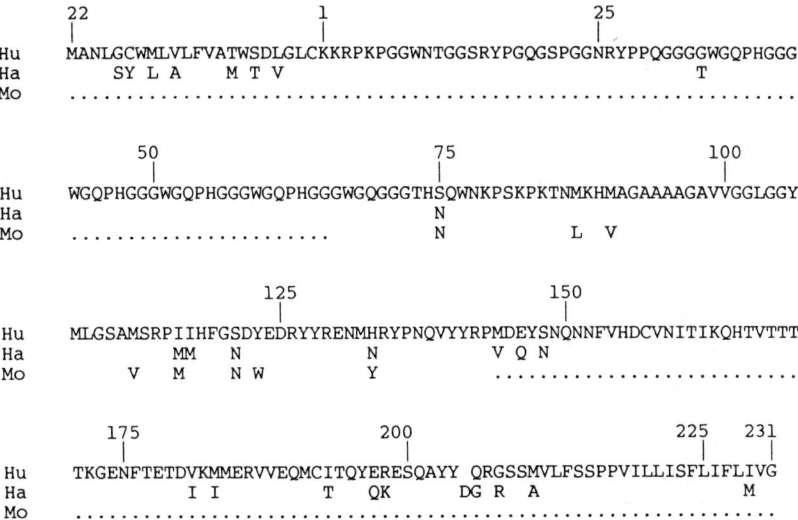

Fig. 3. Comparison of the human PrP sequence (Hu) with the hamster (Ha) (1,21) and the mouse equivalents (Mo) (15). Only amino acid replacements are presented. Unknown parts of the mouse sequence are represented by dots.

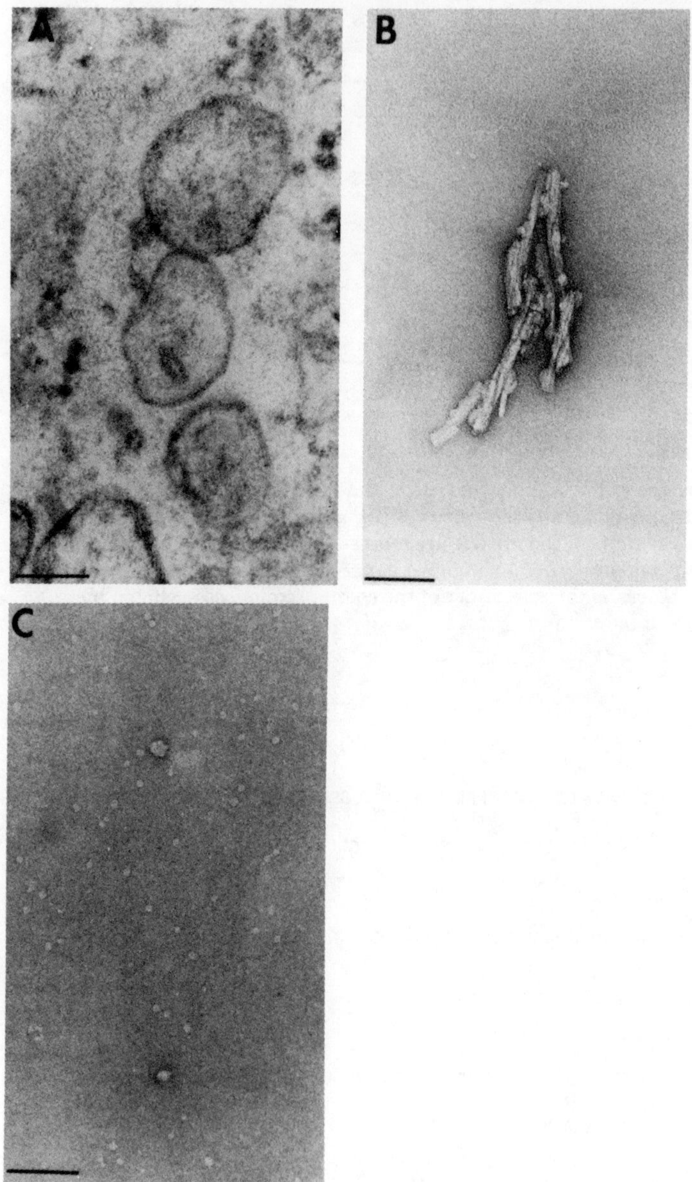

Fig. 4. Multiple forms of scrapie prions isolated from infected hamster brain. (A) Microsomal membranes containing prions. (B) Purified prion rods which are generated upon detergent extraction of membranes from scrapie-infected brain. (C) Prion spheres generated from extensive sonication of rods and isolated by sucrose-gradient sedimentation. All three forms contain high levels of prion infectivity (>10^7 ID_{50}/ml). Bars are 100 nm.

9. Beta Protein: A Possible Marker for Alzheimer's Disease

GEORGE G. GLENNER, M.D.

Department of Pathology (M-012) School of Medicine
University of California, San Diego La Jolla, California 92093

ABSTRACT: Cerebrovascular amyloidosis occurs in 92% of all cases of Alzheimer's disease and in addition to neuritic plaques and neurofibrillary tangles, is pathognomonic of it. It is seen also as a major lesion in hereditary cerebral amyloidosis (Icelandic) and in adult Down's syndrome. The amyloid fibril protein (β protein) from the cerebrovascular amyloidosis of Alzheimer's disease was isolated, purified and amino acid sequence analysis revealed it to have no homology with any other sequenced protein. It was virtually identical in amino acid sequence to the cerebrovascular amyloid fibrils of adult Down's syndrome. This provides the first chemical evidence for a relationship between these two processes and establishes Down's syndrome as a model for Alzheimer's disease. Synthetic peptides of the β protein were used as immuogens and the antibodies obtained localized to amyloid deposits in amyloid-laden cerebral vessels and neuritic plaques in both Alzheimer's disease and adult Down's syndrome. These findings suggest a pathogenetic mechanism for Alzheimer's disease.

Introduction

There is in the literature a recurrent, but often contradictory, theme relating cerebrovascular amyloidosis to Alzheimer's disease (AD). Often this theme is hidden. For example, in the summary descriptions of cerebrovascular amyloidosis of Pantelakis (1) and Surbeck (2), the former noted that all his patients had plaques, whereas the latter noted that they were all demented. In order to clarify the relation between cerebrovascular amyloidosis and AD, a review was undertaken at the Armed Forces Institute of Pathology, Washington, D.C., of cases described as having neuritic plaques, neurofibrillary tangles, cerebral atrophy and dementia. Ninety-two percent of these cases studied by polarization microscopy after Congo red staining had evidence of cerebrovascular amyloidosis (3). A review of other conditions, including Pick's disease and hypertensive encephalopathy, and age-matched normal persons revealed no cerebrovascular amyloidosis. We realize this is contrary to the reports of several other groups (4,5), for which we have no ready explanation other than variations in the Congo red staining technique (6) and polarized light visualization. With this study as baseline, we approached the isolation of the cerebrovascular amyloid from cases of AD. It was necessary first to establish the initial National Alzheimer's Disease Brain Bank at the University of California, San Diego in order to obtain sufficient material for isolation purposes.

There are six pathologic conditions in which amyloid consistently affects vascular walls. Three are systemic (AL, AA and AF) and have an abnormal serum protein which has been isolated. Three are localized to the cerebral vessels: AD (3), adult Down's syndrome (7), and hereditary Icelandic cerebrovascular amyloidosis (HCHWA) (8). The nature (normal or abnormal) of their precursor protein is unknown, although the amyloid fibril protein of HCHWA has been identified as homologous to the serum protein, gamma trace (8).

Applying the concept of the "amyloidogenic" protein precursor to this problem (9), we speculated that all of the characteristic deposits of the cerebrovascular amyloidoses are derived from abnormal serum protein precursors (10). To explain why amyloid was localized to cerebral vessels and not found systemically, we reasoned that, since cerebral vessels are structurally different (tight-junction endothelia, a single arterial elastic lamella), they probably differ metabolically also. In other words, we predicted that the lysosomal enzyme complement of cerebral vessel endothelial cells would differ from that of peripheral vessels. Invoking the proteolytic theory of amyloid fibril pathogenesis (9), we surmised that an abnormal serum protein normally digested by lysosomal enzymes in peripheral vessels would not be similarily cleaved by the different lysosomal enzymes in cerebral vessels, and that cerebrovascular amyloid fibril formation would result. Such a theory suggests that the abnormal precursor serum protein is encoded by a predetermined or acquired abnormal gene or is subjected to abnormal modification, perhaps by an abnormal enzyme or by one that is improperly activated. Indeed, AD is one of the few amyloidotic processes that has both familial and sporadic components, suggesting the existence of an abnormal gene.

Down's syndrome individuals over age 40 have clinical symptoms of dementia or cerebral dysfunction (11). They also have all the pathologic cerebral lesions of AD: plaques, tangles and cerebrovascular amyloidosis (12). No logical explanation for these lesions has been forthcoming except for a gene overdosage due to the trisomy 21. The finding that Down's syndrome occurs in AD families with an incidence three times that in other families (13), thus is striking.

Our hypothesis implicated an abnormal serum protein as the precursor of the cerebrovascular amyloid fibrils (10). This fibrillar lesion causes hemorrhage (14) or stroke-like episodes in about 30% of AD patients as the result of damage to and rupture of vessel walls (7). The vascular amyloid deposition would under any circumstances cause leakage of plasma into the cerebrum, a break in the blood-brain barrier (10). The abnormal or other serum protein would penetrate the neuropil, and as the result of pathoclisis, attach to the neural receptors of specific pyramidal cells. This reaction would perturb the neuronal environment to cause formation from neurofilament proteins of the paired helical filaments (PHF) composing the tangles. These cells would die and their remnants be deposited as plaques, the microglia contributing their lysosomal enzymes to the degradation and amyloid core plaque formation (10). As the result of recent findings reported here, our theory about the origin of plaques has been modified.

Research Results

Amyloid Fibril Isolation and Protein Characterization: It was decided that, since a continuum of amyloid deposits extends between leptomeningeal and intracortical vessels, the amyloid is probably of the same composition in both. Therefore, in order to prevent contamination by parenchymal brain tissue, the leptomeningeal tissue containing abundant amyloidotic vessels was stripped from the cortical surface. Only this leptomeningeal tissue was used for amyloid isolation. The cerebrovascular amyloid fibers were concentrated by previously described methods (15). They were resistant to distilled water suspension (16). To remove or reduce the large quantity of collagen in the leptomeningeal preparation, collagenase treatment was used during monitoring with Congo red under polarization optics. X-ray diffraction revealed clear .476 nm and 1.0 nm d-spacings with little background, consistent with a relatively clean β-pleated sheet fibril preparation. The concentrate was dissolved in 6M guanidine-HCl in the presence of dithiothreitol and centrifuged, and the supernatant fluid was dialyzed against distilled water and lyophilized. This lyophilized sample was dissolved in 1% SDS and applied to a calibrated SDS-urea PAGE gel (17). A protein band at 4,800 daltons appeared only with amyloid preparations from AD patients, and not those from normal controls. It was designated β protein. The sediment was redissolved and placed on a molecular-weight-calibrated G-100 Sephadex column, and the proteins were fractionated. The molecular weight of the β protein was determined to be 4,200 daltons.

We thus isolated from leptomeningeal amyloidotic vessels a unique major protein meeting the standard criteria for an amyloid fibril protein. The β protein was further fractionated by high performance liquid chromatography (HPLC) in 100% acetonitrile to yield three peaks, β_1, β_2, and β_3 (18). Amino acid sequence analysis of the β_2 peak was performed to 28 amino acids (Table 1). Sequence analysis was also performed on the β_1 peak and the sequence found to be identical.

The entire procedure was repeated on leptomeningial vascular amyloidotic tissue from two cases of adult Down's syndrome individuals ages 61 and 62 (18). The Down's profile revealed a lesser quantity of the β_1 peak. No corresponding peaks were noted in three control preparations. In addition these chromatographs resolved from both protein preparations a β_3 peak previously obscured within that of β_2 (18). It was shown that the β_1 protein and the β_2 protein were homologous by amino acid sequence analysis (18). Since β_3 was initially included in β_2 but did not result in sequencing background, β_3 is assumed to be homologous to β_2. Why β protein appears as a doublet or triplet on HPLC is unknown. However, lesser amount of protein initiating with the Ala residue (position 2) and having the identical amino acid sequence to position 28 was found in both the β_1 and β_2 peaks. This is strongly suggestive of proteolytic cleavage of the β protein from a larger precursor, primarily at the N-terminal Asp, but to a lesser extent at the Ala^2 residue. This situation is identical to that described for the amyloid fibril protein AA (19), in which the majority N-terminal sequence is Arg-Ser-Phe-Phe-Ser-Phe but a lesser amount is Ser-Phe-Phe-Ser-Phe, presumably derived by proteolysis from a larger serum protein, SAA.

The amino acid sequence analysis of the Alzheimer's and Down's β_2 protein fraction to residue 28 is presented in reference 29. Their proteins have identical amino acid sequences through position 28 except for a substitution in the Down's protein of a Glu for Gln residue at position 11. The retention of Gln^{15} suggests that Gln^{11} may be a true substitution, rather than the result of an artifactual deamidation. The preparation from the second Down's case gave an HPLC profile with an identical major peak at 36% acetonitrile, but inadequate material was available for sequencing. The β_2 protein is not homologous by computer search to the serum protein gamma trace (8) found to compose the cerebrovascular amyloid protein of an HCHWA (20) nor to any other known sequenced protein (17).

These findings indicate that of the three disease processes most often characterized by cerebrovascular amyloidosis; i.e., AD (3), adult Down's syndrome (7) and HCHWA (20), only AD and adult Down's syndrome share a homologous amyloid protein. This is the first evidence of a chemical relation between AD and Down's syndrome.

Immunohistochemical Localization: Murine polyclonal antibodies were raised to the synthetic peptide (Asp-Ala-Glu-Phe-Arg-His-Asp-Ser-Gly-Tyr) corresponding to the N-terminal decapeptide of β protein coupled to keyhole limpet hemocyanin (KLH). These antibodies (OP1MS1) were demonstrated to be specific for the synthetic β protein homologue and were used immunohistochemically in the peroxidase-antiperoxidase (PAP) method of Sternberger (21) on AD and adult Down's syndrome cerebral tissue.

Tissue from six cases of AD, two cases of adult Down's syndrome, one case of HCHWA and three age-matched normal brains were immunohistochemically studied by the Sternberger PAP method (21) using OP1MS1. Amyloid-laden vascular sites in the leptomeningial and intracortical areas in AD and adult Down's syndrome cases immunostained intensely and corresponded precisely to the areas of Congo red polarization birefringence. This birefringence resulting from Congo red staining is an accepted histochemical marker for the β-pleated sheet structure of amyloid (22). In addition, both diffuse (primitive) and compact (mature) neuritic plaques reacted with OP1MS1 in the PAP procedure in AD and adult Down's syndrome tissue sections. There were rare instances in both conditions in which localized PAP staining appeared in sites resembling small diffuse plaques that did not have corresponding Congo red birefringence. This could be due to the ability of the PAP procedure to detect localized deposits of β protein that either were minute or were not in the β-pleated sheet conformation and thus were non-birefringent.

PAP staining of cerebrovascular amyloid and neuritic plaques could be completely inhibited by preincubating OP1MS1 with OP1. Preincubation of OP1MS1 with a concentration of KLH that eliminated all anti-KLH activity as detected by ELISA had no effect on the PAP staining of cerebrovascular amyloid and neuritic plaques. The specific inhibition with OP1 strongly indicated that the specific PAP staining by OP1MS1 was entirely due to antibodies to OP1.

The normal brain tissue showed no significant PAP staining beyond the slight background also obtained when normal mouse serum was used in place of OP1MS1. This confirms the observation by SDS-polyacrylamide gel electrophoresis and HPLC of the uniqueness of the β protein in cerebral tissues to AD and adult Down's syndrome (17,18). The HCHWA case, though heavily laden with cerebrovascular amyloid as detected by Congo red birefringence, was also unreactive to PAP staining. This is consistent with the fact that HCHWA cerebrovascular amyloid is composed of gamma trace (8), which has no sequence homology with β protein. The lack of reactivityy with the HCHWA case further supports the specificity of OP1MS1 for β protein.

No PAP staining was seen associated with neurofibrillary tangles. This suggests that the etiology and source of neurofibrillary tangles is either distinct from that of cerebrovascular amyloid and neuritic plaques or that the anti-OP1 determinants of neurofibrillary tangles are sterically obscured. Kidd *et al.* (23) and Allsop *et al.* (24) have noted that the amino acid compositions of neuritic plaques, neurofibrillary tangles and cerebrovascular amyloid are similar and suggest that all are composed of the same protein. Our findings support their suggestion that neuritic plaques are composed of β protein but does not confirm their suggestion that neurofibrillary tangles are also. It should be noted that Anderton *et al.* (25) reported that the monoclonal antibodies used by them to identify the immunochemical relations between the 155kd and 210kd neurofilament proteins and neurofibrillary tangles did not react with the amyloid in neuritic plaques. Earlier reports have implicated IgG (26) and prealbumin (27) as the cerebrovascular amyloid and neuritic plaque amyloid protein. We have been unable to duplicate the reported PAP staining of cerebrovascular amyloid and neuritic plaques with anti-human IgG and anti-human-prealbumin antibodies. Furthermore, the amino acid composition of plaque cores and cerebrovascular amyloid are not consistent with the compositions of either IgG or prealbumin.

Discussion

The present studies confirm in part our initial hypothesis about the pathogenesis of AD. It is evident from the electron microscopic and x-ray diffraction data that the amyloid fibrils of the cerebral vessels in AD is composed of proteins in a twisted β-pleated sheet conformation (28). Although they are suspected of being a β-pleated sheet fibril (22) of different protein composition than plaques or cerebrovascular amyloid, the physico-chemical nature of the paired helical filaments of the tangles is still unknown. In this study, antibodies to β protein fail to react with tangles, although those of 155kd and 210kd neurofilament proteins have been reported to do so (25).

The absence of the cerebrovascular amyloid protein, β protein, in vessels of normal individuals and those with HCHWA indicates that β protein is a unique marker for AD. Although it has been known that there are common cerebral lesions, the almost identical amino acid sequence of β protein of the cerebrovascular amyloid fibrils in AD and adult Down's syndrome is the first chemical evidence that Down's syndrome is a pathologic model for AD. Immunohistochemical studies further substantiate the uniqueness of β protein for AD and Down's syndrome.

The HCHWA tissue, although heavily laden with cerebrovascular amyloid as detected by Congo red staining, was unreactive by PAP staining. This was expected, since HCHWA cerebrovascular amyloid fibrils are composed of gamma trace protein (8), which has no homology with β protein. The experiment with the HCHWA case was included as an additional control to demonstrate the specificity of OP1MS1 for β amyloid protein. HCHWA is the only other neuropathologic process known to have cerebrovascular amyloidosis as a significant lesion (8,20). Since our isolation and purification scheme for β protein eliminated contamination by intracerebral tissue, it also eliminated contamination of our original preparations of cerebrovascular amyloid by plaques and tangles. The localization of β protein antibodies to amyloid deposits in cerebral vessels of both AD and Down's syndrome was expected in view of the similarity in amino acid sequence of their β protein (18). Not only was the intended target, cerebrovascular amyloid, stained by OP1MS1, but so also were the neuritic plaques in both AD and adult Down's syndrome. The localization of the β protein antibodies to neuritic plaques in both these conditions indicates that the source of amyloid in plaques and vessels is the same, and it further supports the concept that Down's syndrome is a chemical model for AD (29).

What distinguishes our immunohistochemical work from earlier reports (26,30,31) is that we used antibodies raised to a well-defined, pure synthetic peptide whose sequence was that of the first 10 residues of a purified protein that appears, by three different criteria to be unique to AD and adult Down's syndrome. We do not know if the PAP reaction with OP1MS1 detects the amyloid fibril protein or a non-fibrillary associated component of the plaque: a definite statement on this point can be made only after definitive amino acid sequence analysis of the amyloid fibril protein of the plaque.

The amino acid compositions of plaque amyloid "cores" and cerebrovascular amyloid are similar (23,24). Therefore, it is likely that plaque amyloid fibrils also consist of β protein. This suggests that the amyloid in plaques and cerebrovascular amyloid has a common plasma source. Recently, Masters *et al.* (32) attempted amino acid sequencing of the amyloid plaque cores obtained from cases of AD and Down's syndrome (29). They obtained an inseparable series of at least four polypeptides by HPLC fractionation which had progressive deletions of their N-terminal amino acids. They ordered these according to the amino acid sequence of the β protein of AD and obtained homology with it except for three discrepancies: in positions 11 (Glu for Gln), 27 (Ser for Asn) and 28 (Ala for Lys) (32). It is doubtful that without the knowledge of the sequence of β protein these polypeptides could have been ordered into sequence, since at each cycle at least four amino acids would have been detected.

Using antibodies to peptides 1-11 and 11-23 of β protein, Masters *et al.* (33) found that not only did antibodies to peptides 11-23 react with cerebrovascular amyloid and amyloid plaque core in AD but, contrary to the finding of Wong *et al.* (29), antibodies to peptide 1-11 reacted with neurofibrillary tangles. The finding that cerebrovascular wall and plaque amyloid reacts with antibodies to β protein (29) has been confirmed by several investigators (D. Allsop, D. Selkoc, H. Wisniewski; personal communications). In agreement with our results, there was no reactivity of neurofibrillary tangles with anti-β protein antibodies.

The pathologic implications of our findings strongly support a close association of neuritic plaques with cerebral vessels and/or serum (34). There are six clinical conditions (AL, AA, AF, AD, HCHWA, and adult Down's syndrome) that are associated with vascular amyloid fibril deposits (7,9), and of the three that have been investigated, all have been shown to be derived from an abnormal serum protein precursor (9). On the basis of this precedent, we suggest that the lesions in the three remaining processes (AD, adult Down's syndrome and HCHWA) will be found to have an abnormal serum precursor as well. This finding should lead to the development of a much-needed specific diagnostic serum test for AD.

Down's Syndrome: There is no known spontaneous or experimental animal model for AD. There are mouse models for Down's syndrome (35), but since the trisomic fetuses do not survive beyond term, their value for the study of AD is limited. The human familial cases of AD tend to follow an autosomal dominant pattern of inheritance (13), with the usual statistical prediction of affected progeny. However, the great similarity in the cerebral lesions between adult Down's syndrome and AD (7,12) and the demonstration of chemical homology in the pathologic amyloid fibril β protein strongly suggest that Down's syndrome represents the first truly predictable model for AD.

The presence of a common amyloid protein and a protein synthetic abnormality in both Down's syndrome (trisomy 21) and AD suggests that the genetic defect in AD whether acquired or heritable, is localized to chromosome 21. This makes possible alternative approaches to the non-invasive diagnosis of AD (36,37). One intriguing possibility among many others is that this chemical evidence may signify that a gene defect, in addition to the the trisomic condition, exists in Down's syndrome. Such a defect may signify a specifically labile gene locus on chromosome 21 and might help to explain the statistically significant relation between familial AD and Down's syndrome (13).

The present report fills an important gap in unveiling the pathogenesis of AD and suggests that the formation of neuritic plaques is the result of breaks in the blood-brain barrier (38). Miyakawa *et al.* (39) found that all neuritic plaques were associated with at least one degenerating amyloidotic capillary. We present here evidence that the β protein found in cerebral vessel amyloid is also found in the neuritic plaques. We therefore propose, as a working hypothesis, that cerebrovascular amyloid derives from an isotypic variant of a serum protein precursor (9,19) analogous to the variant prealbumin in familial amyloidotic polyneuropathy (FAP) (40). The cerebrovascular amyloid fibers damage capillary walls (3), causing seepage of β protein precursor along with other plasma substances into the neuropil, leading to the formation of the amyloid of the neuritic plaque via lysosomal (9,10) enzyme degradation by microglia of the precursor of β protein (9,41). We suggest that β protein is also neurotoxic, blocking strategic receptors of specific cortical neurons, perturbing their environment and leading to PHF formation from neurofilament protein.

One of the major objectives of this laboratory is to develop a biochemical assay by which AD can be diagnosed, as no specific diagnostic test short of brain biopsy is now available during the patient's life. The presence of amyloid fibril deposits in vessel walls is indicative of fibrillar derivation from an abnormal serum protein; i.e., a variant or isotype of a normal serum protein. This has been shown for amyloid fibrils derived from the light polypeptide chain of an immunoglobulin protein (42), a prealbumin (Met 30) variant (43) and an SAA protein isotype (44). Therefore, we expect that a protein antigenically related to β protein will be detectable in the serum of normal individuals and persons with AD or adult Down's syndrome. However, the isotypic variant of the normal serum β-related protein should be detected only in AD and Down's serum and should lead to a specific blood test (e.g., by radioimmunoassay) for AD based on the presence of a variant serum protein sharing antigenic determinants with β protein. Furthermore, Down's syndrome individuals may provide a diagnostic pattern of serum β protein concentration levels during aging that might be predictive of eventual diffuse cerebral dysfunction and/or dementia (11,45), and such a pattern might help to detect individuals at risk for AD and lead to a better understanding of the pathogenesis of the cerebral disorder common to AD and Down's syndrome (7). For the present, the diagnosis of AD is made by eliminating all other possible causes of dementia, a method that is costly and time consuming and fraught with a 20% clinical error. If the formation of the cerebrovascular amyloid deposits in AD and adult Down's syndrome is due to an abnormal serum protein precursor, this fact can be exploited to provide a relatively simple serum test. Such a test has already been devised for familial amyloidotic polyneuropathy (46).

With the acquisition of OP1MS1 and its monoclonal antibody counterparts, we are hopeful of being able to use affinity chromatography for purification of the putative serum precursor of the β protein as well as to develop a specific diagnostic radioimmunoassay for AD. In addition, with this antibody it will be possible to utilize molecular cloning technology to identify the genome segment involved in β protein synthesis and to characterize the suspected gene abnormality in AD and adult Down's syndrome (36,37).

Acknowledgments

We wish to express our appreciation to Karen Rasmussen for technical assistance, Dennis Olshefsky for synthesizing the OP1 peptide, Drs. R.M. Peterson and H.L. Wolfinger, Jr. of the San Diego Regional Center for the Developmentally Disabled for Down's syndrome tissues, and Jo-Ann Frisco for her assistance in preparing the manuscript. This study was supported by grants from the National Institutes of Health, AG 056683, The Weingart Foundation, and the John Douglas French Foundation and a contribution from the National Alzheimer's Disease and Related Disorders Association.

Addendum

It has now been established that the cerebrovascular amyloid fibril protein in HCHWA is a variant (isotype) of the serum protein gamma trace (48), thereby substantiating the suggestion made in this article. In addition, an antigenically β protein-related serum protein has been identified in and isolated from sera of patients with AD (Glenner, G. and Wong, C. unpublished observations). Whether this is a serum protein precursor of β protein is under investigation.

References

1. Pantelakis, S. (1954) *Monatschr. Psychiat. Neurol.* **128**, 209-256.
2. Surbek, B. (1961) *Acta Neuropathol. (Berlin)* **1**, 168-197.
3. Glenner, G.G., Henry, J.H. & Fujihara, S. (1981) *Ann. Pathol.* **1**, 105-108.
4. Vinters, H.V. & Gilbert, J.J. (1983) *Stroke* **14**, 924-928.
5. Vanley, C.T., Aguilar, M.J., Kleinbenz, R.J. & Lagios, M.D. (1981) *Hum. Pathol.* **12**, 609-616.

6. Carson, F.L. & Kingsley, W.B. (1980) *Arch. Pathol. Lab. Med.* **104**, 33-335.
7. Glenner, G.G. (1983) *Banbury Report 15: Biological Aspects of Alzheimer's Disease* ed. Katzman, R. (Cold Spring Harbor Symposium, New York) pp. 137-144.
8. Cohen, D.E., Feiner, H., Jensson, H.O. & Frangione, B. (1983) *J. Exp. Med.* **158**, 623-628.
9. Glenner, G.G. (1980) *N. Engl. J. Med.* **302**, 1283-1292; 1333-1343.
10. Glenner, G.G. (1979) *Med. Hypoth.* **5**, 1231-1236.
11. Jarvis, G.A. (1984) *Am. J. Psychiat.* **105**, 102-106.
12. Ellis, W.G., McCulloch, J.R. & Corley, C.L. (1974) *Neurology* **24**, 101-106.
13. Heston, L.L. (1976) *Science* **196**, 322-323.
14. Torack, R.M. (1975) *Am. J. Pathol.* **81**, 349-366.
15. Harada, M., Isersky, C., Cuatrecasas, P., Page, D., Bladen, H.A., Eanes, E.D., Keiser, H.R. & Glenner, G.G. (1971) *J. Histochem. Cytochem.* **19**, 1-15.
16. Pras, M., Zucker-Franklin, D., Rimon, A. & Franklin, E.C. (1969) *J. Exp. Med.* **130**, 777-791.
17. Glenner, G.G. & Wong, C. (1984) *Biochem. Biophys. Res. Commun.* **120**, 885-890.
18. Glenner, G.G. & Wong, C. (1984) *Biochem. Biophys. Res. Commun.* **120**, 1131-1135.
19. Benditt, E.P., Eriksen, N., Hermodson, M.A. & Ericsson, L.H. (1971) *FEBS Lett.* **19**, 169-173.
20. Lofberg, H., Grubb, A.O., Sveger, T. & OLsson, J.E. (1980) *J. Neurol.* **23**, 159-170.
21. Sternberger, L.A. (1979) *Immunocytochemistry* (Wiley, New York), 2nd Ed., pp. 104-169.
22. Glenner, G.G., Eanes, E.D., Bladen, H.A., Linke, R.P. & Termine, J.D. (1974) *J. Histochem. Cytochem.* **22**, 2242-1158.
23. Kidd, M., Allsop, D. & London, M. (1978) *Lancet* **1**, 278.
24. Allsop, D., London, M. & Kidd, M. (1985) *Proceedings of the VIth International Conference on Amyloidosis,* eds. Glenner, G. G. & Osserman, E. (Plenum, New York), pp. 723-732.
25. Anderton, B.H., et al (1982) *Nature* **298**, 84-86.
26. Ishii, T., Haga, S. & Shimizu, F. (1975) *Acta. Neuropath.* (Berlin) **32**, 157-162.
27. Shirahama, T., Skinner, M., Westermark, P., Rubinow, A., Cohen, A.S., Brun, A. & Kemper, R.L. (1982) *Am. J. Pathol.* **107**, 41-50.
28. Eanes, E.D. & Glenner, G.G. (1976) *J. Histochem. Cytochem.* **16**, 673-677.

29. Wong, C.W., Quaranta, V. & Glenner, G.G. (1985) *Proc. Natl. Acad. Sci. USA* **82**, 8729-8732.
30. Cohen, S.A., Said, S.I. & Terry, R.D. (1981) (Abstract) *J. Neuropathol.* **39**, 310.
31. Powers, J.M., Schlaeffer, W.W., Willingham, M.C. & Hall, B.J. (1981) (Abstract) *J. Neuropathol.* **39**, 311.
32. Masters, C.L., Simms, G., Weinman, N.A., Multhaup, G., McDonald, B.L. & Beyreuther, K. (1985) *Proc. Natl. Acad. Sci. USA* **82**, 4245-4249.
33. Masters, C.L., Multhaup, G., Simms, G., Pottgiesser, J., Martins, R.N. & Beyreuther, K. (1985) *EMBO J.* **4**, 2757-2763.
34. Scholz, W. (1938) *Neurol. Psychiatr.* **162**, 694-715.
35. Epstein, C.J. (1983) *Banbury Report 13: Biological Aspects of Alzheimer's Disease,* ed. Katzman, R., (Cold Spring Harbor Symposium, New York) pp. 169-182.
36. Maniatus, T., Fritsch, E.F. & Sambrook, J. (1982) *Molecular Cloning: A Laboratory Manual* (Cold Spring Harbor Symposium, New York), pp. 545.
37. Gusella, J.F., Wexler, N.S. & Conneally, P.M. (1983) *Science* **306**, 234-238.
38. Glenner, G.G. (1981) *J. Clin. Lab. Med.* **98**, 807-810.
39. Miyakawa et al: (1982) *Virchows Arch. (Cell Pathol.)* **40**, 121-129.
40. Dwulet, F.E. & Benson, M.D. (1984) *Proc. Natl. Acad. Sci. USA* **81**, 694-698.
41. Glenner, G.G., Ein, D., Eanes, E.D., Bladen, H.A., Terry, W. & Page, D.L. (1971) *Science* **174**, 712-714.
42. Glenner, G.G., Terry, W., Harada, M., Isersky, C. & Page, D. *Science* **172**, 1150-1151.
43. Benson, M.D. & Dwulet, F.E. (1985) *J. Clin. Invest.* **75**, 71-75.
44. Hoffman, J., Ericsson, L.H., Eriksen, N., Walsh, K.A. & Benditt, E.P. (1984) *J. Exp. Med.* **159**, 641-646.
45. Owens, D., Dawson, J.C. & Losin, S. (1971) *Am. J. Ment. Defic.* **75**, 606-612.
46. Nakazato, M., Kangawa, K., Minamino, N., Tawara, S., Matsuo, H. & Araki, S. (1984) *Biochem. Biophys. Res. Commun.* **122**, 712-718.
47. Ghiso, J., Jensson, & Frangione, B. (1986) *Proc. Natl. Acad. Sci. USA* **83**, 2974-2978.

10. Antibody Staining of Cerebral Amyloid in Alzheimer's Disease, Down's Syndrome, Creutzfeldt-Jakob Disease and Gerstmann-Straussler Syndrome

DAVID ALLSOP, M.D.*

Department of Pathology University of California, San Diego
La Jolla, CA 92093

GARETH ROBERTS,† MICHAEL LANDON,* MICHAEL KIDD,‡ JAMES S. LOWE,§ GAVIN P. REYNOLDS,§ TIMOTHY J. CROW†

ABSTRACT: Four monoclonal antibodies were raised to a synthetic peptide consisting of residues 8-17 of an amino acid sequence reported to be common to the three forms of cerebral amyloid in Alzheimer's disease (AD). These antibodies labeled the cerebrovascular amyloid and all of the senile plaques in sections of brain from cases of AD and Down's syndrome but did not label neurofibrillary tangles. An antiserum to PrP isolated from scrapie-infected hamsters did not label any of the forms of cerebral amyloid associated with AD but did label large numbers of plaques in Gerstmann-Straussler syndrome and Creutzfeldt-Jakob disease. One of the monoclonal antibodies also labeled some of the plaques in the latter disease; dual-labeling studies with both types of antibody revealed minimal co-localization, suggesting the existence of two distinct types of plaque ("Alzheimer" and "prion" plaques): any cerebrovascular amyloid was labeled by the antipeptide monoclonal antibodies but not with the anti-PrP antiserum.

Introduction

The cerebral amyloidoses may be considered as a group of neurological disorders characterized by the deposition of amyloid at one or more of the following sites in the brain: (a) in the neuropil, in the form of discrete amyloid plaques; (b) in some cortical and subcortical neurons, in the form of neurofibrillary tangles; and (c) in the walls of cerebral arterioles and

Departments of *Biochemistry, ‡Human Morphology and §Pathology, The Medical School, Queen's Medical Centre, Nottingham, U.K.; and †Division of Psychiatry, and Clinical Research Centre, Harrow, U.K.

capillaries (Congophilic angiopathy). AD and late Down's syndrome, where amyloid is frequently found at all three sites, are prominent members of this group, which also includes the transmissible subacute spongiform encephalopathies or unconventional slow-virus diseases, in which no significant numbers of tangles have been reported. The latter diseases include scrapie in animals and Creutzfeldt-Jakob disease, Gerstmann-Straussler syndrome and kuru in man.

Considerable progress has been made over the last few years in the protein chemical characterization of the cerebral amyloids in AD and Down's syndrome, due largely to the development of suitable techniques for the isolation of plaque core amyloid (1,2) and also the paired helical filaments (PHF) (3,4), which are the major constituent of neurofibrillary tangles. A considerable impetus to this research was the purification by Glenner and Wong of a novel 4 kd protein β-protein from amyloid-laden meningeal vessels and the determination of the partial amino acid sequence of this protein which established it as unique (5,6). The strikingly similar amino acid compositions of β-protein, plaque core protein and PHF led to the proposal that all three amyloids are composed of a common protein (7,8). Recently, Masters *et al.* reported N-terminal amino acid sequences for plaque core protein (9) and PHF protein (10) that support this proposal.

Advancement toward an understanding of the nature of the cerebral amyloid in the spongiform encephalopathies has been through characterization of the transmissible agent rather than direct isolation of the amyloid. Two research groups have established that subcellular fractions which are enriched for scrapie infectivity contain small fibrous structures, referred to as either "prion rods" (11) or "scrapie-associated fibrils" (12), which yield on dissociation a predominant proteinase-K-resistant protein of molecular weight 27,000-30,000 (PrP [13] or scrapie-associated fibril protein [12]). It is not certain whether the fibrils are themselves infectious: it is possible that they arise as a pathologic response to infection or during the preparative procedures and fortuitously copurify with an as yet undetected agent possibly containing nucleic acid. PrP is encoded on a host gene which is transcribed and translated in a variety of infected and uninfected tissues (14,15) to produce a larger precursor protein (14-16) that is presumably degraded to the smaller protease-resistant form, PrP, only in infected tissues. The implications of this finding for the nature of the infectious agent have been discussed by others (17,18) and will not be considered here. The prion rods exhibit some of the staining characteristics and the ultrastructural appearance of amyloid (11), and antisera to PrP label the rods (19) and also stain amyloid plaques in scrapie (20) and some plaques in Creutzfeldt-Jakob disease in rodents and in Gerstmann-Straussler syndrome and Creutzfeldt-Jakob disease in man (21). This result has added weight to the proposal that the plaque amyloid fibrils in these transmissible diseases are formed from paracrystalline arrays of the infectious agent (11). This hypothesis has also been extended to include AD (22), which so far has not been transmitted to animals.

For the work reported here, monoclonal antibodies were raised to a synthetic peptide corresponding to residues 8-17 of the common amino acid sequence of the three cerebral amyloids in AD. An affinity-purified antiserum to PrP purified from scrapie-infected hamster brain (20) was kindly provided by Dr. S.B. Prusiner. Sections of Formalin-fixed paraffin-embedded human brain tissue from cases of AD, Creutzfeldt-Jakob disease and Gerstmann-Straussler syndrome were stained with each of these two types of antibody; some sections were stained with both antipeptide and antiPrP antibodies using a dual-labeling procedure. Brain tissue from cases of Down's syndrome was stained using one of the monoclonal antibodies only.

Materials and Methods

Materials: A peptide consisting of residues 8-17 of the plaque core protein sequence (9) (Ser-Gly-Tyr-Glu-Val-His-His-Gln-Lys-Leu) with an additional C-terminal cysteine for coupling to carrier protein was purchased from Cambridge Research Biochemicals Ltd., Cambridge, UK. Horse-heart myoglobin, keyhole limpet hemocyanin (KLH), m-maleimidobenzoyl-N-hydroxysuccinimide ester (MBS), N,N-dimethylformamide and 2,2′ -azino-bis-3-ethylbenz-thiazoline sulfonic acid (ABTS) were purchased from Sigma Chemical Co. Ltd., Poole, UK. Tissue culture media, fetal bovine serum (myoclone) and polyvinyl choloride plates (Titertek) were from Flow Laboratories, Irvine, Scotland, UK. Polyethylene glycol 1500 was obtained from BDH Chemicals Ltd., Poole. Immunostaining reagents were purchased from Dako Ltd., High Wycombe, UK or from Amersham International plc, Amersham, UK. Monoclonal antibody subclass determination was carried out using a kit supplied by Serotec Ltd., Bicester, UK.

Coupling of peptide to carrier protein: The synthetic peptide was coupled through the C-terminal cysteine residue to carrier protein (KLH for immunization or myoglobin for enzyme-linked immunosorbent assay [ELISA]) as described by Green *et al.* (23). MBS (1.4 mg in 0.1 ml dimethylformamide) was added dropwise to carrier protein (8 mg in 0.5 ml 10 mM phosphate buffer, pH 7.2) with constant stirring. After 30 min at room temperature, the activated carrier protein was separated from unreacted MBS by gel filtration on a column of Sephadex G-25 eluted with 50 mM phosphate buffer, pH 6.0. Synthetic peptide (10 mg in 2 ml phosphate-buffered saline [PBS]) was added to the pooled fractions containing activated carrier protein, and the mixture (total volume 9-10 ml) was left stirring at room temperature for 3 hr. The efficiency of coupling was not determined. Conjugates were stored at -20° C.

Immunization: A BALB/c mouse was injected intraperitoneally with 0.15 ml KLH-peptide conjugate (containing 0.16 mg peptide) emulsified with an equal volume of Freund's complete adjuvant. Two booster injections using half this amount of protein in Freund's incomplete adjuvant were given at monthly intervals.

Fusion of cells: The mouse myeloma cell line P3 NS1-Ag4 was maintained in RPMI medium supplemented with 10% (v/v) heat-inactivated fetal bovine serum and 8-azaguanine (15 μg/ml). Four days after the final injection, 10^8 mouse spleen cells were fused with 10^7 myeloma cells as described by Mayer and Billett (24) using polyethylene glycol 1500 in RPMI medium as the fusogenic agent. The pellet of fused cells was resuspended directly in HAT medium (15% [v/v] fetal bovine serum, 0.4 μm aminopterin, 0.1 mM hypoxanthine and 16 μM thymidine in RPMI [25]), and the cells were distributed into four 96-well microtiter plates (Titertek) containing 5×10^3 rat peritoneal macrophage feeder cells per well. All media contained streptomycin (60 μg/ml) and penicillin G (100 μg/ml).

Feeder cells: Macrophages were obtained from Wistar rats by peritoneal lavage with 20 ml of RPMI medium containing 10% (v/v) heat-inactivated fetal bovine serum.

Screening of culture fluids: This was performed by solid-phase ELISA in polyvinyl chloride wells previously coated by incubation at 4° C overnight with 10 μl myoglobin-peptide in PBS (0.2 μg peptide/well). The coated wells were washed, incubated with PBS containing 1% bovine serum albumin (BSA) for 4 hr at room temperature to reduce nonspecific binding, and treated with the following: (a) 50 μl culture supernatant fluid overnight at 4° C; (b) 50 μl peroxidase-conjugated rabbit antimouse immunoglobulins (Dako) diluted to 1/1000 with PBS containing 1% BSA for 1 hr at room temperature; (c) 100 μl of ABTS substrate (0.1% ABTS, 0.15% H_2O_2 in 0.1 M citrate buffer, pH 4.0) for 10-20 min at room temperature; and (d) 50 μl stopping reagent (0.01% NaN_3 in 0.1 M citric acid). Between successive steps, the wells were thoroughly washed with PBS containing 0.05% (v/v) Tween 20.

Cloning: Four positive cultures (1D2, 1G10, 3B6, 4D12) were weaned off HAT medium through HT medium (HAT medium without aminopterin) into RPMI medium containing 10% heat-inactivated fetal bovine serum (24). These cultures were cloned twice by limiting dilution on rat peritoneal-exudate feeder cells (24), and stable subclones (1D2/1/2, 1G10/2/3, 3B6/1/1, 4D12/2/6) were obtained. These clones were injected into pristane-primed mice in order to generate ascites fluid. Ouchterlony immunodiffusion analysis of neat culture supernatant fluids with antimouse Ig-subclass-specific antisera showed that all four antibodies were IgG type 1. In each case, a single sharp precipitation line was produced.

Monoclonal antibody purification: Monoclonal antibodies were purified directly from ascites fluid by ion-exchange FPLC (Pharmacia). The ascites fluid was passed through a 0.22-μm filter, and small samples were injected onto a Mono Q column and eluted at 1 ml/min with a 20-min gradient of 0-375 mM NaC1 in 20 mM Tris/HCl buffer, pH 8.0.

Competitive inhibition experiment: ELISA plates were coated by overnight incubation at 4° C with 2 ng uncoupled synthetic peptide per well in 200 μl PBS. Purified monoclonal antibodies (250 ng in 0.5 ml PBS) were mixed with 0.5 ml PBS or 1% BSA or with this same solution containing 5, 10, 50, 100 or 500 ng or 1 μg of peptide and incubated overnight at 4° C. These solutions were then added in 200-μl portions in quadruplicate to individual ELISA plate wells and incubated for an additional 1 hr at room temperature. Bound antibody was detected as described for the screening procedure except that 200-μl volumes were used for steps (b) and (c) and ABTS color development was allowed to proceed for 1 hr. The plates were monitored at 405 nm in a 96-well ELISA plate reader (Titertek).

Immunoperoxidase staining: Sections (10-15 μm) of Formalin-fixed paraffin-embedded cerebrocortical or cerebellar tissue were dewaxed and stained by one of the following methods:

1. Single-antibody method:
   The sections were treated with 3% H_2O_2 in methanol to inhibit endogenous peroxidase, rehydrated, and incubated sequentially at room temperature with (a) 20% normal swine serum in Tris-buffered saline (TBS) for 20 min; (b) monoclonal antibody (neat culture fluid, diluted ascites fluid or ion-exchange-purified antibody at 1-10 μg/ml) for 30 min; (c) peroxidase-conjugated rabbit antimouse immunoglobulins (Dako) diluted to 1/100 with 5% normal swine serum in TBS for 30 min: (d) 0.05% diaminobenzidine, 0.07% imidazole, 0.01% H_2O_2 in TBS for 10 min; and (e) 0.5% $CuSo_4$, 0.9% NaCl in TBS for 10 min.
2. Dual-labeling method:
   The sections were rehydrated and incubated sequentially at room temperature with (a) the first antibody (1 μg/ml purified 1G10/2/3 or 1/500 anti-PrP antiserum) diluted with PBS containing 0.05% BSA, 0.01% Triton X-100 for 0.75-3.00 hr: (b) peroxidase-conjugated antimouse or antirabbit immunoglobulins (Dako) (as appropriate), diluted to 1/200, for 45 min; (c) 0.05% diaminobenzidine, 0.01% H_2O_2

in PBS for 10-15 min; (d) the appropriate second antibody; and (e) β-galactosidase-conjugated antimouse or antirabbit IgG (Amersham), diluted to 1/50, for 45 min. Finally, the sections were treated by the indoxyl method described by Lojda (26) for the localization of β-galactosidase.

Results

Production of monoclonal antibodies: Ten days after fusion, approximately 75% of the wells contained hybridomas, which were screened for antipeptide antibody production by ELISA against bound myoglobin-peptide conjugate. The peptide was presented in this form to facilitate absorption to the wells, although later experiments with the resulting monoclonal antibodies (see below) showed that uncoupled peptide would bind to the ELISA plates. At least 100 positive colonies were detected, and four of the most strongly reactive cultures were cloned twice to produce monoclonal antibody-secreting clones 1D2/1/2, 1G10/2/3, 3B6/1/1 and 4D12/2/6. Further ELISA tests showed that these antibodies did not recognize epitopes on either KLH or myoglobin. The antibodies, all four of which proved to be immunoglobulin subclass IgG_1, were purified from ascites fluid by ion-exchange FPLC using a Mono Q column eluted with a salt gradient; in each case, the antibody was detected as a single prominent peak centering at approximately 200 mM NaC1 (Fig. 1). Reactivity of each of the four monoclonal antibodies with synthetic peptide was confirmed by a competitive inhibition experiement involving preincubation of purified antibody with various amounts of peptide prior to ELISA against solid-phase peptide (Fig. 2).

Immunoperoxidase staining of brain tissue from cases of AD: Sections of cerebral cortex from three cases of histopathologically confirmed AD from the brain collection at The Queen's Medical Centre, Nottingham, were stained by the indirect immunoperoxidase technique (method 1) with the four monoclonal antibodies. All of these antibodies produced clear positive staining of plaque and cerebrovascular amyloid and strong staining of granular material in the peripheral regions of classical plaques (Fig. 3). The latter reaction was unexpected, since extracellular amyloid has not been described as a prominent feature of the periphery, and these antibodies presumably cannot react with the PHF within the dystrophic neurites which are characteristic of this plaque region (see below). Many stained structures had the appearance of primitive plaques, and some more weakly and diffusely stained areas of cortex were observed that could represent very early stages in the genesis of plaques. After counterstaining with Congo red, the typical birefringence of many stained plaques could be observed under the polarizing microscope, although this reaction was sometimes masked by the peroxidase staining product. No Congo red-positive unstained plaques were found. Monoclonal antibody 1G10/2/3 consistently produced more intense staining than the other antibodies at equivalent dilutions. No positive staining was observed with a monoclonal antibody (3D4) raised to rabbit casein (M.C. O'Hare and R.J. Mayer, unpublished data) or in a normal elderly brain, both of which were used as negative controls. These monoclonal antibodies did not label any neurofibrillary tangles.

A further 25 cases of AD from the brain tissue collection at The Clinical Research Centre, Harrow, were stained either with purified 1G10/2/3, which produced results similar to those just described, or with the anti-PrP antiserum provided by Dr. S.B. Prusiner, which produced no positive immunostaining.

Down's syndrome: Cerebrocortical tissue from five cases of Down's syndrome (M2, M3, M4, M5 and M6, aged 34, 64, 52, 59 and 54, respectively) from the MRC Brain Tissue Bank, Addenbrookes Hospital, Cambridge, was stained using purified 1G10/2/3 only. Positive staining of plaque (Fig. 4) and cerebrovascular amyloid was observed in all of these brains except M2. Conventional histopathological examination of M2 subsequently revealed no senile plaques, neurofibrillary tangles or cerebrovascular amyloid, all of which were present in each of the other cases.

Creutzfeldt-Jakob disease: Sections of cerebellum were taken from 14 cases of clinically diagnosed, neuropathologically confirmed Creutzfeldt-Jakob disease obtained from Runwell Hospital, Wickford, and selected for the presence of amyloid plaques in this area of the brain. In nine cases, the plaques were labeled with the anti-PrP antiserum (Fig. 5) but not with 1G10/2/3. In the remaining five cases, all of which were in the senile age range (Table 1), 1G10/2/3 did label some plaques, but the double-labeling technique revealed that in each case, these labeled areas accounted for $<1\%$ of the total stained plaques. Because there was little co-localization of the two stains, nearly all plaques could be clearly categorized as one of two distinct immunoreactive types, referred to here as "Alzheimer" or "prion" plaques. When both types were present, they appeared to be randomly distributed, with no discernible anatomical pattern, except that disproportionately fewer Alzheimer plaques were found in the granule cell layer.

Blocks of frontal cortex were available from case 33/84 (Table 1) and from one additional case of Creutzfeldt-Jakob disease associated with severe amyloid infiltration of cerebral blood vessels (M, aged 62; not shown in Table 1). A clinical and neuropathological description of this latter case is given by Keohane *et al.* (27). Double-stained sections from both blocks showed large numbers of Alzheimer plaques (Fig. 6) with a minority of scattered prion plaques; again, there was little evidence of co-localization of stains. Cerebrovascular amyloid, which was evident in abundance in both cases, was stained by 1G10/2/3 only (Fig. 6); this was also true for the less extensive deposits of vessel amyloid observed in some of the other cases presented in Table 1.

Gerstmann-Straussler syndrome: Sections of frontal cortical tissue and cerebellum were taken from a single case of Gerstmann-Straussler syndrome, a familial transmissible spongiform encephalopathy associated with the presence of numerous amyloid plaques throughout the brain (28). A clinical history and neuropathological assessment of this patient have been presented by Baker *et al.* (29). A large number of prion plaques were observed in this tissue (Fig. 7), but Alzheimer plaques were not seen. Cerebrovascular amyloid was not apparent in the sections examined.

Discussion

Recent amino acid compositional (8) and N-terminal amino acid sequence data (5,6,9,10) indicate that all three cerebral amyloids in AD and Down's syndrome are formed from a similar protein with a molecular weight around 4kd. The immunostaining of the plaque and cerebrovasacular amyloid in these conditions with the monoclonal antipeptide antibodies provides further evidence in support of a close chemical relation between these two amyloids. The inability of the antibodies to recognize neurofibrillary tangles suggests either that the protein chemical data have been misinterpreted, and PHF are in fact composed of an unrelated protein, or, if the "common protein" proposal is correct, that the epitopes recognized by the monoclonal antibodies are not exposed in neurofibrillary tangles, possibly due to protein conformational differences between plaque (and vessel) amyloid fibrils and PHF. Other antisera raised to synthetic peptides corresponding to portions of the common amino acid sequence (10,30) or to purified dissociated components from isolated plaque cores or PHF (10,31) also react with vessel and plaque amyloid but not with neurofibrillary tangles. Selkoe and coworkers see this reactivity pattern as a reflection of contamination of PHF preparations by plaque core protein (31). However, Masters *et al.* have made the significant observation that an antiserum to a synthetic peptide consisting of residues 1-11 of the common amino acid sequence labels some neurofibrillary tangles (10), thus demonstrating that part of the common sequence does form an exposed epitope in these structures. This finding is apparently contradicted by the observation of Wong *et al.* that an antiserum to residues 1-10 labeled plaque and vessel amyloid but not PHF (30). However, this peptide was linked to KLH through an additional C-terminal cysteine residue, whereas the peptide of Masters *et al.* was linked to KLH via the N-terminus, which would generate an antiserum directed against a different region of the peptide.

An alternative approach to the identification of components of PHF has been based on the immunoreactivity of neurofibrillary tangles and isolated PHF with antibodies to cytoskeletal elements, in particular neurofilaments (32-37) and microtubule-associated proteins (38,39). This approach has helped to reinforce the widely held view that PHF are abnormal neurofilaments. Mammalian neurofilaments are composed of three subunits, NF-L (68 kd), NF-M (150 kd) and NF-H (200 kd), which all possess a central α-helical rod region flanked by nonhelical head and tail domains (40). To date, all of the well-characterized antineurofilament monoclonal antibodies that label neurofibrillary tangles (33-35) are directed against the C-terminal tail extensions of either NF-M or NF-H. These regions are thought to be involved in the formation of sidearms connecting adjacent filaments (40). Whereas the complete sequence of porcine NF-L is known (41), only partial sequences are available for NF-M (42) and NF-H (40), and these sequences do not include the C-terminal tail regions. It is possible, therefore, that the common 4 kd protein is a proteolytic fragment of one of these unsequenced regions. An alternative explanation for the neurofilament-like immunoreactivity of neurofibrillary tangles is that these are heterogeneous structures containing a distinct predominant PHF protein together with epitopes derived from partially degraded neurofilament proteins. In a healthy neuron, these proteins are synthesized in the cell body and transported orthogradely into the axon (43); this transport system could not be expected to function effectively in the presence of a large perinuclear bundle of PHF. Thus it is possible that in the pathologically affected neurons, any newly synthesized neurofilament protein is degraded, leaving the most-resistant epitopes to become incorporated into the tangle. Neurofilaments are known to be susceptible to an endogenous calcium-activated protease (44), and the sidearms show some resistance to proteolytic attack (45). Furthermore, antineurofilament antibodies label structures that are probably polyribosomes located within neurofibrillary tangles (37), and in immunogold-labeling studies testing these antibodies against isolated PHF, the gold particles are located on amorphous-looking material adhering to the PHF rather than on the filament shafts (33,34,36). This finding suggests that some neurofilament-like immunoreactive material may be tightly associated with PHF and retained even after extraction with sodium dodecylsulfate. Microtubule-associated protein 2 (38) and tau (39) epitopes are also present within some neurofibrillary tangles but, again, there is no convincing evidence to equate these with PHF *per se*. It is interesting to note that "ghost" or "tombstone" tangles, where the surrounding cell appears to have degenerated completely, leaving behind naked PHF, do not react with any of the antibodies to cytoskeletal elements (36,39). A cytoskeletal origin for PHF is therefore unproved.

The failure of the anti-PrP antiserum to react with any of the forms of cerebral amyloid in AD is not surprising since the partial amino acid sequence of the common 4 kd protein shows no homology with the sequence deduced from the PrP gene (14). This fact, coupled with the inability to find scrapie-associated fibrils in this disease (46), argues against an unconventional slow-viral (or "prion") etiology of AD.

In contrast, numerous anti-PrP-positive (prion) plaques were observed in the cerebellar tissue from patients with Creutzfeldt-Jakob disease or Gerstmann-Straussler syndrome, confirming the report of Kitamoto *et al.* (21) and suggesting that the proposal of Prusiner—that the plaque amyloid fibrils in these diseases are composed of aggregates of PrP-like molecules (11)—may well be correct, although isolation and chemical characterization of the amyloid is required to confirm this. In some of the cases of Creutzfeldt-Jakob disease, small numbers of 1G10/2/3-positive (Alzheimer) plaques were also present in the cerebellum, and the dual-labeling procedure resulted in minimal co-localization of staining. Thus it appears that two distinct types of plaque, which differ in their pathogenesis, can coexist in this disease; only a few plaques are hybrids. Any cerebrovascular amyloid was stained only by 1G10/2/3 and so is likely to be formed from β-protein. Most of the observations of cerebrovascular amyloid and Alzheimer plaques in these Creutzfeldt-Jakob cases are explicable in terms of the limited Alzheimer changes which occur as a consequence of "normal" aging, since these lesions were found in the older cases. Case 33/84 and the case described described by Keohane *et al.* (27) may reflect the coexistence of the two diseases; the abundant cortical plaques and the cerebrovascular amyloid in these cases are fully supportive of a diagnosis of AD, whereas the prion plaques in the cerebellum and the spongiform changes are characteristic of Creutzfeldt-Jakob disease. Whether this coexistence is fortuitous or whether there are closer links between these two diseases deserves further investigation.

Finally, it should be noted that the cerebral amyloidoses include a condition, hereditary cerebral hemorrhage with amyloidosis (47), that is associated with the deposition of a third type of cerebral amyloid. These amyloid deposits are composed of proteolytic fragments of a small basic serum protein, gamma trace (48), that is distinct from both PrP and β-protein.

Acknowledgments

We are grateful to Prof. L.W. Duchen for providing brain tissue from the case of Gerstmann-Straussler syndrome; R. Brown, R. Lofthouse, W. Tomlinson and A. Gardner for technical assistance; Dr. Ellen Billett for advice on the production of monoclonal antibodies; and A. Tomlinson for help with some of the figures. This work was supported by The Wellcome Trust and the MRC.

References

1. Allsop, D., Landon, M. & Kidd, M. (1983) *Brain Res.* **259**, 348-352.
2. Kidd, M., Allsop, D. & Landon, M. (1985) In: *Modern Approaches to the Dementias: Etiology and Pathophysiology,* ed. R.F. Clifford (Karger, Basel) pp. 114-126.
3. Selkoe, D.J., Ihara, Y. & Salazar, F.J. (1982) *Science* **215**, 1243-1245.
4. Ihara, Y., Abraham, C. & Selkoe, D.J. (1983) *Nature* **304**, 727-730.
5. Glenner, G.G. & Wong, C.W. (1984) *Biochem. Biophys. Res. Commun.* **120**, 885-890.
6. Glenner, G.G. & Wong, C.W. (1984) *Biochem. Biophys. Res. Commun.* **122**, 1131-1135.
7. Allsop, D., Landon, M. & Kidd, M. (1986) In: *Proceedings of the IVth International Symposium on Amyloidosis,* ed. G.G. Glenner & E. Osserman. (Plenum, New York) pp. 723-732.
8. Kidd, M., Allsop, D. & Landon, M. (1985) *Lancet* **1**, 278.
9. Masters, C.L., Simms, G., Weinman, N.A., Multhaup, G., McDonald, B.L. & Beyreuther, K. (1985) *Proc. Natl. Acad. Sci. USA* **82**, 4245-4249.
10. Masters, C.L., Multhaup, G., Simms, G., Pottgeisser, J., Martins, N.R. & Beyreuther, K. (1985) *EMBO J.* **4**, 2757-2763.
11. Prusiner, S.B., McKinley, M.P., Bowman, K.A., Bolton, D.C., Bendheim, P.E., Groth, D.F. & Glenner, G.G. (1983) *Cell* **35**, 349-358.
12. Diringer, H., Gelderblom, H., Hilmert, H., Ozel, M., Edelbluth, C. & Kimberlin, R.H. (1983) *Nature* **306**, 476-478.
13. Bolton, D.C., McKinley, M.P. & Prusiner, S.B. (1982) *Science* **218**, 1309-1311.
14. Oesch, B., Westaway, D., Walchli, M., McKinley, M.P., Kent, S.B.H., Aebersold, R., Barry, R.A., Tempst, P., Teplow, D.B., Hood, L.E., Prusiner, S.B. & Weissmann, C. (1985) *Cell* **40**, 735-746.
15. Chesebro, B., Race, R., Wehrly, K., Nishio, J., Bloom, M., Lechner,

D., Bergstrom, S., Robbins, K., Mayer, L., Keith, J.M., Garon, C. & Haase, A. (1985) *Nature* **315**, 331-333.
16. Bendheim, P.E. & Bolton, D.C. (1986) *Proc. Natl. Acad. Sci. USA* **83**, 2214-2218.
17. Harris, T. (1985) *Nature* **315**, 275.
18. Robertson, H.D., Branch, A.D. & Dahlberg, J.E. (1985) *Cell* **40**, 725-727.
19. Barry, R.A., McKinley, M.P., Bendheim, P.E., Lewis, G.K., DeArmond, S.J. & Prusiner, S.B. (1985) *J. Immunol.* **135**, 603-613.
20. DeArmond, S.J., McKinley, M.P., Barry, R.A., Braunfeld, M.B., McColloch, J.R. & Prusiner, S.B. (1985) *Cell* **41**, 221-235.
21. Kitamoto, T., Tateishi, J., Tashima, T., Takeshita, I., Barry, R.A., DeArmond, S.J. & Prusiner, S.B. *Ann. Neurol.* (in press).
22. Prusiner, S.B. (1984) *N. Engl. J. Med.* **310**, 661-663.
23. Green, N., Alexander, H., Olson, A., Alexander, S., Shinnick, T.M., Sutcliffe, J.G. & Lerner, R.S. (1982) *Cell* **28**, 477-487.
24. Mayer, R.J. & Billett, E.E. (1985) In: *Techniques in the Life Sciences: Techniques in Protein and Enzyme Biochemistry,* ed. K.F. Tipton (Elsevier, Amsterdam) pp. 1-55.
25. Littlefield, J.W. (1974) *Science* **145**, 709-710.
26. Lojda, Z. (1970) *Histochemie* **23**, 266-288.
27. Keohane, C., Peatfield, R. & Duchen, L.W. (1985) *J. Neurol. Neurosurg. Psychiatr.* **48**, 1175-1178.
28. Masters, C.L., Bajdusek, D.C. & Gibbs, C.J. (1981) *Brain* **104**, 559-588.
29. Baker, H.F., Ridley, R.M. & Crow, T.J. (1985) *Br. Med. J.* **291**, 299-302.
30. Wong, C.W., Quaranta, V. & Glenner, G.G. (1985) *Proc. Natl. Acad. Sci. USA* **82**, 8729-8732.
31. Selkoe, D.J., Abraham, C.R., Podlisny, M.B. & Duffy, L.K. *J. Neurochem.* (in press).
32. Anderton, B.H., Breinburg, D., Downes, M.J., Green, P.J., Tomlinson, B.E., Ulrich, J., Wood, J.N. & Kahn, J. (1982) *Nature* **298**, 84-86.
33. Miller, C.C.J., Brion, J-P., Calvert, R., Chin, T.K., Eagles, P.A.M., Downes, M.J., Flament-Durand, J., Haugh, M., Kahn, J., Probst, A., Ulrich, J. & Anderton, B.H. (1986) *EMBO J.* **5**, 269-276.
34. Miller, C.C.J., Haugh, M. & Anderton, B.H. (1986) *Trends Neurol. Sci.* **9**, 76-81.
35. Cork, L.C., Sternberger, N.H., Sternberger, L.A., Casanova, M.F., Struble, R.G. & Price, D.L. (1986) *J. Neuropathol. Exp. Neurol.* **45**, 56-64.

36. Rasool, C.G., Abraham, C., Anderton, B.H., Haugh, M., Kahn, J. & Selkoe, D.J. (1984) *Brain Res.* **310**, 249-260.
37. Perry, G., Rizzuto, N., Autilio-Gambetti, L. & Gambetti, P. (1985) *Proc. Natl. Acad. Sci. USA* **82**, 3916-3920.
38. Kosik, K.S., Duffy, L.K., Dowling, M.M., Abraham, C., McCluskey, A. & Selkoe, D.J. (1984) *Proc. Natl. Acad. Sci. USA* **81**, 7941-7945.
39. Kosik, K.S., Joachim, C.L. & Selkoe, D.J. *Proc. Natl. Acad. Sci. USA* (in press).
40. Geisler, N., Fischer, S., Vandekerckhove, J., Van Damme, J., Plessmann, U. & Weber, K. (1985) *EMBO J.* **4**, 57-63.
41. Geisler, N., Plessmann, U. & Weber, K. (1985) *FEBS Lett.* **182**, 475-478.
42. Geisler, N., Fischer, S., Vandekerckhove, J., Plessman, U. & Weber, K. (1984) *EMBO J.* **3**, 2701-2706.
43. Grafstein, B. & Forman, D.S. (1980) *Physiol. Rev.* **60**, 1167-1283.
44. Nixon, R.A., Brown, B.A. & Marotta, C.A. (1981) *J. Cell Biol.* **94**, 150-158.
45. Geisler, N., Kaufmann, E., Fischer, S., Plessmann, U. & Weber, K. (1983) *EMBO J.* **2**, 1295-1302.
46. Merz, P.A., Rohwer, R.G., Kascsak, R., Wisniewski, H.M., Somerville, R.A., Gibbs, C.J. & Gajdusek, D.C. (1984) *Science* **225**, 437-440.
47. Gudmundsson, G., Hallgrimsson, J., Jonasson, T.A. & Bjornason, O. (1972) *Brain* **95**, 387-404.
48. Cohen, D.H., Feiner, H., Jensson, O. & Frangione, B. (1983) *J. Exp. Med.* **158**, 623-628.

TABLE 1. Immunoreactivity of cerebellum sections from patients with confirmed Creutzfeldt-Jakob disease

Case No.	*Age*	*Sex*	*1G10/2/3 immunoreactivity*
201/81	56	F	—
71/82	56	M	—
136/71	57	F	—
42/79	58	F	—
217/81	60	M	—
247/79	64	F	—
57/70	67	F	—
116/76	68	F	+
33/83	72	M	—
248/79	72	F	+
171/83	73	F	—
67/77	75	F	+
33/84	79	F	+*
21/83	81	M	+

* Sections of frontal cortex of this patient also contained numerous Alzheimer plaques.

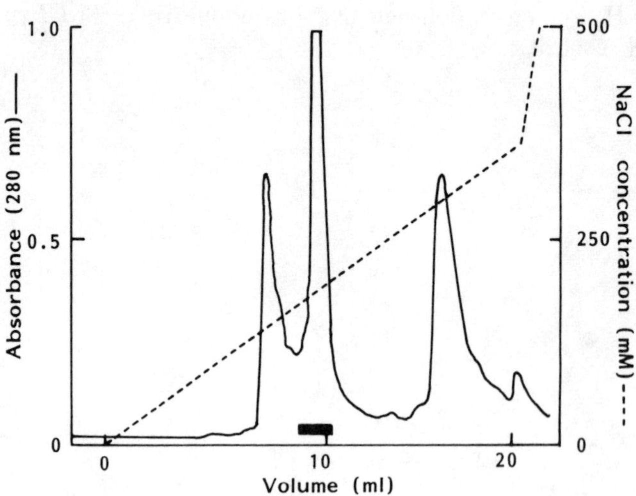

Fig. 1. Purification of monoclonal antibody 4D12/2/6 from 100 μl ascites fluid by ion-exchange FPLC on a Mono Q column. Bar indicates fractions with antipeptide activity.

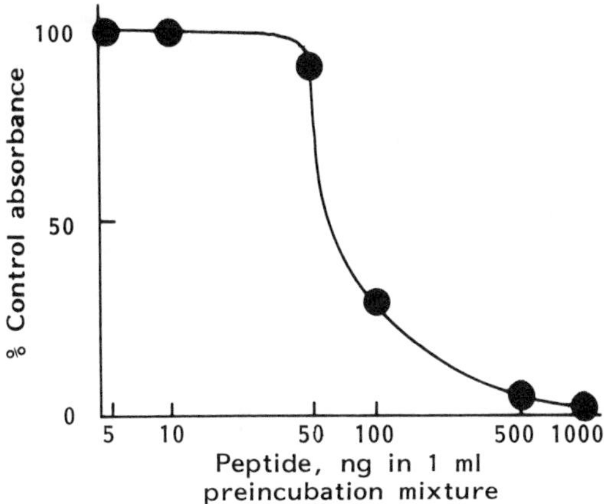

Fig. 2. Inhibition curve demonstrating reactivity of monoclonal antibody 1G10/2/3 to synthetic peptide. When no peptide is present in preincubation mixture, value obtained (control absorbance) is defined as 100%. Each point is the mean of four values.

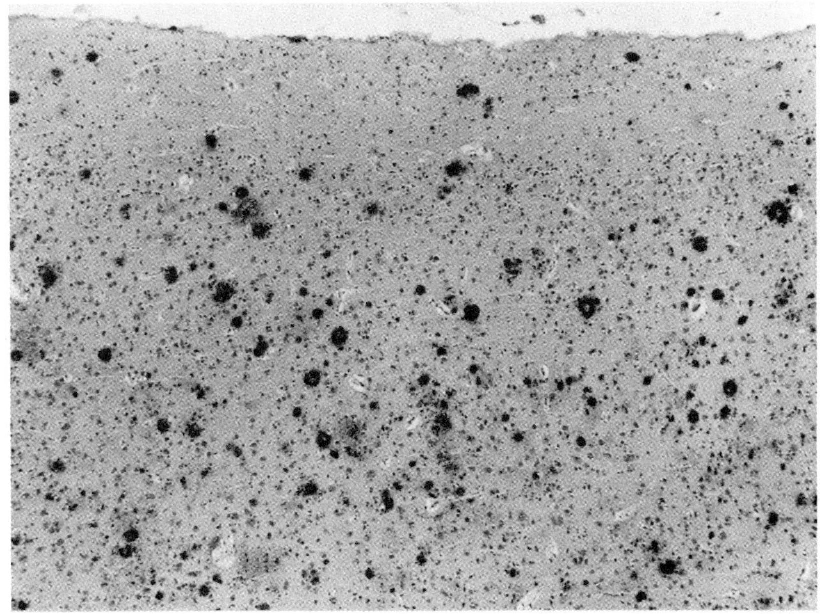

Fig. 3. Cortical senile plaques in a case of AD stained using FPLC-purified monoclonal antibody 1G10/2/3 (5 μg/ml). Section was counterstained with hematoxylin. (x 90).

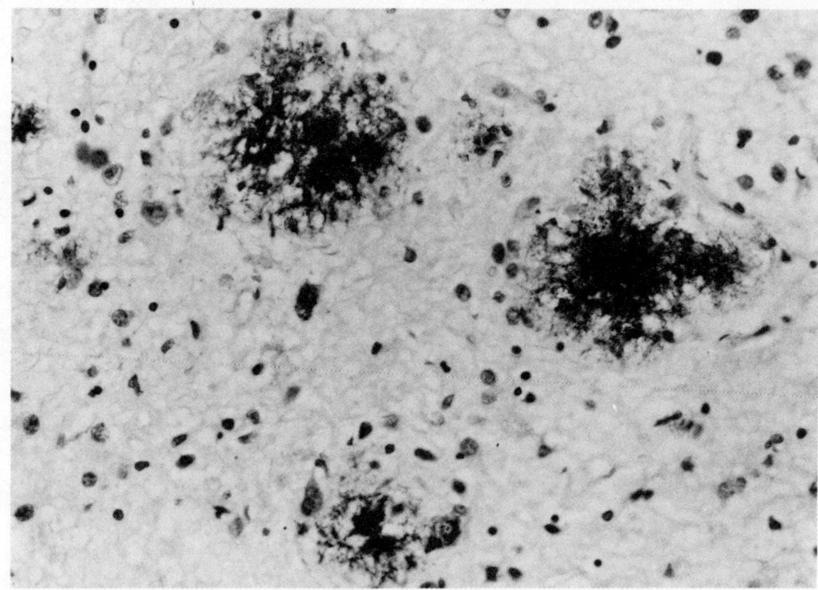

Fig. 4. Plaques in Down's syndrome (case M6) stained using purified 1G10/2/3 (5 μg/ml). (x 345).

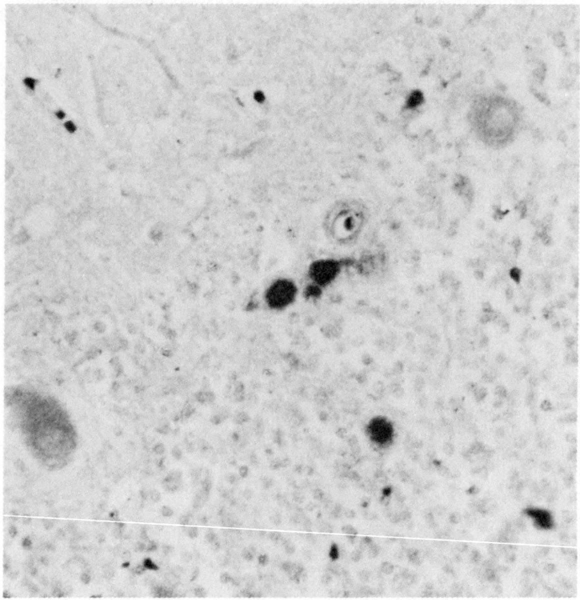

Fig. 5. Cerebellar anti-PrP-positive (prion) plaques in a case of Creutzfeldt-Jakob disease. (x 275).

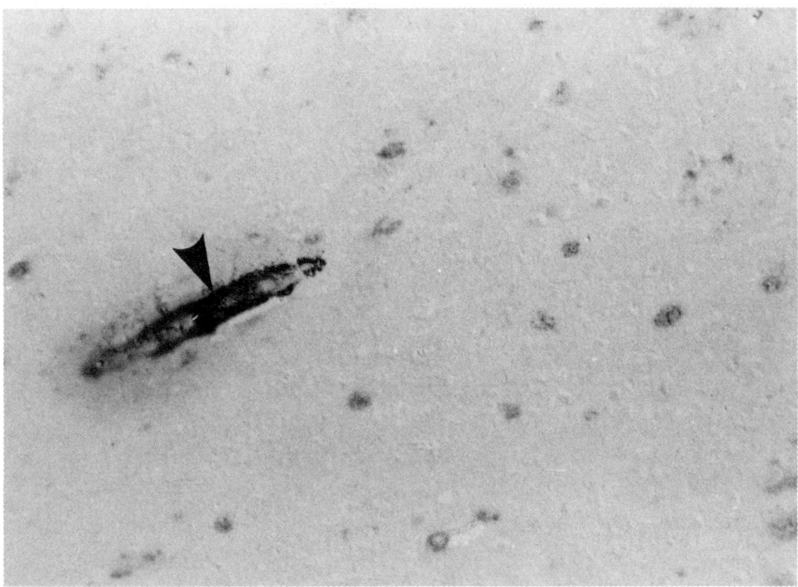

Fig. 6. Section of frontal cortex from case of Creutzfeldt-Jakob disease described by Keohane *et al.* (27) stained by purified 1G10/2/3 (1 μg/ml). Note cerebrovascular amyloid (arrow) and numerous Alzheimer plaques. (x 100).

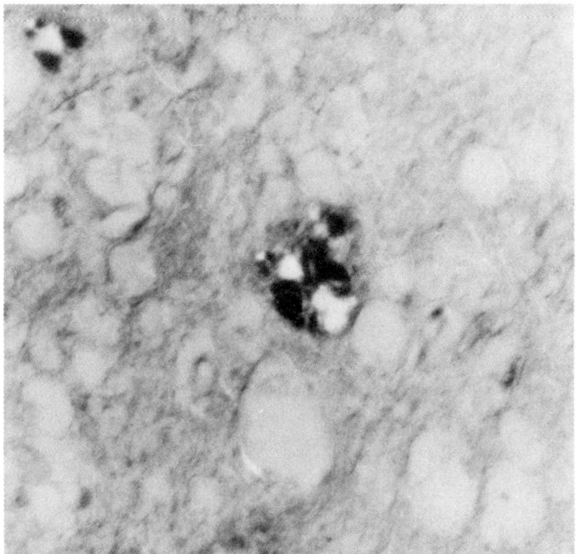

Fig. 7. Prion plaques in cerebellum from case of GerstmannStraussler syndrome. These plaques were positively stained using anti-PrP antiserum, counterstained with Congo red and photographed between crossed polarizers. (x 350).

11. Down's Syndrome and Alzheimer's Disease: What Is the Relation?

CHARLES J. EPSTEIN, Ph.D.

Departments of Pediatrics and of Biochemistry and Biophysics
University of California San Francisco, CA 94143

ABSTRACT: Several lines of evidence indicate that Alzheimer's disease (AD) occurs in individuals with Down's syndrome (DS). Morphological studies have demonstrated that the brains of adults with DS have degenerative changes and neuronal losses that are qualitatively, quantitatively, and geographically similar, if not indistinguishable, from those present in individuals with AD alone. Numerous other neurotransmitter, biochemical, and metabolic similarities also exist. However, despite the presence of the pathology of AD, not all adults with DS develop the clinical signs of dementia, although a gradual loss of cognitive function does appear to affect most or all indivudals with DS eventually. Two approaches can be used for unraveling the relation between AD and DS. One starts with the fact that DS is a disorder of gene dosage and is based on an examination of the consequences of having a 1.5-fold increase in the amounts of known chromosome 21 gene products. The other approach is based on a consideration of the manifold phenotypic abnormalities known to result from trisomy 21. Of particular interest in this regard is whether the DS brain is intrinsically defective from early in life and thereby predisposed to degenerative changes later. Although some family studies of AD have suggested that there is an increased frequency of DS in relatives of affected individuals, this does not appear to be a general phenomenon, and its significance with regard to the pathogenesis of AD in DS individuals is unclear. An animal model for human trisomy 21 has been developed: mouse fetuses with trisomy 16 have many somatic and nervous system abnormalities similar to those present in DS, notably the decreased cell proliferation and deficits of neurons in the cortex and cerebellum, and others which will be discussed. These animals, especially in the form of chimeras, can be used for investigations of whether trisomic neurons are intrinsically more sensitive to injurious exogenous agents.

Introduction

The relation between Alzheimer's disease (AD) and Down's syndrome (DS) has recently become the subject of intense interest to both the AD and DS research and patient/family communities. Those primarily concerned with AD are intrigued by the virtually invariant occurrence of the pathological changes of AD in the brains of DS adults in the fourth and later decades of life. They suspect, not unreasonably, that important clues concerning the pathogenesis of AD may be obtained by studying the high-risk DS population (1,2). On the other hand, the families of individuals with DS are concerned about the threat that AD poses to their relatives at a time in life when it would be hoped that such a potentially devastating problem would not have to be dealt with. Furthermore, an understanding of how DS predisposes to or causes the development of AD could shed light on how the presence of the extra chromosome 21 in DS leads to other of the phenotypic features in DS and, in particular, to the mental retardation which is so characteristic of the syndrome.

In this article, I consider two major issues bearing on the relation between AD and DS. The first is the evidence that the pathological and clinical condition found in DS is, in fact, AD; the second is the possible pathogenetic mechanisms by which DS leads to the development of AD. I conclude with discussions of some genetic issues raised by the relation of AD and DS and of how an animal model for DS can be used to investigate some of the mechanisms that have been or might be proposed. For earlier reviews and a fuller discussion of several of the points to be considered, the reader is referred to references 3-5.

The Evidence That Alzheimer's Disease Is Present in Individuals with Down's Syndrome

Pathology and Neurochemistry: Several lines of evidence have been brought together to establish that AD does actually occur in DS (Table 1). Many of the studies are primarily morphological, based on light and electron microscopic observations, and demonstrate that the brains of adults with DS possess granuovacular cytoplasmic changes, senile plaques, and neurofibrillary tangles which are qualitatively, quantitatively, and geographically indistinguishable from those present in individuals with AD alone (2,6-11). These lesions may appear as early as the second and third decades of life (9) and are virtually always present by the fourth and fifth decades (7,9,12). Similar patterns of nerve cell loss have also been observed in DS and AD (13).

In support of the morphological observations have been descriptions of chemical similarities between the brains of individuals with AD and adults with DS. These include decreases in various parts of the brain of the enzymes acetylcholinesterase and choline acetyltransferase (14) and of the monoamines norepinephrine, dopamine, and 5-hydroxytryptamine (15-17). Furthermore, Glenner and Wong (18) and Wong *et al.* (19) have shown that the partial amino acid sequences of β_2 proteins from cerebrovascular amyloid fibrils (or amyloid cerebral/Congophilic angiopathy) obtained from brains of elderly individuals with DS are virtually identical to those from patients with AD. Masters *et al.* obtained the same results with the identical or very closely related amyloid plaque cores derived from the neuritic plaques themselves (20). Finally, a 68,000 dalton protein antigen, found to be increased 15- to 30-fold in the temporal cortices of individuals with AD and recognized by the monoclonal antibody Alz-50 (21), was also increased in amount in the brain of an adult with DS (22).

The one significant neurochemical discrepancy between AD and DS described to date is the approximately 2-fold elevation of neurotensin concentrations in the caudate nucleus, temporal cortex and frontal cortex of adults with DS but not of individuals with AD (23). However, these increases were unrelated to the presence of AD-type degenerative changes and were also observed in the brains of two infants with DS, suggesting that they represent some process independent of that involved in the pathology of AD in DS.

The development of positron emission tomography (PET) with injection of [^{18}F]2-fluoro-2-deoxy-D-glucose has made it possible to study cerebral metabolism in individuals with DS and with AD. A decreased rate of glucose utilization has been documented in AD (24-26), and a ≈23% decrease from young adult levels has recently been found in older adults (47 to 63 years of age) with DS (27). This decrease in the older individuals with DS occurs after a period in young adulthood (19 to 33 years of age) during which persons with DS have a ≈30% higher than normal rate of glucose utilization, so that overall rates of metabolism for older DS and control individuals are similar. Thus, it is the age-dependent pattern of change, rather than the absolute values of cerebral glucose utilization, that makes the older DS population resemble the population of individuals with AD.

Taken together, the morphological, chemical and metabolic data indicate that the pathological process occurring in the brains of adults with DS is indistinguishable from that which occurs in the brains of individuals with AD. What has been more perplexing and controversial, however, is the relation between these abnormalities and the psychological and behavioral changes which may or may not take place in older individuals with DS.

Neuropsychology: Wisniewski and Rabe (28) recently reviewed in detail the discrepancy between Alzheimer-type neuropathology and dementia in people with DS and concluded that "we do not yet know the prevalence of Alzheimer type dementia among DS persons." In part, the problem may be methodological and related to difficulties in diagnosing dementia on a background of moderate to severe mental retardation, but this does not appear to be the whole explanation. A significant proportion of adult DS individuals simply do not have dementia by any criterion. The best estimate at present is that only ≈25% are in fact demented (9), although numbers as high as 45% have been suggested (29). Wisniewski and Rabe (28) reject the notion that this absence of dementia in all DS individuals with the pathology of AD indicates that the pathology and the development of psychological and behavioral changes are unrelated. Rather, they believe, both in AD that occurs in the non-DS population and in adults with DS, that the appearance of dementia is dependent on the pathological abnormalities (as measured by numbers of plaques and tangles) exceeding some threshold value, a value which, they suggest, is higher in DS than in non-DS individuals. In support of this idea, they present data, taken from the studies of Wisniewski *et al.* (9) on DS and Blessed *et al.* (30) and Wilcock and Esiri (31) for non-DS AD, which show that demented individuals in either group have higher densities of plaques and tangles than do nondemented individuals. These data, which really are not directly comparable, suggest that the putative threshold density of plaques and tangles for dementia is higher in DS than in the non-DS group (28). This hypothesis would provide a convenient explanation for why only a fraction of adults with DS are clinically demented and thereby have both the pathological and clinical characteristics of AD, but why it should be so is not obvious. In fact, we might have suspected just the opposite—that a brain which is already functionally compromised should have a lower, rather than a higher, threshold for the development of dementia.

Before leaving the subject of dementia and related clinical abnormalities in adults with DS, one additional point needs to be made. Increasing evidence is being accumulated which suggests that a loss of a variety of intellectual functions occurs in older individuals with DS, irrespective of whether frank dementia occurs. Two of the more recent studies are worthy of note. One is that of Thase *et al.* (29,32), who compared institutionalized adults with DS with a control group of institutionalized mentally retarded individuals with the same IQ distribution. Using several psychological tests, including digit span recall, object identification, and visual memory (5- and 30-sec delay), those investigators demonstrated significantly lower scores in the DS group. Of greater interest was the progressive decline with age in the scores of the DS group so that, for example, visual memory (5-sec delay) scores dropped progressively from 4.5 in the 25- to 34-year-old group to 2.0 in the 55- to 64-year-old group, whereas in the control group scores rose from 3.4 to 4.5. Additional evidence for progressive loss of function in DS adults has been presented by Schapiro *et al.* (27). In neuropsychological tests carried out on the "young" and "old" groups of DS individuals already discussed with regard to cerebral metabolism, Schapiro's group found significant decreases in performance on a large battery of language, visuospatial, attention, and visual recognition memory tasks. Even though three of the six older patients were considered to be demented, the scores of the nondemented patients in the "old" group were similar to those of the demented subjects in the group and did not significantly overlap with the scores of the "young" group.

It thus appears that the situation in adults with DS can be summarized as follows. Starting in the third decade of life, the pathological changes of AD begin to appear; and by the fourth decade, all or nearly all DS individuals have this pathology and its associated chemical and metabolic consequences. During and beyond the same period of time, there is a slowly progressive loss of a variety of cognitive functions which probably affects most if not all individuals with DS. In addition, approximately 25% of DS adults develop other neurological abnormalities, including loss of the skills of daily living and of vocational skills, impaired abstract thinking or judgment, disturbances of higher cortical function, and personality changes (27), which permit a clinical diagnosis of dementia and, therefore, of AD in all of its manifestations.

The Pathogenetic Relation of Down's Syndrome to the Pathology of Alzheimer's Disease

As was pointed out in an earlier review (3), the critical fact that must be kept in mind when considering the effects of trisomy 21 in the causation of DS and its phenotypic features, including AD, is that the basic problem stems from the presence of an extra but normal chromosome. Therefore, the abnormalities must be related to the presence of an extra set of *normal* genes rather than to genes that are in some way abnormal. A trisomy is, therefore, a disorder of gene dosage, and all available evidence indicates, not only for genes on human chromosome 21, but also for the more than 40 other human and mouse genes that have been examined, that the presence of three rather than two copies of a gene results in the synthesis of 150% of the normal amount of the gene product

(4) (Table 2). Gene products can, of course, be of any kind, and the confirmed or provisionally identified loci on chromosome 21 include genes for several enzymes, a receptor, several cell-surface molecules or antigens, a structural protein, and an unknown product induced by estrogen, as well as a proto-oncogene (Table 2). Among the possible classes of gene products (4), all that are still lacking on chromosome 21 are known growth factors, transport proteins and regulatory molecules, but given that chromosome 21 contains anywhere from 50 to 1000 active loci (33), it is likely that representatives of all types of gene products will be encoded on this chromosome.

The Effects of Imbalance of Loci on Human Chromosome 21: There are two approaches that might be used to unravel the pathogenetic relation between DS and AD. One is to start with each of the genes known to be located on chromosome 21 and to determine experimentally, or at least to predict on theoretical grounds, the consequences of having an extra copy of the gene and 1.5 times as much gene product. This type of exercise has been carried out for two of the known chromosome 21 loci, SOD-1 and IFNRA (or IFRC), and a detailed discussion is presented in reference 4.

For the interferon-α (IFN-α) receptor, trisomy 21 fibroblasts have the expected 1.5 times the normal amount of receptor and demonstrate proportional increases in the induction by IFN-α of the enzyme (2′-5′)oligoisoadenylate synthetase and of eight intracellular peptides of as yet unknown function (4,34-36). However, when the physiological effects of interferon treatment are examined, the responsiveness or sensitivity of trisomic cells to the antiviral effect of IFN-α is increased from 3- to 15-fold (mean = 6.3) and to all effects about 5-fold (4). Although we have attributed this functional amplification to the extra dose of the IFN-α receptor, this remains to be proved. Furthermore, whatever the cause of the amplified response in trisomic cells, it is not possible, because of the multitudinous and often contradictory actions of the interferons, to predict what effect this enchanced sensitivity will have on the nervous system during development and normal physiological functioning or in response to exogenous toxins or infectious agents.

Much has been written about the increased concentration of superoxide dismutase-1 (SOD-1) in trisomic cells and tissues and its potential role in the pathogenesis of both the mental retardation and AD associated with DS (37,38). SOD-1 catalyzes the conversion (dismutation) of O_2-(superoxide) radicals to H_2O_2 and O_2, and H_2O_2 and O_2 can further react to form the highly reactive and injurious hydroxyl radical (OH·). Direct evidence for functional alterations in the metabolism of oxygen as a result of increased SOD-1 activity is quite limited. However, Groner *et al.* have found that cells overexpressing

SOD-1 2- to 6-fold after transfection with cloned SOD-1 genes are more *resistant* to the lethal effects of Paraquat, an agent which leads to the generation of superoxide radicals (39). By contrast, it has been claimed that trisomic fibroblasts, with only 1.5 times the normal amount of SOD-1, are more *sensitive* to the toxic effects of 95% oxygen, which are also attributed to increased superoxide generation, in terms of both decreased survival and increased lipid peroxidation (40).

If increased activity of SOD-1 is injurious to the brain, it would be expected that this would manifest itself as an increase in lipid peroxidation. And, in fact, Brooksbank and Balazs did observe such an increase in brains of fetuses with trisomy 21 (41). However, those investigators also found significant alterations in the composition of polyunsaturated fatty acids in the trisomic brains, which could explain, in whole or in part, the increase in lipid peroxidation (42). In studies of an animal model system (see below), no increase in lipid peroxidation was found in fetal brains in which SOD-1 activity was increased 1.5-fold. It must be concluded, therefore, that a relation between increased SOD-1 activity and the pathogenesis of AD in DS must be considered entirely speculative at this time.

Our failure to obtain any strong leads from a consideration of the loci now known to be on chromosome 21 should not be discouraging, since, as has already been pointed out, relatively few of the genes in the DS region of chromosome 21 have as yet been identified. Ultimately, the locus or loci involved, whether by their direct action or by increasing susceptibility to some other agent or event, will be identified. The reasons for this conviction are outlined at length in reference 4.

Schweber has taken the concept just advanced, of a connection between specific chromosome 21 loci and AD, a bit further and has suggested that AD in the non-DS population could be the result of a minute duplication of a region of chromosome 21, resulting in the presence of three copies of the region (43). How this would occur in the sporadic cases of AD is not clear, but it could be supposed that such could be the case in familial AD. However, were such a duplication actually present in familial AD, it might be expected that the time of appearance of the disease in such families, both pathologically and clinically, would resemble that found in DS, yet this does not appear to be the case. For example, in the very large pedigree studies by Nee *et al.* (44), the age of onset ranged from 47 to 59 years. But, rather than speculate on the matter, we would be better advised to wait for the results of linkage studies apparently in progress (45). If a gene for familial AD were found to be linked to a chromosome 21 molecular marker (a restriction-fragment-length polymorphism or RFLP) this would constitute a persuasive reason to look for the postulated minute duplications or for other types of mutations on chromosome 21 which could have the same functional effect. The only linkage study published to date, that involving the family described by Nee *et al.* (44), reports data "consistent with the possibility that genes in the *HLA* region of chromosome 6 and perhaps also in the *Gm* region of chromosome 14 are determinants of susceptibility" (46), but chromosome 21 markers were not available when that study was performed.

Indirect Effects of Trisomy 21: Another way to explore the possible pathogenetic relation between DS and AD is to look at the phenotypic features of DS. Although the molecular mechanisms (in terms of known loci on chromosome 21) of such features are still largely unknown, it is still possible to consider how they might be involved in the pathogenesis of AD. A list of such features is given in Table 3. The features in this list, which does not include the major congenital cardiac and gastrointestinal anomalies and the many minor dysmorphic features that characterize DS, point to a variety of abnormalities in cellular responses, membrane function, and susceptibility to external infectious agents which could be relevant to the pathogenesis of AD (3). However, once again, it is not now clear how any of these cellular and functional abnormalities can be implicated. The notion of premature aging has deliberately been omitted from the list, since there is little evidence to support its existence in DS, and claims for its relation to the occurrence of AD in DS generally represent exercises in circular reasoning (see refs. 3 and 4).

As was noted earlier (3), one possibility worthy of further consideration is that the neurons of individuals with DS are intrinsically defective and predisposed to degenerative changes from the beginning of life. That the nervous system in DS is abnormal from early in life is obvious from the neonatal hypotonia and early onset of developmental delay and mental retardation. But is there anything different about the nervous system in DS that distinguishes it from other causes of mental retardation which are not associated with the development of AD later in life? Some studies have pointed to abnormalities in the number and structure of dendritic spines (47,48), but the specificity of these abnormalities is questionable. More recent investigations have focused on decreases in neuronal density and synaptogenesis in the brains of infants and children with DS. Thus, Ross *et al.* studied the brain of a 6-year-old girl with DS and found a "poverty" of granular cells, which was particularly striking (with decreases of 20% to 80%) in certain regions of the brain, such as areas 3, 17, and 41 (49). They suspect that a particular cell type, the aspinous stellate, may be especially affected. Similarly, McGeer *et al.* studied the brain of a 5.5-month-old infant with DS and found a 50% reduction in the number of cells of the basal forebrain cholinergic system; there was a normal complement of cells in the noradrenergic system of the locus ceruleus (50). Sylvester studied the brains of 20 DS adults between 18 and 70 years of age and found the areas of the dentate gyrus and the pyramidal cell layer of the hippocampus to be significantly below those found in controls (51). Despite the finding of "senile changes" in all but three cases, he concluded that the small sizes of these structures in all individuals with DS is "likely to be largely due to congenital malformation."

The most detailed studies of neuronal density and synaptogenesis in the early DS brain have been carried out by Wisniewski *et al.* (52). They studied 73 DS brains from individuals between birth and 14 years of age and found neuronal densities to be decreased by 10% to 50% in several areas, including the visual, parahippocampal, and visual cortices. Granular layers II and IV seemed to be particularly affected. Synaptic density was decreased 24% at birth in the DS visual cortex, but the values were normal between 8 months and 4 years of age. However, the mean surface area per synaptic contact zone was reduced 20% to 35% over the entire period of development. On the basis of these observations, Wisniewski *et al.* concluded that there is an arrest of prenatal neurogenesis and of prenatal and postnatal synaptogenesis in DS (52).

None of the observations just cited proves that abnormalities of the early development of the DS brain predispose it to the degenerative changes of AD later in life. Unless accompanied by chemical or functional alterations that could compromise neuronal integrity, deficiencies in cell number should not, in themselves, lead to premature cell degeneration. However, examples of chemical and functional abnormalities in the DS nervous sytem have already been mentioned—for example, altered composition of polyunsaturated fatty acids in fetal DS membranes (42) and abnormal electrical properties in cultured fetal DS dorsal root ganglion cells (53,54)—so it is conceivable that these derangements, superimposed on an existing deficiency of neurons, could well play a role in the development of AD. However, whether this is actually the case or not, there is a bit of a paradox operating here: if loss of neurons and neuronal connections is responsible for the development of dementia, why should there be the discrepancy between the pathology and the appearance of the clinical manifestations of dementia that is observed in DS? As previously noted, just the opposite might be expected when the nervous system is compromised to start with.

The Genetic Relation Between Down's Syndrome and Alzheimer's Disease

All of the foregoing discussion has been predicated on the premise that, from the genetic point of view, the starting point for discussion is the presence of the extra chromosome 21 in individuals with DS and that the important issue is how this extra chromosome leads to the development of AD. In this approach, the fact that non-DS-related AD may or may not be inherited (for a recent review, see ref. 55) is relevant only insofar as one wishes to postulate and to search for chromosome 21 loci that may be implicated in familial or sporadic AD. However, a peculiar circumstance has led to a curious reversal of thinking—that there is a common genetic factor that may be responsible both for the development of AD in familial cases and for the birth of individuals with DS (*i.e.*, for the occurrence of meiotic nondisjunction). This notion is based on the observation of Heston *et al.* that there is, in the families of 125 probands that they studied, an excess in the number of individuals born with DS (Table 4) as well as in the frequency of lymphoproliferative disorders (56). Although stating that "these relationships seem too remote to make any sense genetically," Heston *et al.* nonetheless went on to suggest a "unitary genetic etiology" in which a postulated genetic defect of microtubules and microfilaments leads severally to the neurofibrillary tangles and other degenerative changes of AD, meiotic abnormalities causing trisomy 21 and DS, and immunological abnormalities leading to lymphoproliferative malignancies (56).

As I stated elsewhere (3), I find these suggested connections unconvincing and conceptually unhelpful, and review of several other studies (Table 4) supports this view. In the only other comparable family study (57), a familial association between AD and lymphoproliferative disorders was not found, although the calculated incidence of DS (including one case of a transmissible translocation) was slightly elevated to 3.6 per 1000, as opposed to an expected but not independently ascertained rate of 1.3 per 1000. In another study in which only first-degree relatives were considered, there was no increase in hematological malignancies, and no cases of DS were found in 329 relatives at risk (58). These two investigations, like those of Heston and his collaborators (56), were carried out on multiple families of individually ascertained probands. However, three additional studies have appeared in which six large families with a total of 121 affected individuals are described (44,59,60) (Table 4). Among 474 first- to third-degree relatives at risk, there is only one case of DS in a second-degree relative. Heston *et al.* have suggested that the frequency of DS would be expected to be most increased in families with the highest genetic risk for developing AD, and they quote a figure as high as 10.6 cases/1000 in births observed after 1950 (for all families, not just those with more than one case of AD) (56). If this suggestion were correct, then I would expect a higher than observed frequency of DS among members of families in which there is strong evidence for a highly penetrant gene inherited in an autosomal dominant manner. Furthermore, looking at all of the studies listed in Table 4, only 1 of the total of 15 cases of DS (excluding the translocation case) occurred in a first-degree relative, a somewhat surprising result, since the likelihood of the putative genetic factor predisposing to both AD and to DS being present would be greatest in first-degree relatives. Since we are still dealing with quite small numbers, both of affected and at risk, more extensive data will be required before any firm conclusions can be drawn.

Just as work is now in progress to search for an AD "locus" on chromosome 21, investigators are also searching for loci or regions on chromosome 21 that predispose to the occurrence of nondisjunction. Were both types of loci/regions actually to be found, then the hypothesis of Heston and his collaborators would certainly warrant reconsideration and further study. For the moment, we can just wait for more information.

An Animal Model for Human Trisomy 21

Over the past several years, my collaborators and I have been developing a mouse model for human trisomy 21 (61-63). This model is based on the identification on mouse chromosome 16 of several loci located on human chromosome 21: SOD-1, IFNRA, PRGS, and ETS2, (64,65), with three of these loci localized to the distal region of the mouse chromosome (64). These results have been interpreted as indicating that a significant region of mouse chromosome 16 is homologous to the distal part of human chromosome 21, in which the DS region is located (66), and that mouse trisomy 16 will be genetically similar to human trisomy 21 insofar as those loci present on both chromosomes are concerned. Mouse fetuses with trisomy 16 have been bred and studied in detail, and several similarities with human trisomy 21 have been noted (4, 63). Adult Ts16 ↔ 2n chimeric mice containing both trisomic (Ts) and diploid (2n) cells have also been prepared and can be considered as models for human trisomy 21/2n mosaics (62).

In the context of the present discussion, the trisomy 16 mouse is of interest because it reproduces many, if not all, of the genetic imbalance found in DS. As such, its study is relevant to both the mental retardation found early in the life of individuals with DS and to the AD which develops later. The principal findings concerning the nervous system of trisomy 16 mouse fetuses and of adult Ts16 ↔ 2n chimeras are summarized in Table 5, and the anatomic, neurotransmitter, and behavioral studies (on chimeras) have recently been reviewed in detail by Oster-Granite *et al.* (67) and Coyle *et al.* (68).

In its present form, the trisomy 16 mouse model is best suited for studies of the effects of the aneuploid state on early development of the nervous system, and some interesting parallels with DS have emerged. Most notable are the decreased cell proliferation and deficits of neurons in the cortex and cerebellum (67) (as compared with the results of Wisniewski *et al.* [52] in DS), the abnormalities of electrical conduction in cultured spinal cord dorsal root ganglion (DRG) neurons (69,70; Orozco *et al.*, submitted) (as compared with the observations of Scott *et al.* [53] on fetal DRG neurons in DS) and the presence of normal brain glutathione peroxidase activity and lipid peroxide concentration in the face of elevated SOD-1 activity (Anneren and Epstein, submitted) (as compared with the findings of normal glutathione peroxidase and elevated lipid peroxidation in fetal DS brains [41,42]). The last of these observations indicates that, at least during the period of gestation, increased SOD-1 activity is not necessarily accompanied by increased lipid peroxidation. Although they do not disprove the notion that the 1.5-fold increase in SOD-1 can be injurious to the brain, these findings do not lend any support to it.

For investigations more directly relevant to the pathogenesis of AD, it is necessary to have adult trisomic animals. At present, the best that we can do is to make animals that are chimeric and have both trisomy 16 and diploid cells in the brain and other tissues. Oster-Granite *et al.* have proposed a method for preparing chimeras in which all of the central nervous system neurons will be trisomic in genotype (67). In either case, useful results concerning the central nervous lesions of AD will be obtained only if the predisposition for the development of such abnormalities resides within the neurons themselves, whether because of some intrinsic abnormality or of an enchanced susceptibility to external toxic or infectious agents. If this predisposition operates through some more general susceptibility factor; *e.g.*, an impaired immune response, then the animals with somatic chimerism would not be expected to display the abnormality since the presence of normal diploid cells would correct the somatic defect. As an example of how the chimeric animal model can be used, experiments proposed in an earlier article (3) are in progress to determine whether Ts16 ↔ 2n chimeras are more susceptible than control animals to the development of scrapie after intracerebral inoculation of the scrapie prion (Prusiner *et al.*, unpublished data).

Although it would have been desirable to be able to come to a positive conclusion concerning the relation and DS and AD, it must be admitted that this relation remains as obscure as ever. Nevertheless, there are many avenues of investigation that can be pursued from both sides of the question, and it is not unreasonable to hope that useful insights will eventually emerge.

Acknowledgments

This work was supported by grants from the National Institutes of Health (HD-17001 and GM-24309).

References

1. Burger, P.C. & Vogel, F.S. (1973) *Am. J. Pathol.* **73**, 457-476.
2. Ball, M.J. & Nuttal, K. (1981) *Neuropathol. Appl. Neurobiol.* **7**, 13-20.
3. Epstein, C.J. (1983) In: *Biological Aspects of Alzheimer's Disease*, Banbury Report 15, ed. Katzman, R. (Cold Spring Harbor Laboratory, Cold Spring Harbor, NY) pp. 169-178.
4. Epstein, C.J., (1986) *The Consequences of Chromosome Imbalance: Principles, Mechanisms, and Models* (Cambridge University Press, Cambridge and New York).
5. Epstein, C.J., ed. (1986) *The Neurobiology of Down Syndrome* (Raven Press, New York).
6. Ellis, W.G., McCulloch, J.R. & Corley, C.L. (1979) *Neurology* **24**, 101-106.
7. Whalley, L.B. & Buckton, K.E. (1979) In: *Alzheimer's Disease: Early Recognition of Potentially Reversible Defects*, eds. Glen, A.I.M. & Whalley, L.J. (Churchill Livingstone, Edinburgh) pp. 36-41.
8. Ball, M.J. & Nuttall, K. (1980) *Ann. Neurol.* **7**, 462-465.
9. Wisniewski, K.E., Wisniewski, H.M. & Wen, G.Y. (1985) *Ann. Neurol.* **17**, 278-282.
10. Wisniewski, K.E., Dalton, A.J., Crapper McLachlan, D.R., Wen, G.Y. & Wisniewski, H.M. (1985) *Neurology* **35**, 957-961.
11. Ball, M.J., Schapiro, M.B. & Rapoport, S.I. (1986) In: *The Neurology of Down Syndrome,* ed. Epstein, C.J. (Raven Press, New York) (in press).
12. Malamud, N. (1972) In: *Aging and the Brain,* ed. Gartz, C.M. (Plenum Press, New York) pp. 63-87.
13. Mann, D.M.A., Yates, P.O. & Marcyniuk, B. (1984) *Neuropathol. Appl. Neurobiol.* **10**, 185-207.
14. Yates, C.M., Simpson, S., Maloney, A.J.F., Gordon, A. & Reid, A.H. (1980) *Lancet* **2**, 979.
15. Yates, C.M., Ritchie, I.M., Simpson, J., Maloney, A.J.F. & Gordon, A. (1981) *Lancet* **2**, 39-40.

16. Nyberg, P., Carlsson, A. & Winblad, B. (1982) *J. Neural Transm.* **55**, 289-299.
17. Reynolds, G.R. & Godridge, H. (1985) *Lancet* **1**, 1368-1369.
18. Glenner, G.G. & Wong, C.W. (1984) *Biochem. Biophys. Res. Commun.* **122**, 1131-1135.
19. Wong, C.W., Quaranta, V. & Glenner, G.G. (1985) *Proc. Natl. Acad. Sci. USA* **82**, 8729-8732.
20. Masters, C.L., Simms, G., Weinman, N.A., Multhaup, G., McDonald, B.L. & Beyreuther, K. (1985) *Proc. Natl. Acad. Sci. USA* **82**, 4245-4249.
21. Wolozin, B.L., Pruchnicki, A., Dickson, D.W. & Davies, P. (1986) *Science* **232**, 648-650.
22. Davies, P. quoted in Schmeck, H.M. Jr. (1986) *New York Times,* April 25, p. 15.
23. Yates, C.M., Fink, G., Bennie, J.G., Gordon, A., Simpson, J. & Eskay, R.L. (1985) *J. Neurol. Sci.* **67**, 327-335.
24. Cutler, N.R. (moderator) (1985) *Ann. Intern. Med.* **103**, 566-578.
25. de Leon, M.J., Ferris, S.H., George, A.E., Reisberg, B., Christman, D.R., Kricheff, I.I. & Wolf, A.P. (1983) *J. Cereb. Blood Flow Metab.* **3**, 391-394.
26. Foster, N.L., Chase, T.N., Mansi, L., Brooks, R., Fedio, P., Patronas, N.J. & Di Chiro, G. (1984) *Ann. Neurol.* **16**, 649-654.
27. Schapiro, M.B., Haxby, J.V., Grady, C.L. & Rapoport, S.I. (1986) In: *The Neurology of Down Syndrome,* ed. Epstein, C.J. (Raven Press, New York) (in press).
28. Wisniewski, H.M. & Rabe, A. (1986). *Ann. NY Acad. Sci.* (in press).
29. Thase, M.E., Liss, L., Smeltzer, D. & Maloon, J. (1982) *J. Ment. Defic. Res.* **26**, 239-244.
30. Blessed, G., Tomlinson, B.E. & Roth, M. (1968) *Br. J. Psychiatr.* **114**, 797-817.
31. Wilcock, G.K. & Esiri, M.M. (1982) *J. Neurol. Sci.* **56**, 343-356.
32. Thase, M.E., Tigner, R., Smeltzer, D.J. & Liss, L. (1984) *Biol. Psychiatr.* **19**, 571-585.
33. Epstein, C.J. (1986) In: *The Neurobiology of Down Syndrome,*ed. Epstein, C.J. (Raven Press, New York) (in press).
34. Weil, J., Epstein, C.J., Epstein, L.B., van Blerkon, J. & Xuong, N.H. (1983) *Antiviral Res.* **3**, 303-314.
35. Weil, J., Tucker, G., Epstein, L.B. & Epstein, C.J. (1983) *Hum. Genet.* **65**, 108-111.
36. Epstein, C.J. & Epstein, L.B. (1983) *Lymphokines* **8**, 277-301.
37. Sinet, P.M (1982) *Ann. NY Acad. Sci.* **396**, 83-94.
38. Sinet, P.M., Lejeune, J. & Jerome, H. (1979) *Life Sci.* **24**, 29-34.
39. Groner, Y., Lieman-Hurwitz, J., Dafni, N., Sherman, L., Levanon,

D., Bernstein, Y., Danciger, E. & Elroy-Stein, O. (1985) *Ann. NY Acad. Sci.* **450**, 133-156.
40. Mayes, J., Muneer, R. & Sifers, M. (1984) *Am. J. Hum. Genet.* **36**, 15S.
41. Brooksbank, B.W.L. & Balazs, R. (1984) *Dev. Brain Res.* **16**, 37-44.
42. Balazs, R. & Brooksbank, B.W.L. (1986) In: *The Neurobiology of Down Syndrome*, ed. Epstein, C.J. (Raven Press, New York) (in press).
43. Schweber, M. (1985) *Ann. NY Acad. Sci.* **450**, 223-238.
44. Nee, L.E., Polinsky, R.J., Eldridge, R., Weingartner, H., Smallberg, S. & Ebert, M. (1983) *Arch. Neurol.* **40**, 203-208.
45. Kolata, G. (1986) *Science* **232**, 248-250.
46. Weitkamp, L.R., Nee, L., Keats, B., Polinsky, R.J. & Guttormsen, S. (1983) *Am. J. Hum. Genet.* **35**, 443-453.
47. Suetsuga, M. & Mehraein, P. (1980) *Acta Neuropathol.* **50**, 207-210.
48. Marin-Padilla, M. (1976) *J. Comp. Neurol.* **167**, 63-82.
49. Ross, M.H., Galaburda, A.M. & Kemper, T.L. (1984) *Neurology* **34**, 909-916.
50. McGeer, E.G., Norman, M., Boyes, B., O'Kusky, J., Suzuki, J. & McGeer, P.L. (1985) *Exp. Neurol.* **87**, 557-570.
51. Sylvester, P.E. (1983) *J. Ment. Defic. Res.* **27**, 227-236.
52. Wisniewski, K.E. Laure-Kamionowska, M., Connell, F. & Wen, G.Y. (1986) In: *The Neurobiology of Down Syndrome*, ed. Epstein, C.J. (Raven Press, New York) (in press).
53. Scott, B.S., Becker, L.E. & Petit, T.L. (1983) *Prog. Neurobiol.* **21**, 199-237.
54. Scott, B.S. (1986) In: *The Neurobiology of Down Syndrome*, ed. Epstein, C.J. (Raven Press, New York) (in press).
55. Kay, D.W.K. (1986) *Br. Med. Bull.* **42**, 19-23.
56. Heston, L.L., Mastri, A.R., Anderson, A.R. & Anderson, V.E. (1981) *Arch. Gen. Psychiatr.* **38**, 1085-1090.
57. Heyman, A., Wilkinson, W.E., Hurwitz, B.J., Schmechel, D., Sigmon, A.H., Weinberg, T., Helms, M.J. & Swift, M. (1983) *Ann. Neurol.* **14**, 507-515.
58. Whalley, L.J., Carothers, A.D., Collyer, S., DeMey, R. & Frackiewicz, A. (1982) *Br. J. Psychiatr.* **140**, 249-256.
59. Cook, R.H., Ward, B.E. & Austin, J.H. (1979) *Neurology* **29**, 1402-1412.
60. Goutsmit, J., White, B.J. Weitkamp, L.R., Keats, B.J.B., Morrow, C.H. & Gajdusek, D.C. (1981) *J. Neurol. Sci.* **49**, 79-89.
61. Cox, D.R., Epstein, L.B. & Epstein, C.J. (1980) *Proc. Natl. Acad. Sci. USA* **77**, 2168-2172.

62. Cox, D.R., Smith, S.A., Epstein, L.B. & Epstein, C.J. (1984) *Dev. Biol.* **101**, 416-424.
63. Epstein, C.J., Cox, D.R. & Epstein, L.B. (1985) *Ann. NY Acad. Sci.* **450**, 157-168.
64. Cox, D.R. & Epstein, C.J. (1985) *Ann. NY Acad. Sci.* **450**, 169-177.
65. Watson, D.K., McWilliams-Smith, M.J., Kozak, C., Reeves, R., Gearhart, J., Nunn, M.F., Nash, W., Fowle, J.R. III, Duesberg, P., Papas, T.S. & O'Brien, S.J. (1986) *Proc. Natl. Acad. Sci. USA* **83**, 1792-1796.
66. Summitt, R.L. (1981) In: *Trisomy 21 (Down Syndrome): Research Perspectives*, eds. de la Cruz, F.F. & Gerald, P.S. (University Park Press, Baltimore) pp. 225-235.
67. Oster-Granite, M.L., Gearhart, J.D. & Reeves, R.H. (1986) In: *The Neurobiology of Down Syndrome*, ed. Epstein, C.J. (Raven Press, New York) (in press).
68. Coyle, J.T., Gearhart, J.D., Oster-Granite, M.L., Singer, H.S. & Moran, T.H. (1986) In: *The Neurobiology of Down Syndrome*, ed. Epstein, C.J. (Raven Press, New York) (in press).
69. Orozco, C., Epstein, C.J., Smith, S. & Rapoport, S. (1985) *Soc. Neurosci. Abstr.* **11**, 398.
70. Orozco, C.B., Smith, S.A., Latker, C.H., Epstein, C.J. & Rapoport, S. (1986) *Soc. Neurosci. Abstr.* **12**, (in press).

TABLE 1. Similarities between the brains of adults with Down's syndrome and of patients with Alzheimer's disease*

Neuropathology
Similar qualitative and quantitative appearance and geographical distribution of granulovacuolar changes, senile plaques, neurofibrillary tangles, and neuronal loss.

Neurochemistry
Enzymes: decreased choline acetyltransferase and acetylcholinesterase

Monoamines: decreased norepinephrine, dopamine, and serotonin (5-HT)

Similar/identical structure(s) of β_2 protein of cerebrovascular amyloid fibrils and of amyloid plaque core protein

Elevation in concentration of Alz-50 (67K) protein antigen

Cerebral metabolism
Reduction in cerebral glucose metabolism from premorbid levels

*See text for references.

TABLE 2. Genes mapped to human chromosome 21 and their dosage effects*

Regional assignment	*Gene symbol*	*Gene name*	*Ts/2n*†
Confirmed			
q21-q22.1	*CBS*	Cystathionine β-synthase	1.61
q21-qter	*IFNRA*‡	Interferon-α/β receptor	1.57
q22	*ETS2*	Proto-oncogene Ets-2	
q22	*PFKL*	Phosphofructokinase, liver type	1.47
q22.1	*PRGS*	Phosphoribosylglycinamide synthetase	1.56
q22.1	*SOD1*	Superoxide dismutase-1	1.52
q22.3	*BCE1*	Breast cancer, estrogen-inducible gene	
Provisional			
	PAIS	Phosphoribosylaminoimidazole synthetase	
	CRYA1	Crystallin, alpha-A_2 polypeptide	
	MF13	Antigen (glycoprotein, MW 86kd)	
	MF14	Antigen (glycoprotein, MW 145kd)	
	MF17	Leukocyte-cell adhesion molecule (phorbol ester-induced, MW 90kd)	
	S14	Surface antigen	

*From Tables 2 and 3 of ref. 33. † Ratio of activities or concentrations in trisomic (Ts) and diploid (2n) cells. ‡ Formerly IFRC.

TABLE 3. Certain phenotypic features of trisomy 21*

Frequency or amount	*Features*
10- to 18-fold	Increased frequency of leukemia (also leukemoid responses)
3- to 15-fold	Enchanced cellular sensitivity to interferon
5- to 9-fold	Exaggerated fibroblast cAMP response to β-adrenergic agonists
3- to 5-fold	Increased adhesiveness of fetal lung and heart fibroblasts
1.4- to 6-fold	Increased cellular sensitivity to viral transformation
$\leq$2-fold	Increased cellular sensitivity to radiation
0.4-fold	Decreased platelet serotonin
	Altered immune response, particularly of T-lymphocyte system
	Growth retardation
	Decreased neuronal density and synaptogenesis
	Abnormal membrane properties of cultured fetal dorsal root ganglia

* See text and ref. 4 for references.

TABLE 4. Occurrence of Down's syndrome in families of individuals with Alzheimer's disease

Number of probands or families	*Incidence of DS in relatives*	*Degree of relation of DS cases to proband*	*Ref.*
Families identified through single probands:			
125	0.0036 (11/3044)	1°,2°,3° x 9	56
	0.0106 (births after 1950)		
74	0	0/329, 1° only)	58
68	0.0036 (4/1125)	2° × 3; t(15;21)*	57
Large pedigrees with multiple affected individuals:			
3 families with 33 cases of AD	0/203 non-AD 1°-3° relatives in 1 family		59
2 families with 37 cases of AD	1/148 non-AD 1°-3° relatives	2°	60
1 family with 51 cases of AD	0/123 non-AD 1°-3° relatives		44

* Resulting from transmissible (familial) translocation.

TABLE 5. The nervous system in mouse trisomy 16 and in Ts16 ↔ 2n chimeras*

Anatomic
Reduced brain weight (to as little as 32% to 38% that of controls)
Decreased cell proliferation in the ventricular zone with impaired tangential and radial growth of the pallium
Retarded development of cerebellar foliation and hippocampal fissure formation
Retarded development of the basicranium and craniofacial apparatus
Structural alteration of the cochlear and vestibular portions of the inner ear
Neurotransmitter
Decreased catecholaminergic system markers, except for increased DOPA decarboxylase and catechol-O-methyl transferase
Decreased or normal cholinergic system markers
Decreased serotonergic system markers
Normal GABAergic system marker (glutamate decarboxylase)
Behavioral
Increased spontaneous activity in Ts16 ↔ 2n chimeras (65)
Physiological
Altered action potentials and sodium channels in cultured fetal dorsal root ganglion cells (69,70; Orozco *et al.*, submitted)
Neurochemical
Elevated superoxide dismutase-1 activity (1.5 times normal), but normal glutathione peroxidase activity and concentration of lipid peroxides (Anneren and Epstein, submitted)
Transmissible agents
Altered susceptibility of Ts16 ↔ 2n chimeras to scrapie prion (Prusiner *et al.*, unpublished data)

*Taken from ref. 63 except as noted. All studies were carried out on fully trisomic fetuses except as noted.

12. New Technologies for Noninvasive Imaging in Aging and Dementia

THOMAS F. BUDINGER, M.D., Ph.D.

Donner Laboratory and Lawrence Berkeley Laboratory
University of California, Berkeley, CA 94720 and
Department of Radiology University of California, San Francisco

ABSTRACT: Nuclear magnetic resonance (NMR) imaging and spectroscopy has the potential for revealing pathological changes *in vivo* but has not as yet revealed changes in patients with Alzheimer's disease. Both single-photon tomography and positron tomography have shown a pattern of decreased glucose metabolism and flow in the temporoparietal region of Alzheimer's patients. The physical concepts and near-future potentials of NMR and emission techniques are presented, with the conclusion that significant new insights into the etiology of central nervous system aging and dementia can be expected from these new technologies.

Introduction

The quest for noninvasive methods of evaluating dementia has followed the general evolution shown in Figure 1. X-ray computed tomography (CT) studies showed by the late 1970's that brain atrophy and hydrocephalus associated with advanced stages of dementia of all types could be diagnosed easily. However, there was nothing specific in the X-ray CT pattern that would give the diagnosis of Alzheimer's disease (AD) as an entity separate from other dementias such as multiple-infarct dementia (MID).

In the late '70's, tracers specific for brain metabolism and blood flow became available, along with adequate instrumentation for emission tomography. It was not until early 1980 that a particular pattern of metabolic defect was discovered as specific for AD (1-3). We now know that both flow and metabolism are depressed in the temporoparietal region in AD (Fig. 2).

Nuclear magnetic resonance proton imaging developed almost in parallel with emission tomography and perhaps because of the attractiveness of its potential and the visual impact of NMR images (4), interest and use has far surpassed that of emission tomography even though NMR cannot detect the pattern of AD seen readily by both positron emission tomography (PET) (5) and single-photon emission CT (SPECT) (see chapter by Jagust, *et al.*). However, NMR does provide a method for evaluating multiple sclerosis and, of relevance to this book, has revealed a remarkably high prevalence of white-matter lesions in asymptomatic elderly subjects (6,7).

This chapter discusses the fundamentals of NMR and emission tomography (PET and SPECT), with the goal of explaining the techniques, limitations and potentials for studies of dementia and aging of the central nervous system. Jagust, *et al.* review recent results using SPECT to study AD.

Nuclear Magnetic Resonance

The theory of NMR is reviewed in a number of recent sources (8-10). Most chemical elements have at least one reasonably abundant isotope whose nucleus is magnetic. The magnetic nuclei or nuclear spins of high abundance in biological material are ^{1}H, ^{13}C, ^{23}Na, ^{31}P and ^{39}K. The hydrogen nucleus (proton) is especially abundant in the body because of the high water content of nonbony tissues. In an external magnetic field, these nuclear spins behave like small magnets and assume a low-energy state aligned with the field or a higher-energy state aligned against the field. When the body is immersed in a static magnetic field of 0.25 T (2500 gauss), the difference between these aligned populations of about one proton in a million produces a net magnetization. A rapidly alternating magnetic field at an appropriate radiofrequency (RF), applied by a coil near the subject or specimen in the static magnetic field, changes the orientation of the nuclear spins relative to the direction of the strong static magnetic field (Fig. 3). The changes are accompanied by absorption of energy by protons which undergo the transition from a lower energy state to the higher energy state. When the alternating field is turned off, the nuclei return to the equilibrium state with the emission of energy at the same frequency as that of the stimulating alternating field (RF). That frequency is the resonance or Larmor frequency, given by

$$F = (\gamma/2\pi)B \qquad (1)$$

where γ is the characteristic gyromagnetic ratio of the nucleus and B is the static magnetic field. The nuclei of different elements, and even of different isotopes of the same element, have very different resonance frequencies. For a field of 0.1 T (1000 gauss), the resonance frequency of protons is 4.2 MHz and that of phosphorus is 1.7 MHz. Thus, the magnetic nuclei in the body, when placed in a static magnetic field, can be made to act as receivers and transmitters of RF energy.

Relaxation parameters: The physicochemical properties of the tissue and the molecular environment of the nuclei are reflected in the time variation in the amplitude of the RF signal. This variation is a consequence of the interaction of the nuclear spins with a fluctuating magnetic field produced by nearby magnetic moments, including other similar and dissimilar nuclei as well as paramagnetic ions. The imposed RF energy is designed to perturb the thermal equilibrium of the magnetized nuclear spins, and the time dependence of the received signal is determined by the manner in which this system of spins returns to its equilibrium magnetization. The return is characterized by two parameters: T_1, the longitudinal relaxation time, describes the behavior of the component of the magnetization vector parallel to the applied static field B_0; and T_2, the transverse relaxation time, describes the behavior of the component of the magnetization vector transverse to B_0 (Fig. 3). Each component "relaxes" to its equilibrium value; the first is precisely the equilibrium magnetization, which is along B_0, and the second is zero at equilibrium. One can think of T_2 as a time for the nuclear spins to lose coherence (dephase) (Fig. 3).

The T_2 and T_1 values of pure water are about 2 seconds at 25° C and are nearly independent of B_0 for the field strengths considered here. Addition of solutes such as proteins shortens these times considerably to an extent that is a function of B_0. This has been investigated extensively for solutions of diamagnetic proteins and for proteins containing paramagnetic ions. The results and insights gained by studying solutions of known composition can be transferred readily to investigations of the relaxation times of tissue, including the effects of paramagnetic ions (11).

To the extent that T_1 and T_2 are tissue specific, these differences can be exploited to delineate different tissues in NMR images. The dependence of the image contrast on these differences and the ability to bring out the differences by tailoring the timing and energy of RF pulses are shown by Figures 4 and 5. One of the early discoveries of NMR imaging was the ability to detect the plaques of multiple sclerosis. The T_2 of these plaques is longer than that of white matter; thus by using a particular NMR pulsing technique, one can create an image with more signal from the long T_2 regions than the signal from the shorter T_2 regions (Fig. 6). The reasons for the differences in relaxation behavior of different tissues are not yet known, but it is known that the variation in water content, although it can affect relaxation, is not sufficient to explain all the differences observed. Among the fundamental factors influencing the differences will be the distribution of protein size in any tissue as well as the presence of fixed surfaces and interfaces (membranes, cytoskeletons and so on) with which tissue water can interact.

Relaxation times can be measured at each point of an image. Because differences in tissue relaxation times determine image contrast, data on the relaxation behavior of different tissues as a function of static field strength B_0 are important in the selection of the optimal field strength and RF pulse sequence (for instance, spin-echo or inversion recovery) for acquisition of NMR images.

For spin-echo imaging, a commonly used imaging technique, the signal amplitude is given by

$$S \simeq Nf(v)(e^{-TE/T_2})\,(1 - e^{-TR/T_1}) \qquad (2)$$

where N is the concentration of nuclei (local spin density), f(v) is the signal modulation due to moving nuclei (blood flow), TE is the elapsed time between the 90° RF pulse and the reception of a spin-echo signal; and TR is the repetition rate between successive spin-echo sequences. In accord with Eq. (2), we note that a decrease in T_1 or an increase in T_2 results in an increase in the NMR signal. Fat has a shorter T_1 and a longer T_2 than other soft tissues; thus the NMR signals from fat produce the strongest signals in proton imaging. Cerebrospinal fluid has a long T_1 and a long T_2; thus, with long TR we can overcome the loss of signal due to long T_1, and with long TE (*e.g.*, "second echo" of Fig. 4) we obtain a relatively high signal from the cerebrospinal fluid.

The T_2 of the brain gray matter is higher than that of white matter. Thus if we acquire data using different TE's (times between the stimulating RF pulse and the echo signal from another stimulation pulse) we see from Eq. (2) that the tissues with short T_2 will give less and less signal as the TE is increased. The rate of decline in signal is less for tissue of relatively larger T_2. A general ranking of T_2's is given in Table 1. Tumors and abscesses with T_1's and T_2's longer than those of the normal tissues can be demonstrated with good contrast by choosing a pulse sequence which takes the best advantages of the differences between the relaxation parameters of the diseased tissue and those of the normal tissue.

The inversion-recovery NMR RF-pulse method is frequently used when differences in T_1 are being imaged. For inversion recovery, high contrast is accomplished by first inverting the magnetization with a 180° pulse and then allowing the magnetization to recover toward equilibrium for a time interval (TI) before applying a 90° RF pulse. Only the absolute value of the signal, which is positive whether the magnetization is along or against B_0, is usually detected. The contrast differences will depend on the T_1 differences and the TI chosen for imaging.

The ability to quantify relaxation rates accurately *in vivo* is important for understanding and optimizing image contrast. Pure T_1 and pure T_2

images can be computed from data acquired with more than one RF pulse sequence (14), and these representations can be combined to reconstitute computed images which retrospectively optimize the contrast between normal and abnormal tissues. Unfortunately, measurement of T_1 and T_2 are subject to large errors from blood-flow artifacts, patient motion, RF field inhomogeneity, RF pulse sequence effects, variation in tip angle and the multiexponential relaxation behavior of many tissues. Thus, the conditions for accurate measurements of relaxation times will not in general be satisfied throughout the volume of the slice.

Another contrast mechanism is flow (Fig. 7). The concentration of excited spins in a region selected for imaging will change because of the movement of spins out of the region and the movement of unsaturated spins into the region of selection. In addition, there are phase changes within the image elements which can cause a decrease in signal and, for some pulse sequences (*e.g.*, multiple echo), can result in an increase or return of signal (Fig. 7).

Imaging strategies: The frequency of the NMR signal is proportional to the magnetic field strength. Thus, if the field is varied across an object, the signal frequency will depend on the position of the transmitting nuclei in the object. The strength of the signal at each frequency can be interpreted as the nuclear magnetization in a plane within the object where the magnetic field corresponds to that frequency:

$$F(x) = \gamma/2\pi\,(B_0 + \Delta B/\Delta x \cdot x) \qquad (3)$$

In order to obtain spatial information, some early systems employed a-c magnetic gradients to define "sensitive lines" or "sensitive points," which were translated electronically or mechanically through the image space to obtain the corresponding information. These early methods have been supplanted by other methods made practical by recent advances in digital electronics and computer hardware.

Combinations of gradients in different directions can be used to select points, lines or planes within the body. Selection of planes, or "slices," such as the transverse section of Figure 5, is most commonly used in imaging strategies. These sections can be oriented in any direction, in contrast to the usual transaxial slice orientation of x-ray CT. By application of a gradient during the application of a narrow RF band, the protons are excited in a plane whose position and thickness depend on the RF pulse shape. Once the plane has been selected, for example, by a z gradient, then x and y gradients are employed to determine the location within the selected x-y plane of the spin density and relaxation parameters. In the well-known projection method, the NMR signal is encoded by using magnetic field gradients applied in different directions, so that the NMR spectrum corresponds directly to spatial projections. If broadband pulses are used to excite the system in the presence of a linear gradient, the Fourier transform of the received signal is equal to the projection of the signals from all nuclei within the planes perpendicular to the line. Two-and three-dimensional images are created using algorithms somewhat similar to those used for x-ray CT. Since all of the nuclei in the tissue volume (or plane, in the two-dimensional case) being imaged are excited during each pulse, this technique is capable of achieving the highest signal-to-noise ratio possible for a given resolution per unit acquisition time. Because time must be allowed for the spins to relax at least partially after each pulse, there are limits to the minimum performance time required to produce an image.

Another class of methods, known as two-dimensional Fourier transform or spinwarp or echo planar, use gradients of varying magnitude to phase-encode the detected signals and thereby provide spatial information after multiple Fourier transformation of the encoded signals. Echo planar imaging offers faster image acquisition than other techniques and has been used to produce images of the beating heart. This technique employs multiple spin echoes produced in oscillating gradients during the single transient signal known as the free induction decay (FID) following one pulse.

NMR spectroscopy and chemical shift spectroscopy: We have seen that the frequency of the NMR signal is proportional to the field in accord with the basic Larmor theorem given in Eq. (3). This fact was used to acquire spatial imaging data because imposed small changes, $\Delta B/\Delta x$, in fields have corresponding frequency changes, and these frequencies are directly related to the spatial position of the field. Another change in frequency of the signal from a specimen in a particular B_0 field is due to the small reduction in field near various nuclei from electronic shielding. Electrons encircling a nucleus and electrons involved in chemical bonding will give different amounts of shielding to nuclei, depending on the position in the molecule of the nuclei. In accord with the basic Larmor equation, there will be corresponding frequencies for each shielded nuclear species.

The small differences in NMR frequencies from the various molecular groups are called chemical shifts, and their separations are proportional to the strength of the applied magnetic field. These electrons very slightly shield the nuclei from the applied magnetic field. For example, the protons surrounding each of the three carbon atoms of alcohol experience a slightly different field by a few parts per million. That is, the electron distribution in the CH_3 group is different from that in the CH_2 or OH groups. Consequently, the protons in the various chemical groups experience slightly different field values and respond at slightly different NMR frequencies.

The NMR signal following a 90° NMR pulse consists of three superimposed frequencies which the computer of the NMR spectrometer sorts out by Fourier transformation to give the spectrum of three discrete lines (Fig. 8). The relative intensities of the three spectral lines are 3, 2, 1 which gives us a good clue where they come from. The line of intensity 3 comes from the three protons in the methyl (CH_3) groups, the line of intensity 2 comes from the two protons in the methylene (CH_2) groups and the line of intensity 1 comes from the single protons in the hydroxyl (OH) groups. Thus the protons do not all have exactly the same NMR frequency but differ by a few parts per million. These three lines from ethyl alcohol provide an example of a simple NMR spectrum. The spectrum can be used to identify chemicals and ascertain abundance if adequate standards are used.

Next, suppose we put a human body in a magnetic field and apply a resonant NMR pulse (Fig. 8). The proton NMR response usually observed is two frequencies corresponding to water and fat, separated by about three parts per million. The electronic environment of the protons in water molecules is different from that in the methylene groups in the fat. The stronger response usually comes from the water, since there is more water in most tissues. At the higher resolution usually provided by a higher field, additional resonant frequencies corresponding to protons on different atoms of molecules such as lactate, Nacetylaspartate and creatine can be identified.

These chemical shift effects are found with all nuclei, not just with protons. Moreover, the effects are larger with other nuclei. The hydrogen atom has only one electron, but, for example, phosphorus atoms have 15 electrons, and their chemical shifts are an order of magnitude larger. The phosphorus spectrum is the most popular because spectral peaks associated with energy metabolism are readily identified.

Spatial resolution of spectroscopy: The potential of NMR for revealing chemical composition is hampered by its inherent insensitivity. Because protons are abundant in tissue, the sensitivity problem is not too great for conventional magnetic resonance imaging nor for creating images of predominantly fat protons and images of predominantly water protons (Fig. 9). But, as shown in Table 2, the abundance and NMR sensitivity of other nuclei are orders of magnitude less than for protons. Thus, measurement of spectral peak abundance in small tissue volumes is not practical at fields commonly used. The approach is to obtain spectra from selected regions within the body or organ of interest using either a surface coil which has a selective response over the area of the coil and to a depth of about the coil radius, or, by using a series of imposed magnetic field gradients, to stimulate nuclei from only specific regions, usually 30 cc or greater. Selected-region spectroscopy has not been used as yet for *in vivo* studies in dementia, but limited studies have been reported on tissue samples (12).

Emission Tomography

As with x-ray CT, energetic photons are detected as part of the tomographic procedure. The basic physical difference between x-ray tomographic imaging and emission tomographic imaging is that in the latter the information sought is the source and intensity of the gamma radiation emitted by the isotope, whereas in x-ray transmission tomography, the measurements reflect the tissue densities or physical attenuation coefficients. In this respect, NMR is somewhat similar to x-ray CT in that NMR proton imaging shows the anatomy of different tissue properties. Additionally, NMR *in vivo* spectroscopy can provide information about the chemical constituents of tissues in selected regions of about 30-cc volumes. However, NMR cannot show tissue blood flow; metabolism of amino acids, sugars and fats or the concentration of receptor molecules in the central nervous system. In that the measurements in emission reflect tissue flow, permeability, metabolism and receptor density, both PET and SPECT studies have a unique role in studies of dementia.

Positron emission tomography has become a major tool for the study of mental disorders in the last few years. The position of a positron-emitting radionuclide can be determined because the two photons produced upon the annihilation of the positive electron (positron) with a negative electron are emitted 180° from one another (Fig. 10). Therefore, by positioning detectors around a patient, it is possible to determine the line along which a disintegration occurred. The availability of physiologically interesting positron-emitting radiopharmaceuticals and of suitable instrumentation, as well as the development of algorithms for CT image reconstruction, provided the impetus for PET advancement over the last 10 years. Single-photon emission tomography involves the detection of gamma photons released from certain radionuclides during radioactive decay. As the back-to-back emission seen in PET is not available, a mechanical focusing system known as a collimator is necessary to determine the path along which the radionuclide photon arose.

The earliest clinical use of emission transverse-section tomography was the work of Kuhl and Edwards in the early 1960's (13). This procedure involved single-photon emitters as distinct from positron emitters and for the past 10 years has been dormant due to the unavailability of appropriate isotopes and instruments (14). This section discusses the principal physical attributes of both PET and SPECT.

An advantage of PET over SPECT is its much greater sensitivity in detecting radiopharmaceuticals, because in the single-photon technique, physical collimation results in the loss of many available photons. The ability to label compounds with positronemitting isotopes of carbon, nitrogen, oxygen and fluorine is the basis for the biochemical potentials of PET. To produce radiopharmaceuticals containing these radionuclides, it is necessary to have a cyclotron or, for some positron emitters, a portable generator. By contrast, single-photon emitters, for instance, ^{99m}Tc and ^{123}I, can be obtained from noncyclotron or remote sources, and they are easier to work with because of their longer half-lives. Thus, as discussed in Jagust *et al.*, SPECT has a practical and clinically efficacious role in the detection and characterization of mental disorders.

The first positron imaging system was developed by Massachusetts General Hospital in 1953 and the first positron camera in 1954. For 25 years, instrument development rested in the hands of only a few universities in the United States and Japan. Now, there is increasing interest mainly because of the sensitivity of emission tomography in differentiating disorders or physiological processes, and PET instrumentation is available from commercial sources. All commercial systems have the same general characteristics. They have rings of bismuth germanate ($Bi_4Ge_3O_{12}$) detectors individually coupled or coded to photomultiplier tubes. Employment of cross-coincidences between rings results in more image levels than the number of individual rings of crystals; thus a four-ring system can give data for seven planes.

Recent trends in positron instrumentation have been in two directions: toward high resolution and toward the use of time-of-flight to improve image statistics. High resolution is achieved by using many thin detectors in a ring configuration. Since photoelectron tubes have relatively large dimensions, various coding schemes have been proposed to identify the individual detectors.

The sensitivity of PET and SPECT systems: The sensitivity of these systems is usually given in terms of the number of events per second for a phantom 20 cm in diameter uniformly filled with a water solution containing 1 μCi of a positron emitter per cubic centimeter; it is denoted here by S^{-1}. This unit is convenient for expressing sensitivity, particularly for brain imaging devices.

For PET, sensitivity ranges from 1×10^4 to 5×10^5 S^{-1}. For SPECT, the sensitivity is $<1 \times 10^4$ and, as shown in Figure 11, the sensitivity varies with the same factors as with PET but decreases as the square of the resolution decreases.

As shown in Figure 12, the overall disadvantage in sensitivity of SPECT *vs.* PET is a factor of 15 for 10-mm resolution and 30 for 5-mm resolution. These factors are less than is generally believed because frequently expectations were based on comparisons between a solid ring of detectors in PET and a single gamma camera in SPECT. Systems designed especially for SPECT (Fig. 13) can incorporate as much as four times more detector surface than is associated with a single camera. In addition, the use of focusing collimators with SPECT might improve sensitivity further.

Spatial imaging resolution: Many factors limit the practical resolution of emission imaging systems. For SPECT, the limit is the sensitivity, because improvement in resolution requires finer collimation with a commensurate loss in sensitivity. However, for positron systems, if we merely improve resolution in two dimensions (*e.g.*, in plane resolution), the sensitivity will not decrease. Figures 11 and 12 refer to resolution in three dimensions. For positron systems, the most important factors affecting resolution limits are the distance the positron travels through tissues before annihilation, the angular deviation of ±0.25° from 180° for the two photons emitted on annihilation and the finite detector dimensions. Depending on the radionuclides and the PET detector-ring dimensions, the first two factors set a limit of a few millimeters on the resolution, defined as full width at half-maximum (FWHM), which is the smallest separation at which two signal sources can be placed and still be detected.

The major deterrent to improved resolution is the construction of efficient detectors with adequate time and energy resolution for PET. Improvement in scintillation detectors involves development of a detector with the high efficiency of bismuth germanate but increased speed and the light output. Fast detectors are needed to faciliate separation of true coincident events from false coincidences, which occur at high data rates, and better light output improves detection reliability.

As the three-dimensional resolution requirements ultimately affect the sensitivity of both SPECT and PET, the statistical uncertainty in reconstruction resulting from the finite number of detected events is the principal factor limiting the resolution of positron tomographs (Fig. 14). Most current instruments produce images with a resolution of 10-to 20-mm FWHM. Resolutions to 5 mm are claimed for commercial instruments. The best resolution is the Donner 600-crystal system, which has a resolution of 2.3 mm (15).

The limit for improving sampling resolution does not rest solely on sensitivity and statistical certainty questions. No matter how good the statistics, a poor resolution relative to the size of objects being measured will lead to significant errors in the observed concentration (15). The problem of relatively low resolution is that image data are spread over areas larger than the actual region from which the data originated (Fig.

15). Good-resolution systems will confine data into a smaller number of picture elements than a poor-resolution system. This will lead to an effective improvement in statistical uncertainty, because the uncertainty is dependent on the area occupied by the data as well as on the total number of data points collected (Fig. 14). A third argument for improving resolution is one analogous to that for improving the resolution of any imaging system. Detection is dependent on contrast, but low resolution blurs the signal; thus, the contrast is lowered, and at some level of blurring (resolution relative to the size of the object being detected), the signal is lowered to a value near that of the surrounding background.

Attenuation, scattering, variable resolution and sampling: It is important to recognize that attenuation of the emitted photons by the material they pass through is a problem for which both PET and SPECT must compensate. Scattered radiation, part of the attenuation process, results in erroneous photon trajectories for both techniques as well. Variable resolution throughout the image region is not as great a problem for PET as it is for SPECT except for the moving focused collimator design. Another physical attribute of emission tomography is the requirement for adequate angular and linear sampling. In both PET and SPECT, the number of detector channels should be two times greater than the number of resolution elements across the image. Of greater importance, fine sampling leads to an accurate description of the true concentration. These observations are particularly relevant when considering the prospects of imaging activity in the basal nuclei, substantia nigra, locus cereleus, etc. It is this potential for noninvasive *in vivo* metabolism studies of central nervous system structures <5 mm in dimension which leads to the conclusion that increased resolution of PET systems is a requirement for future studies whereas lower-resolution instruments of practical availability are the realm for SPECT.

Summary

Whereas NMR has not revealed a pattern diagnostic for AD, it has demonstrated detection sensitivity for the white-matter lesions associated with dementia and for unique multiple sclerosis plaques. However, the potentials of NMR imaging and selective-region spectroscopy have not yet been fully explored. Selective-region proton, phosphorus and carbon spectroscopy have great potential but will probably require fields >2 T and even as high as 10 T for tissue composition identification because of the expected signal-to-noise increases with the field and the improved line separation.

Emission tomography has had recent achievements in Alzheimer's studies, and the prospects for the near future in the study of AD include investigation of the role of brain nuclei in the etiology of this disease, the possibility of abnormal protein interactions as causative and the evaluation of brain metabolism in response to various proposed therapies. The possibility for development of new tracers and expected improvements in instrument resolution make this approach attractive for *in vivo* studies and critical experiments on the etiology of AD.

Acknowledgments

This work was supported in part by the Director, Office of Energy Research, Office of Basic Energy Sciences, Biology and Medicine Division of the U.S. Department of Energy under Contract No. DE-AC03-76SF00098 and also by the National Institute of Health, National Heart, Lung, and Blood Institute under Grant No. PO1 HL25840.

References

1. Benson, D.F., Kuhl, D.E., Hawkins, R.A., Phelps, M.E., Cummings, J.L. & Tsai, S.Y. (1983) *Arch. Neurol.* **40**, 711-714.
2. Friedland, R.P., Budinger, T.F., Ganz, E. *et al.* (1983) *J. Comp. Assist. Tomogr.* **7**, 590-598.
3. Chase, T.N., Foster, N.L., Fedio, P., Brooks, R., Mansi, L. and DiChiro, G. (1984) *Ann. Neurol.* **15 (suppl)**, S170-S174.
4. Bottomley, P.A., Hart, H.R., Edelstein, W.A. *et al.* (1984) *Radiology* **150**, 441-446.
5. Friedland, R.P., Budinger, T.F., Brant-Zawadski, M. & Jagust, W. (1984) *JAMA* **252**, 2750-2752.
6. Bradley, W.G., Walch, V., Brant-Zawadzki, M. *et al.* (1984) *Noninvas. Med. Imaging* **1**, 35-41.
7. Brant-Zawadzki, M., Fein, G., Van Dyke, C., Kiernan, R., Davenport, L. & DeGroot, J. (1985) *AJNR* **6**, 675-682.
8. Budinger, T.F. & Lauterbur, P.C. (1984) *Science* **226**, 288-298.
9. James, T.L. (1984) *Biomed. Mag. Reson.* **2**, 7-22.
10. Maudsley, A. Physics. Medical magnetic resonance imaging & spectroscopy. In: *Proc. Soc. Mag. Res. Med.* Fifth Annual Meeting, Montreal, Canada, 17-22 Aug. 1986 (in press).
11. Koenig, S.H., Brown, R.D. III, Adams, D., Emerson, D. & Harrison, C.G. (1984) *Invest. Radiol.* **19**, 76, and Koenig, S.H. & Brown, R.D. III *Mag. Res. Med.* (in press).
12. Barany, M., Chang, Y.C., Arus, C., Rustan, T. & Frey, W.H. (1985) *Lancet* **1**, 517.

13. Kuhl, D. & Edward, R.O. (1963) *Radiology* **80**, 653-662.
14. Budinger, T.F. (1981) *J. Nucl. Med.* **22**, 1094-1097.
15. Derenzo, S.E., Huesman, R.H., Vuletich, T.W., Cahoon, J.L., Geyer, A. & Budinger T.F. High resolution 600-crystal dynamic PET tomograph. IEEE NS (in press).
16. Budinger, T.F., Derenzo, D.E. & Huesman, R.H. (1984) *Ann. Neurol.* **15 (suppl)**, S35-S43.

TABLE 1. Typical NMR signal intensities in T_2-weighted imaging, decreasing top to bottom*

Fat
Marrow
Gray matter
White matter
Liver, spleen, pancreas
Muscle, kidney
Ligaments, tendons
Blood vessels with rapid flow
Compact bone
Air

*Depends on tissue hydration, T_1, and TR of pulse sequence as per equation (2) on page 178.

TABLE 2. Nuclei usable for *in vivo* spectroscopic studies

Element	Relative sensitivity at constant field for equal numbers of nuclei	Tissue concentration (molar)	Relative detection sensitivity
^{1}H	1.0	90*	1.0
^{19}F	0.83	2.6†	2.4×10^{-2}
^{23}Na	0.09	0.14‡	1.4×10^{-4}
^{31}P	0.07	0.008§	6.2×10^{-6}
^{13}C (storage lipid)	0.016	0.45‖	8.0×10^{-5}
^{13}C (endogenous lactate)	0.016	0.00005¶	8.9×10^{-9}**

*Hydrogen from 80 percent water in tissues. †Blood concentration after injection of 500 ml of fluorocarbon. ‡Blood and extracellular fluid. §Concentration of tissue phosphorus associated with ATP or creatine phosphate. ‖Assuming 7.3 mg of ^{13}C per gram of adipose fat tissue at the natural abundance of 1.1 percent ^{13}C. ¶Natural abundance of ^{13}C for a lactate concentration of 5 m*M*. (^{13}C-methyl is 0.05 m*M*). **Theoretically, 60 times greater relative sensitivity can be achieved by spin-spin heteronuclear double-resonance techniques. Presently achieved threshold for detection of enriched ^{13}C-lactate in vivo is 0.5 m*M* per minute (*46*). Proton spectroscopy using homonuclear double-resonance techniques or spin-echo methods is capable of detecting endogenous lactate at normal and pathological concentrations.

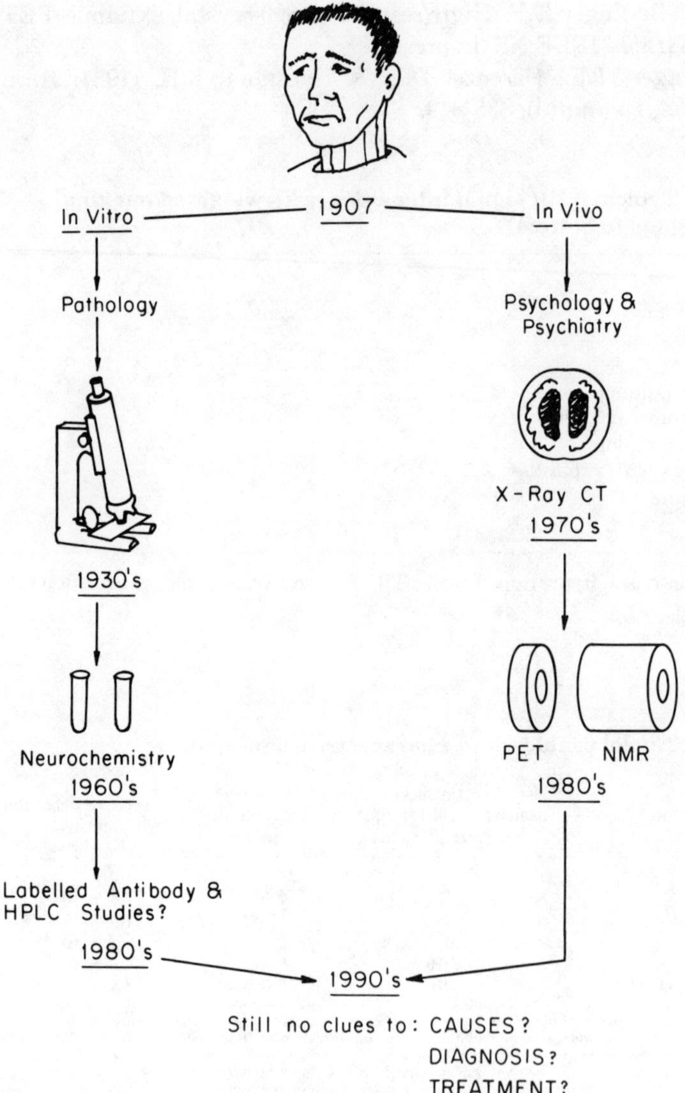

Fig. 1. Scientific inquiries regarding AD can be considered in the two categories of *in vitro* and *in vivo* investigations. The *in vivo* studies of emission tomography and NMR studies are the subject of this chapter.

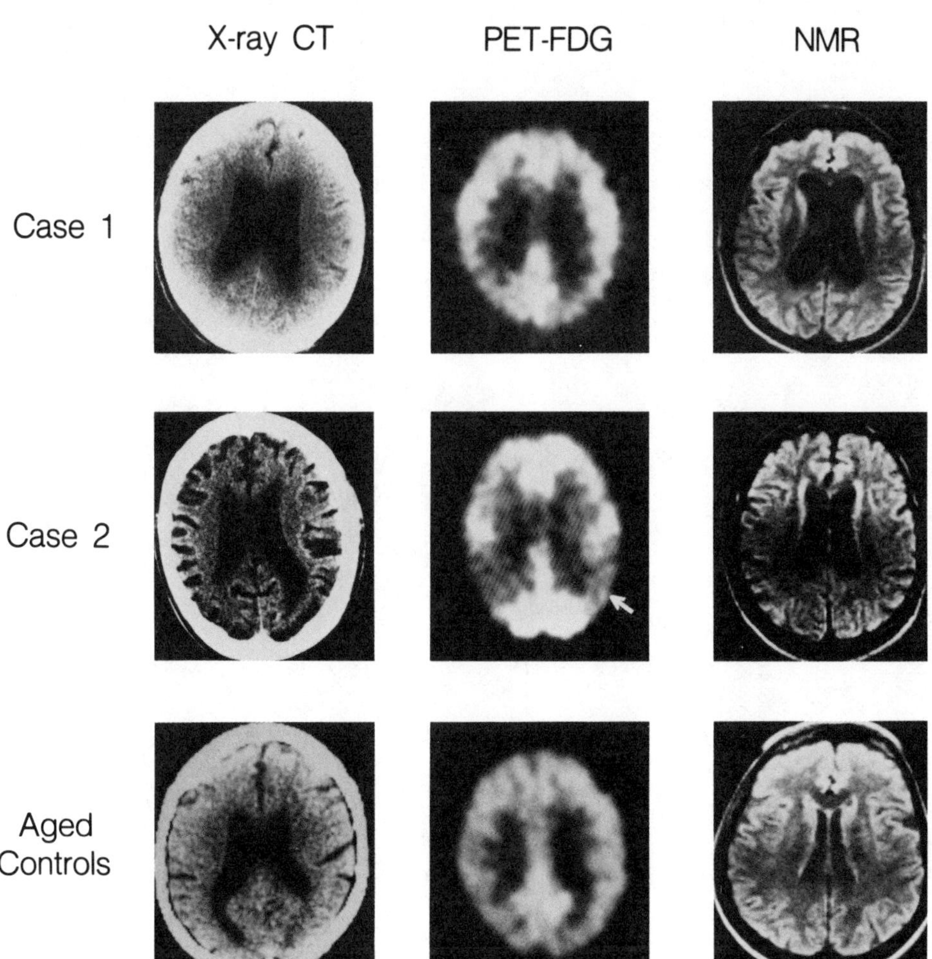

Fig. 2. CT (left), PET (middle), and NMR spin-echo images (right) in cases 1 (top) and 2 (middle) and healthy, aged controls (bottom). The CT and PET studies on the bottom row were performed on healthy 63-year-old control subject; the NMR image is from different healthy 82-year-old subject. In all images, subject's left is on viewer's right. The CT images are not contrast enhanced. The PET images are of 2-[^{18}F]-2-deoxy-D-glucose (FDG) accumulation, and NMR images are of spin-echo images, second echo (TE 56 ms). Arrow indicates location of right temporoparietal cortex.

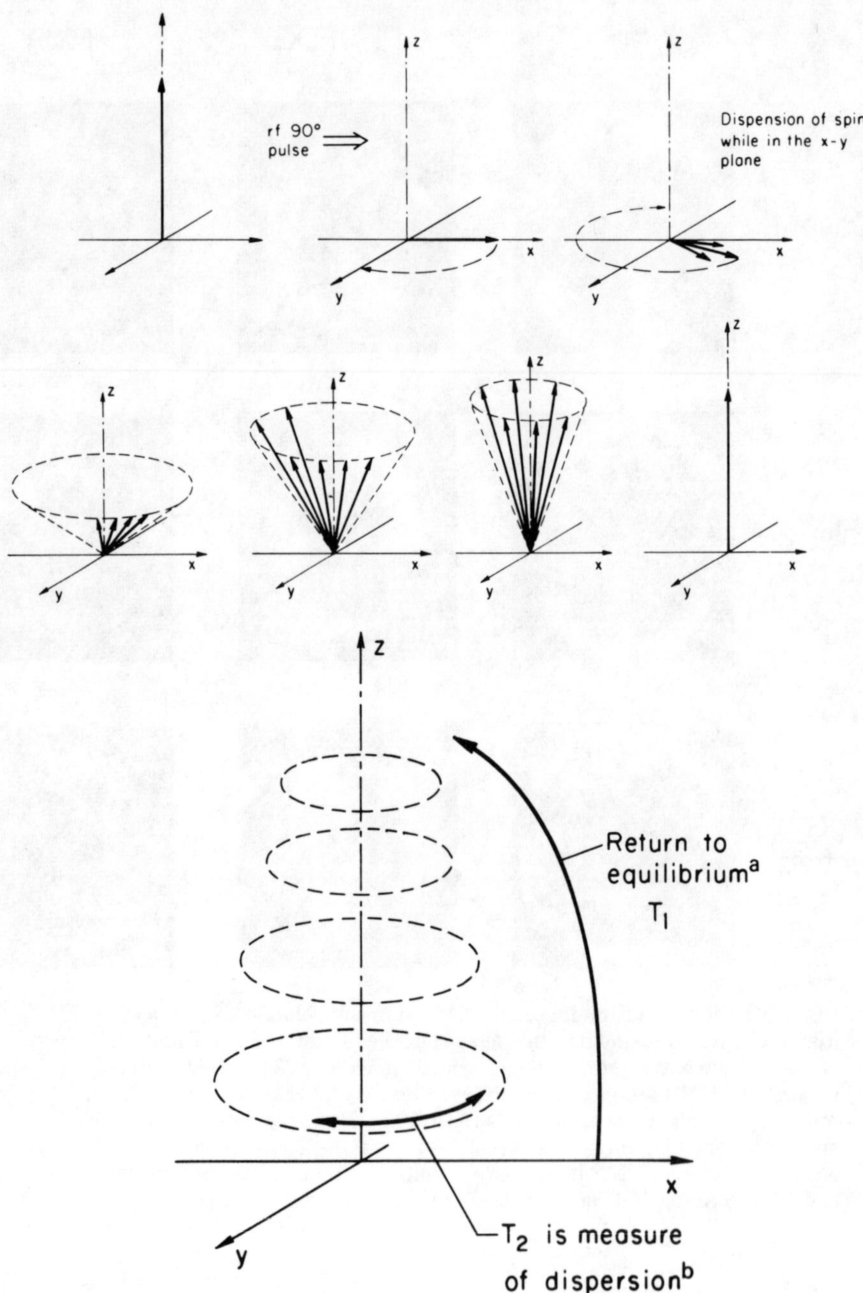

Fig. 3. Upper diagram (left to right): the tipping of the net magnetization vector by a radiofrequency pulse, the dispersion of spins (T_2) and recovery to equilibrium (T_1) after the RF pulse is switched off.

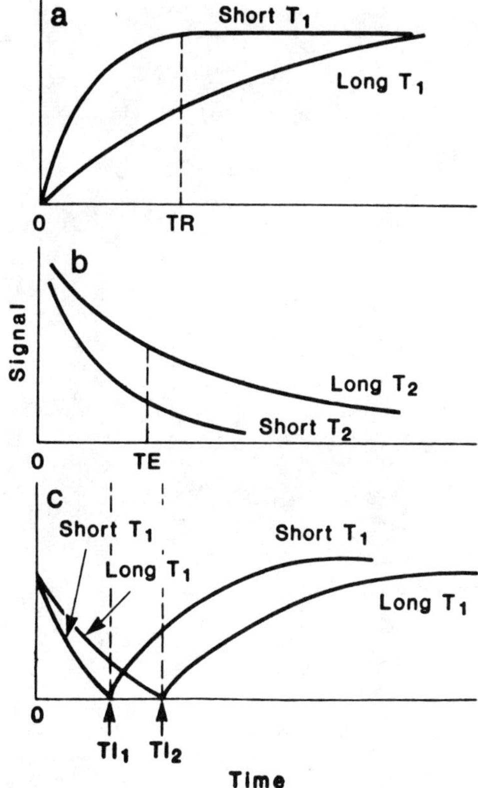

Fig. 4. The NMR proton-image contrast between normal and pathological tissue depends on differences in T_1 and T_2 relaxation times and, to a lesser extent, on differences in spin density. Optimal contrast is dependent on the particular pulse sequence timing. A. For spin-echo imaging, the interval between pulses TR will dictate the contrast between tissues with different T_1's. B. Spin-echo timing TE will control the contrast between tissues with different T_2's. C. Inversion recovery sequences are useful for demonstration of T_1 differences. The direction of the difference depends on the difference in T_1's as well as on the time interval T_1 between the 180° and 90° RF pulses. For example, changing the interval between TI_1 and TI_2 would reverse the contrast for tissues with the T_1's shown in C.

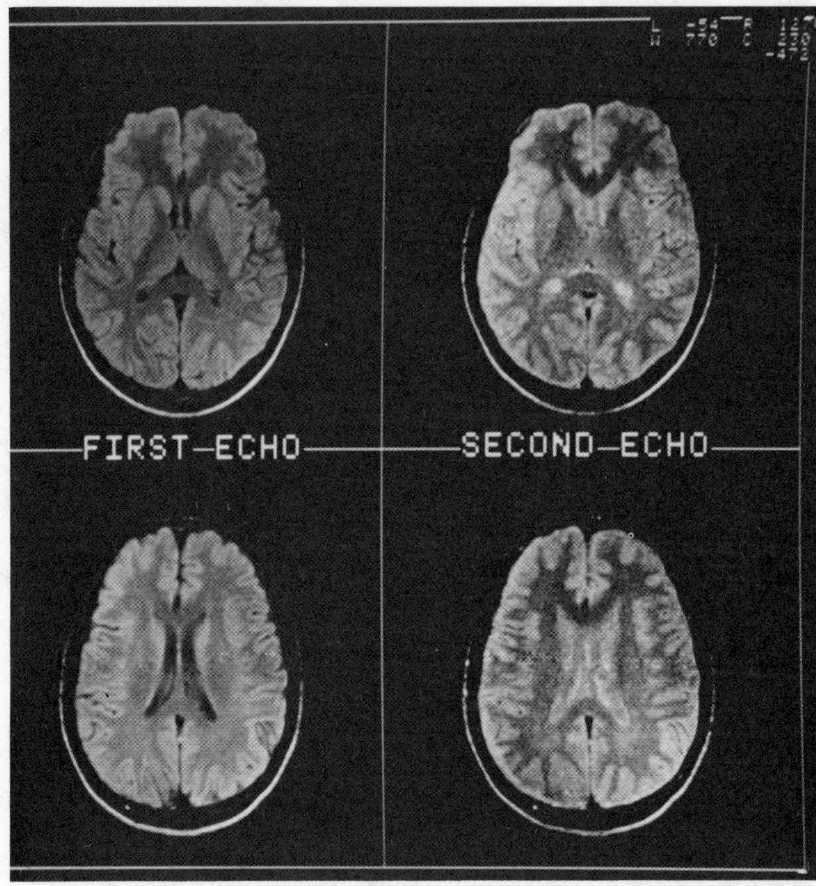

Fig. 5. Spin-echo RF pulses provide a means of obtaining image contrast when there is a variation of either T_1 or T_2 between tissues. A short period between stimulating pulses and a long time for the echo pulse will encance T_2 differences. In this series of two contiguous brain levels of 5-mm thickness, a TR of 1.5 sec was used with the first echo of 60 msec and the second echo for 120 msec. The principal difference between the images on the left and those on the right is the appearance of a bright signal from the cerebrospinal fluid.

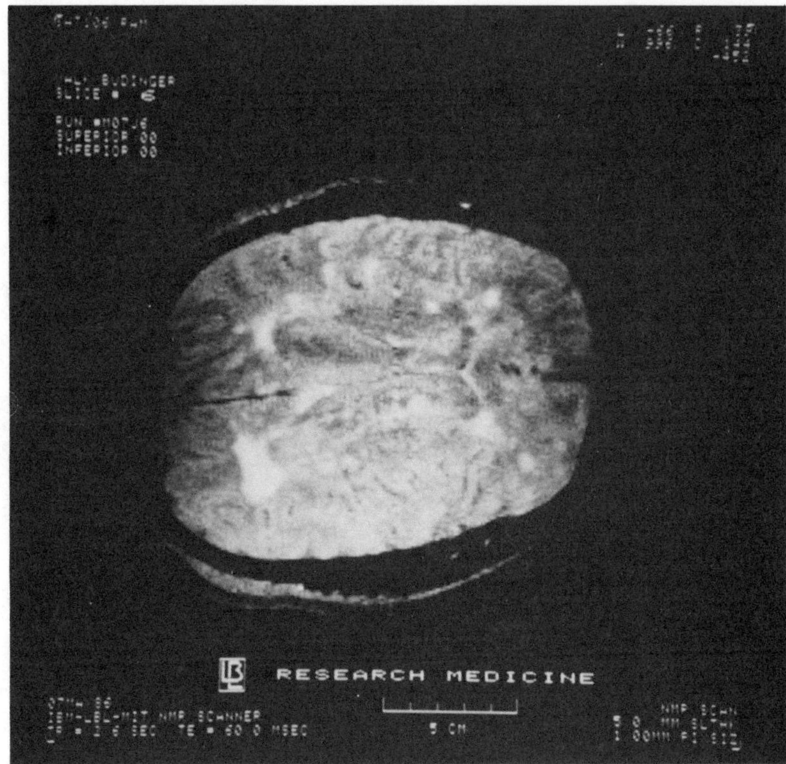

Fig. 6. Spin-echo NMR study in multiple sclerosis. The plaques have a high signal because T_2 value is higher than that of surrounding normal brain. Ventricles do not show dark contrast because the TR and TE of the pulse sequence was not optimized to give contrast between brain tissue and ventricular fluid.

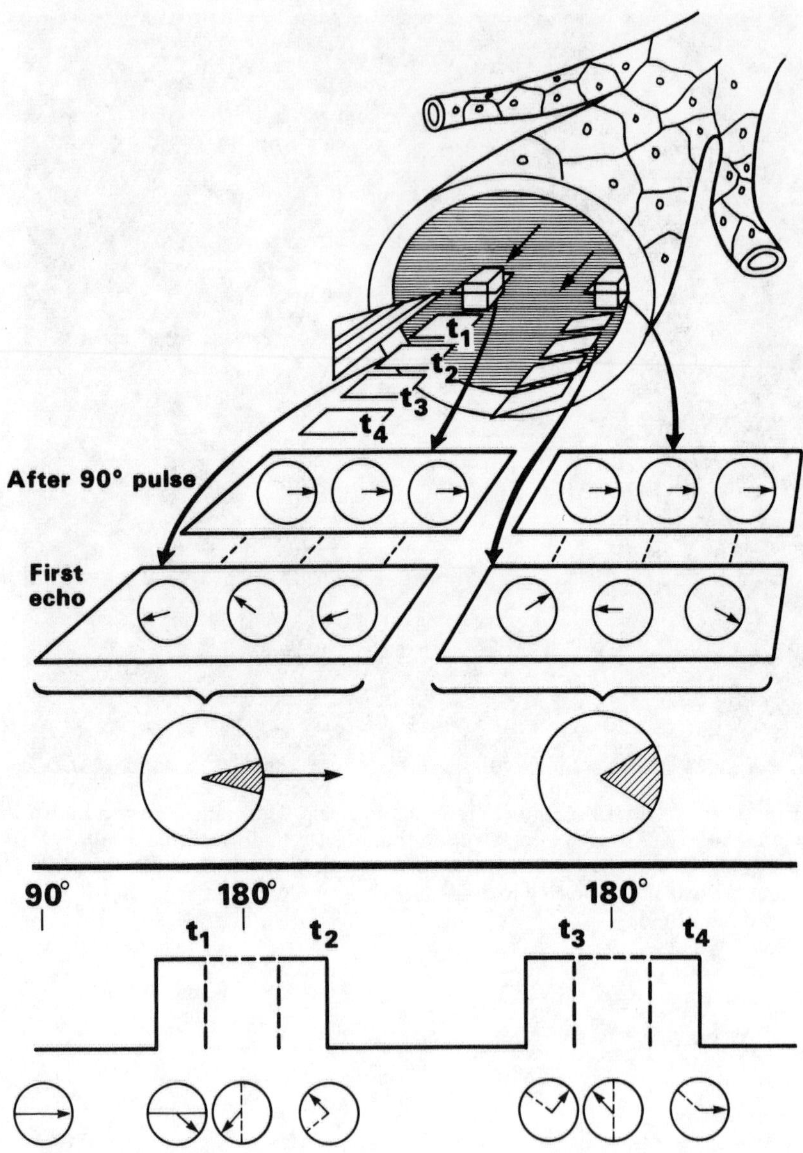

Fig. 7. Movement of excited spins (protons) out of the region being imaged results in a decreased signal and definition of vascular spaces. Other effects are explained by the demonstration of the mixture of spin phases within regions of a vessel and the evolution of the transverse magnetization for the first and second echos of a spin-echo pulse sequence.

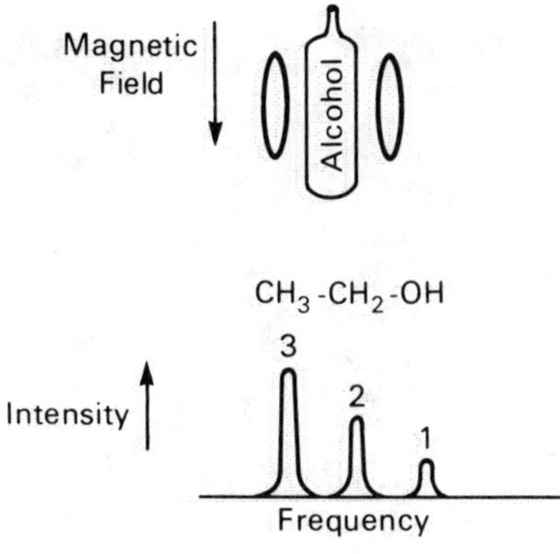

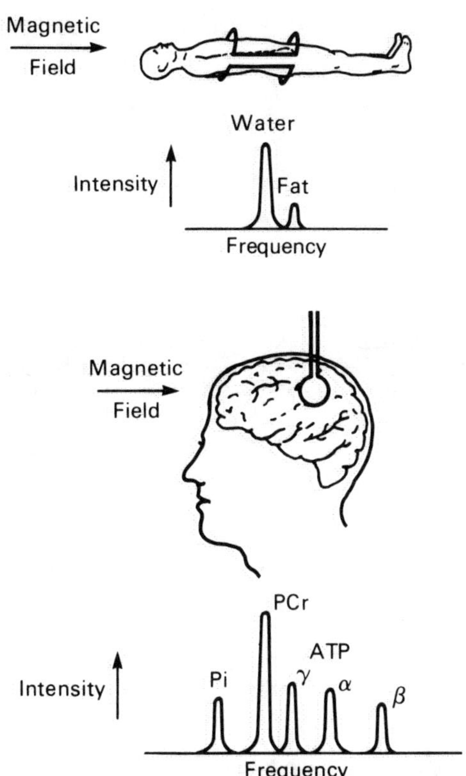

Fig. 8. NMR spectroscopy relies on the slightly different resonant frequencies of nuclei due to the chemical environment. From top to bottom: the expected proton spectra of alcohol, fat and phosphorus from muscle.

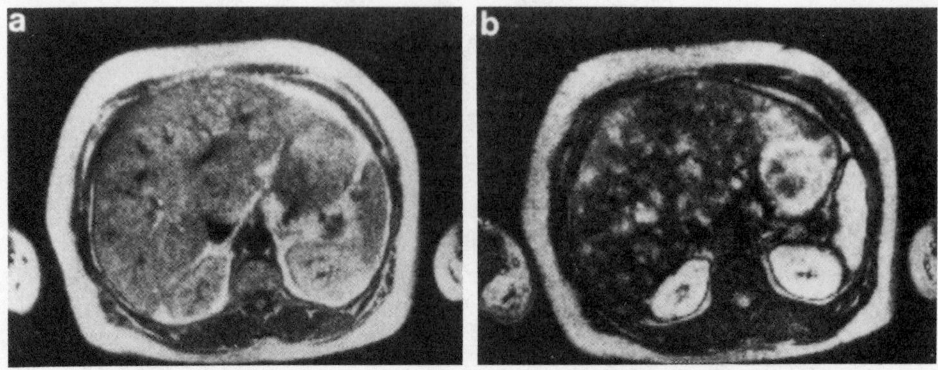

Fig. 9. Proton NMR images obtained with a spin-echo pulse sequence (40-msec TE, 1.5-sec TR). A. Conventional spin-echo sequence. B. Spin-echo sequence modified so that lipid spins are 180° out of phase with water spins. Courtesy of W.T. Dixon, Washington University.

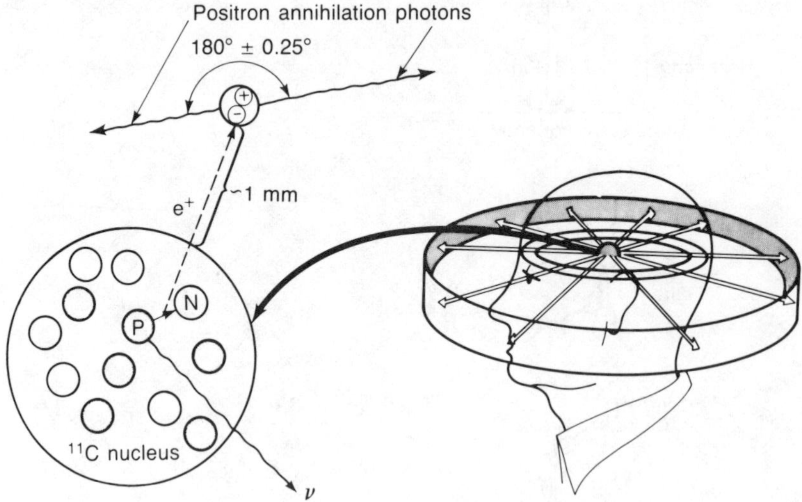

Fig. 10. The positron encounters an electron within millimeters of the nucleus. The combination of these two particles (antimatter and matter) results in annihilation with the emission of two gamma photons, each with 511 keV of energy, 180° from each other. Positron decay is involved in nuclei that have fewer photons than neutrons. When a nuclear proton becomes a neutron, the positron is ejected.

SENSITIVITY

$$S_{Tc-99m} \propto \frac{(detectors)(resolution)^2(packing)(efficiency)(atten(\gamma))}{4\pi R_1^2}$$

$$S_{\beta+} \propto \frac{(2\pi R_2)(resolution)(packing)(efficiency)^2(atten(\beta^+))}{4\pi R_2^2}$$

Radius of detector array:

$$R_1 = 200mm$$
$$R_2 = 300mm$$

Attenuation:

$$Tc - 99m \sim e^{-\mu d/2}$$
$$\beta^+ \sim e^{-\mu d}$$

Fig. 11. Sensitivity of SPECT and PET depends on the area of the detectors, the resolution efficiency and attenuation by different factors.

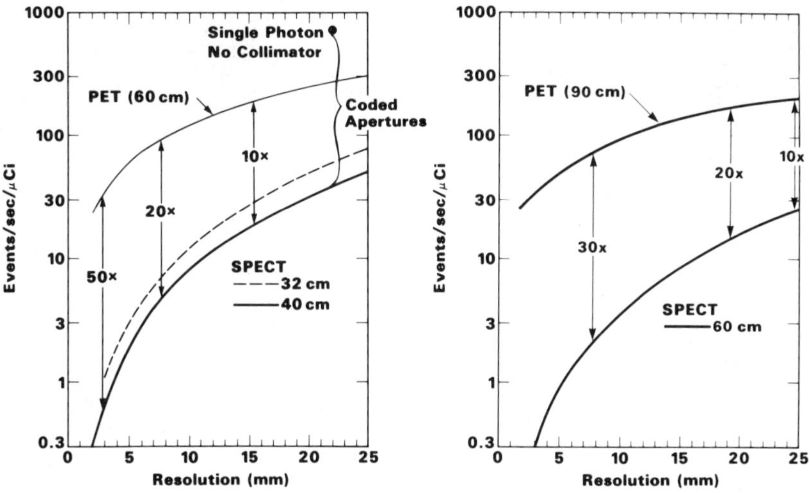

Fig. 12. Comparison of sensitivity between PET and SPECT as a function of resolution. Four banks of detectors are assumed for the SPECT system. If a single camera is used with an optimum collimator, the SPECT sensitivity will decrease by a factor of 4.

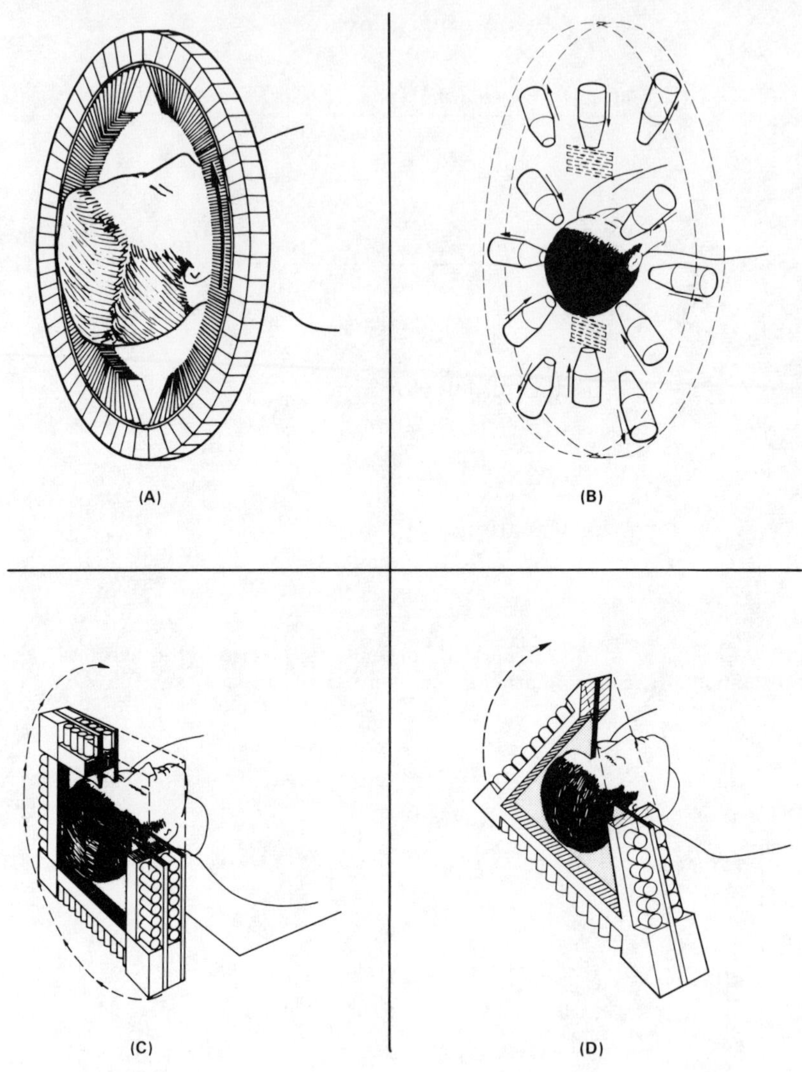

Fig. 13. Four configurations for improving the sensitivity of SPECT compared to one or two gamma cameras.

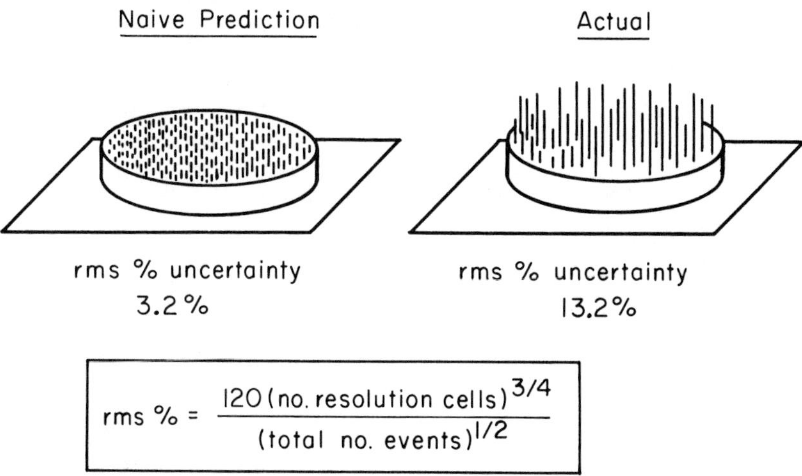

Fig. 14. Statistical uncertainty in tomography depends on the number of resolution elements as well as on the number of events detected.

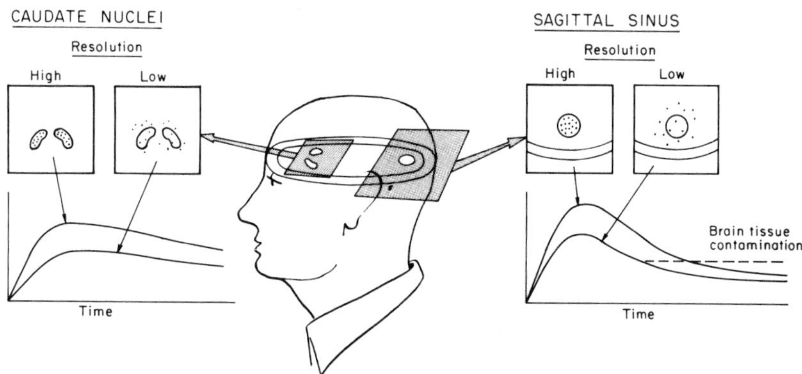

Fig. 15. Poor-resolution systems spread data over a region larger than the actual area or volume in which the tracer accumulated. This results in an erroneous decrease in activity, which affects the quantitative accuracy of both dynamic and static emission tomography.

13. Transmitter Alterations in Alzheimer's Disease: Relation to Cortical Dysfunction as Suggested by Positron Emission Tomography

THOMAS N. CHASE, M.D.
CAROL A. TAMMINGA, M.D.

Experimental Therapeutics Branch National Institute of Neurological and Communicative Disorders and Stroke Bethesda, Maryland 20892

ABSTRACT: The cause of the neuronal degeneration in AD remains unknown. While the search for etiologic factors continues, the application of classical transmitter pharmacology may facilitate rational development of drugs to afford symptomatic relief. This approach is based on the possibility that a linkage can be established between a particular set of neurologic signs and dysfunction in a particular transmitter system. Once such a relation has been established, drugs can be developed which will selectively modify the critical system in the appropriate direction. This pharmacologic strategy led to the discovery of drugs which alleviate symptoms of Parkinson's disease and might be no less successful in the search for drugs to ameliorate the dementia of Alzheimer's disease.

Introduction

Abnormalities in several cerebral transmitter systems have been observed in Alzheimer's disease (AD) (1). For certain of these systems; for example, cortical cholinergic projections from the basal forebrain nuclei, there is convincing documentation of a characteristic deficit (2,3). For several other systems; for example, those containing GABA or substance P, inconsistent results have been reported (1). Finally, a number of cortical neuronal systems, including those containing cholecystokinin or vasoactive intestinal peptide, appear to be entirely normal (1), lending support to the suggestion that neuronal degeneration in AD is characteristically selective.

Until now, most biochemical studies of central transmitters in postmortem tissues from patients with AD have been based on a more or less random sampling of cerebral regions. In view of the considerable heterogeneity of the human brain and the possibility of regional as well as neuronal selectivity, this approach may not yield meaningful results. Thus, the ability to localize changes in the living brain with the aid of positron emission tomography (PET) promises increased understanding of AD.

Positron Emission Tomography

The estimation of local rates of glucose utilization with PET provides an important approach to the noninvasive mapping of human brain dysfunction (4). Following intravenous administration of ^{18}F-fluorodeoxyglucose (FDG), its phosphorylated metabolite accumulates in central neuronal tissues in proportion to the rate of glucose utilization (5). Since fluorine-18 is a positron-emitting radionuclide, a PET scanner can quantitate local FDG concentrations throughout the brain and mathematical models are available to convert these isotope concentrations into the local metabolic rates for glucose, which in turn may serve as an index of the functional activity of neuronal tissues (5,6). The PET-FDG technique has now been applied to the clinical study of various aspects of normal and disordered brain function (7-9) and could help focus biochemical probes for the identification of critical transmitter alterations in patients with AD.

Alzheimer's disease has often been considered a rather uniformly diffuse cortical degenerative disorder associated with a global decline in cognitive function. Unfortunately, much of our knowledge of this disorder derives from the study of postmortem specimens from individuals with advanced disease, when the initial, critical changes may be obscured by later, secondary alterations. PET avoids this limitation by allowing examination of brain function at earlier stages. Application of this technique has suggested a relatively focal pattern of cortical involvement (10-12). Although glucose utilization is markedly reduced in the cerebral cortex, ranging from 10% to 49% below control levels, the pattern of hypometabolism is not uniform (13). The posterior parietal region (especially Brodmann area 39) evidences the most profound metabolic reduction, twice that found in a representative area of the frontal cortex (Brodmann area 10). Portions of the anterior occipital and posterior temporal cortex adjoining the parietal lobe are also severely affected, whereas the frontal and primary motor-sensory cortical areas appear relatively spared.

Comparison of patients judged clinically to be mildly demented with those considered to be severely affected has revealed substantial differences in cognitive test performance (13). For example, relative to values obtained from normal persons, Wechsler Adult Intelligence Scale (WAIS) IQ scores were reduced by 26% in the mild, and by 44% in the severe, cases of AD ($p<.001$). Mean overall cortical glucose metabolism was significantly below normal rates in both patient groups ($p<.01$); the reductions averaged 25% in mild and 30% in severe AD. Nevertheless, comparison of glucose metabolic rates between the mild and severely demented patients, whether in the entire cerebral cortex or only in selected Brodmann areas, revealed no statistically significant differences. In both the mildly and the severely affected patients, the posterior parietotemporal cortex was most profoundly hypometabolic, although the metabolic decrement between the two patient groups appeared to affect the frontal lobe at least as much as the posterior cortical areas. Thus, with increasing severity of dementia, small decrements in glucose utilization are associated with substantially greater declines in cognitive ability.

Whether the metabolic deterioration found in our patients can be attributed to a loss of intrinsic cortical neurons or to their hypofunction due to partial degeneration or deafferentation remains to be determined. Preponderant involvement of the parietal association cortex, a site of integration of somatosensory, visual, and auditory inputs to the cortex, is consistent with the major clinical features of AD, most notably aphasia, apraxia and agnosia. Unfortunately, portions of the medial temporal lobe such as the amygdala and hippocampus which have been implicated in memory function cannot be assessed reliably by the scanning methods employed. Consistent with the results of this study, some neuropathologic studies suggest that the neurodegenerative process in AD may primarily affect portions of the parietal and temporal lobes (14,15).

Cholinergic System

These PET-FDG results suggesting a relatively focal cortical distribution of neuronal dysfunction in AD provide a basis for biochemical studies directed toward the identification of critical transmitter abnormalities. It is now well established that cortical choline acetyltransferase (CAT) activity and rates of acetylcholine (ACh) synthesis are substantially reduced in Alzheimer patients, most likely because of degeneration of cholinergic projections from the nucleus basalis and other ventral forebrain nuclei (2,3,16). The possibility that dysfunction of this cholinergic pathway contributes to Alzheimer dementia is suggested by the close relation between the decline in cortical CAT activity and the degree of intellectual impairment (17) as well as by the tendency of cholinomimetics to improve, and anticholinergics to impair, cognitive function in normal individuals (18,19).

To evaluate the contribution of cholinergic system dysfunction to the dementia of AD and to the cortical glucose utilization pattern found in this disorder, the activity of the cholinergic marker CAT was compared in cortical areas evidencing the least and the most *in vivo* metabolic change (20). Cerebral tissues were obtained at autopsy from 10 individuals with AD and eight neurologically normal control individuals matched for age, sex and postmortem conditions. The diagnosis of AD was made according to generally accepted gross and microscopic criteria. Radiochemical assay indicated a reduction in cortical CAT activity by an overall mean of 40% in Alzheimer patients as compared with control individuals. A significant decrease was present in all cortical areas examined. Parietal cortex did not, however, evidence a significantly greater reduction in CAT activity than did frontal areas.

The foregoing results, although confirming numerous previous reports of a reduction in cortical CAT activity, failed to localize the CAT deficit to the area of maximal hypometabolism disclosed by the PET-FDG technique. Indeed, reductions in the activity of this cholinergic marker were similar throughout the cortical areas examined. Other investigators also have reported a relatively uniform decrement in CAT activity throughout the cerebral cortex in AD (11,21). Given these data, it is difficult to propose that the degeneration of cholinergic projections to the cerebral cortex could account for the disproportionate FDG reductions in the parietal association area.

Notwithstanding the close association between cholinergic dysfunction and Alzheimer dementia, numerous attempts to provide symptomatic relief to these patients through the administration of either ACh precursors, such as choline or lecithin (23,24), or degradation inhibitors, such as physostigmine (25,26), have yielded generally disappointing results. Drugs which directly stimulate postsynaptic ACh receptors provide an alternative approach to the augumentation of central cholinergic function. Such agents have the advantage of acting independently of presynaptic cholinergic neurons. Although parenteral administration of the selective muscarinic agonist arecoline has been reported to improve memory in some Alzheimer patients, its short duration of action and high incidence of adverse effects limits clinical usefulness (27). RS-86 (2-ethyl-8-methyl-2,8-diazospiro-(4,5)-decane-1,3-dione hydrobromide), on the other hand, is a highly selective and potent muscarinic (mixed M_1 and M_2 receptor) agonist, with a considerable duration of central action following oral administration and comparatively few peripherally mediated effects (28). The drug displaces ^{3}H-QNB from rodent forebrain binding sites but has no effect on central esterases. Behaviorally, RS-86 induces tremor, EEG arousal, and an atropine-sensitive hypothermia with a potency comparable to that of arecoline or oxotremorine.

Eight patients (three men and five women ages 62 ± 1.5 years) with clinically diagnosed AD have been treated with RS-86 (29). Symptom duration ranged from 1 to 5 years, and dementia ranged from mild to moderately severe. The drug was administered orally in a double-blind, placebo-controlled design. An initial RS-86 dose of 0.5 mg per day was increased daily until either 5 mg per day was reached or significant adverse effects developed, most notably diaphoresis or hypersalivation. Therapeutic efficacy was then evaluated at the highest dose free of significant untoward effects (mean 4.6 mg per day). Patients received RS-86 and placebo, each for 8 days, in random order. Comparison of the average neuropsychological scores between persons receiving placebo or the maximum tolerated RS-86 dose suggested slight improvement in three tests of verbal cognitive function (Story Recall, Word Learning and Dichotic Listening) and two tests of visuospatial functioning (Visual Form Discrimination-Copy and Pictorial Memory). All other tests, including the evaluation of attention, showed either no alteration or even a slight performance decrement. None of these changes attained statistical significance. When evaluating individual patients no significant change in aggregate cognitive test performance emerged. Moreover, no relation could be discerned between the overall pretreatment dementia severity and the average drug-induced change in all test scores, or between any individual pretreatment test score and the magnitude of change during drug administration.

The failure to find any consistent effect of RS-86 on cognitive function in Alzheimer patients contrasts with the somewhat more favorable results of earlier studies of arecoline (27) and could reflect nothing more than an inadequate RS-86 dose or treatment duration. On the other hand, each patient did receive the maximum individually tolerated dose of RS-86, and there is no obvious pharmacologic rationale for a long delay in response. However, coadministration of an anticholinergic drug with limited central nervous system access might have reduced the signs of peripheral parasympathetic activation and thus allowed higher RS-86 dosage.

The general interpretation of the results of the administration of cholinomimetics to Alzheimer patients is complicated by various theoretical uncertainties. For example, the marginal clinical efficacy of drugs which increase synaptic ACh levels by stimulating synthesis or blocking degradation of this transmitter might simply reflect the paucity of residual cholinergic terminals in the cerebral cortex. On the other hand, therapeutic attempts with postsynaptic receptor agonists such as RS-86 might be equally inappropriate, since these agents tonically stimulate a system which is presumably phasically active. None of the cholinomimetics used to date may thus have provided a definitive test of the validity of this therapeutic strategy.

The pharmacologic activity of all cholinomimetics depends on the integrity of the postsynaptic cholinergic receptors. Most studies have found no significant alteration in cortical muscarinic receptors in AD, especially those receptors considered to be situated postsynaptically (30,31). On the other hand, as already noted, there is ample neuropathologic and biochemical evidence to indicate that neurons intrinsic to the cerebral cortex also degenerate in AD. Presumably, neurons which lie distal to the cortical cholinergic projections characteristically become dysfunctional. It may thus be unlikely that ACh replacement alone could substantially reverse the cognitive deficits of this disorder. Indeed, a therapy directed towards the restoration of synaptic function at downstream sites might confer a higher probability of therapeutic benefit.

GABA System

γ-aminobutyric acid (GABA) is a major inhibitory neurotransmitter in the human cerebral cortex. Some biochemical evidence suggests that an abnormality in cortical GABA-containing neurons may occur in AD. Spinal fluid GABA concentrations are characteristically reduced (32-34), and several studies of postmortem cortical tissues have shown a decrement in GABA concentrations as well as in the activity of the GABA-synthesizing enzyme, glutamic acid decarboxylase (1,35,36). Loss of GABA neurons, possibly situated postsynaptically to cortical cholinergic projections, might contribute to the cognitive decline in Alzheimer patients and account for the limited ability of cholinomimetics to ameliorate the dementia.

The foregoing considerations support the view that pharmacologic stimulation of GABA-mediated synaptic function might confer symptomatic benefit to individuals with AD. To evaluate this possibility, a controlled clinical trial of the potent selective GABA agonist (37) THIP (4,5,6,7-tetrahydroisoxazolo(5,4-c)pyridin-3-ol) was carried out in patients with mild to moderately advanced symptoms. Six men with clinically diagnosed AD age 58 $\pm$ 2.0 years were studied (34). Symptom duration averaged 4.5 years and severity ranged from mild to moderately advanced. THIP was administered orally in a double-blind, placebo-controlled, crossover design. An initial THIP dose of 20 mg per day was gradually increased until clinically significant adverse effects were observed; these occurred at an average daily dose of 116 mg given in four equal doses. Patients were then randomly assigned to either a THIP-placebo treatment sequence or the reverse. When administered at maximum tolerated doses (mean 65 mg/day; range 30-140 mg/day) THIP had no consistent effect on any of the psychologic measures tested (34). Although the results of some verbal tests improved slightly, others showed virtually no change or even a small decline. Reaction time, used here as a measure of attention, also changed insignificantly. Informal observations recorded by the ward staff gave no indication of any THIP-induced alteration in the ability of these patients to perform the activities of daily living.

All patients admitted to this study had relatively low GABA levels in their lumbar spinal fluid (38 ± 6.2 pmol/ml). GABA values not only averaged 77% (range 60% to 82%) below those found in normal controls but also were 64% below those found (106 ± 7.8 pmol/ml) in an otherwise unselected group of 22 age-matched, untreated Alzheimer patients ($p<.001$). There was no correlation between the degree of reduction of pretreatment GABA levels and the response to THIP therapy. Moreover, THIP failed to influence GABA concentrations in spinal fluid.

The foregoing results suggest that the short-term administration of THIP, at maximum tolerated doses exerts no clinically significant effect on cognitive function in patients with AD. Adverse effects occurring at the highest doses attained during the dose-finding portion of this study, including somnolence, incoordination, confusion, anxiety and involuntary movements, appeared centrally mediated and resembled those associated with other central GABA agonists (38). Although no significant change in spinal fluid GABA levels could be documented, this result is not inconsistent with findings in experimental animals receiving pharmacologically active doses of other GABA agonists. Accordingly, it may be reasonable to assume that THIP doses sufficient to stimulate central GABA receptors were administered and thus that GABA agonists generally are unlikely to confer substantial clinical benefit to patients with Alzheimer dementia.

The results of this clinical trial also cast some doubt on the possibility that a loss of cortical GABA interneurons contributes significantly to the cognitive decline in AD. The assumption was made that Alzheimer patients with the most marked evidence of a central GABA deficit would benefit most from replacement therapy. Thus, patients selected for this study had significant reductions in spinal fluid GABA levels, not only in comparison with normal control individuals, but also in comparison with an otherwise unselected group of Alzheimer patients. Nevertheless, the group as a whole failed to respond to THIP therapy, and no relation could be found between pretreatment GABA levels in lumbar spinal fluid and either baseline cognitive function or THIP-induced changes in neuropsychological test performance. Although a loss of postsynaptic

GABA receptors could account for the observed failure of THIP to benefit patients with Alzheimer dementia, no consistent abnormalities of this type have been reported (39,40). On the other hand, not all investigations of AD have found biochemical evidence of a GABA system abnormality; the reliability of postmortem assays for the GABA system, especially those measuring glutamic acid decarboxylase activity, is open to question (2,41,42). Furthermore, brain GABA levels in Alzheimer patients correlate poorly with neuropathological findings (43). The distribution of GABA abnormalities in relation to those suggested by PET-FDG has not been explored in postmortem tissues.

Neuropeptide Y System

The finding that neuropeptide Y (NPY) occurs in extraordinarily high concentrations in the human cerebral cortex (44), and that it is co-localized with somatostatin in certain cortical neurons (45) prompted a comparison of this putative transmitter in PET-FDG-identified areas of cortical dysfunction in AD (20). Cerebral material was obtained at autopsy from 10 individuals with histologically verified disease and eight control individuals matched for age, sex and postmortem conditions. There was no significant difference in cortical NPY concentrations between the Alzheimer and control groups in any brain region sampled: frontal lobe 22 ± 6.1 vs 25 ± 6.5; parietal lobe 18 ± 4.3 vs 18 ± 4.2 pg/μg protein in Alzheimer patients and normal controls, respectively. Moreover, in neither patients nor controls could any appreciable difference in NPY concentrations be discerned between the frontal and parietal cortices.

These findings confirm and extend earlier reports suggesting that cortical NPY-containing neurons are not abnormal in AD (46,47). The apparent sparing of the NPY system is interesting in view of the alterations in somatostatin in this disorder and the coexistence of these two neuropeptides in normal human cortical neurons. Although many cortical neurons contain both NPY and somatostatin, there is a population of neurons which contain only somatostatin and another population which contain only NPY (45). Conceivably, only neurons which have somatostatin, alone or together with other transmitters other than NPY, degenerate in AD. Reported increases in NPY concentrations in the substantia innominata (46) may be due to alterations in turnover or to sprouting on NPY-containing neurons.

Somatostatin System

Another neurochemical abnormality found consistently in AD is a reduction in cortical somatostatin (21,22,49,50). Little is known, however, about the relation of this change to the symptomatology, PET-FDG abnormalities or histologic features which characterize this disorder.

Spinal fluid somatostatin concentrations from 24 Alzheimer patients were found to average 39% below the age-matched controls ($p<.001$) (50). The degree of somatostatin reduction was stable in seven patients who had repeat lumbar punctures at intervals exceeding 9 months; initial somatostatin values (25 ± 3.6 pg/ml) did not differ significantly from repeat values (33 ± 4.3 pg/ml). There was no correlation between the CSF content of somatostatin and the duration of dementia, which ranged from 1 to 5 years. Significant positive correlations were obtained between CSF somatostatin concentrations and cognitive function, including various tests of verbal, visual, visuospatial and general memory function. However, WAIS Verbal IQ and Performance IQ scores did not correlate with CSF somatostatin levels. The CSF somatostatin values also correlated positively with overall cortical glucose utilization rates in the cerebral hemispheres ($r = .44$; $p<.04$) as determined by PET-FDG. The pattern of correlations was not uniform: the relation was closest in parietal ($r = .54$; $p<.01$) and temporal ($r = .44$; $p<.04$) cortices but was not significant in frontal or occipital areas.

Postmortem tissues were obtained for study from eight Alzheimer subjects (three men and five women age 75 ± 3.2 years) with histologically verified disease and from nine neurologically normal individuals (six men and three women age 74 ± 3.2 years) (50). In frontal and parietal cortex, somatostatin was reduced by 54% in the two posterior parietal areas sampled (Brodmann 39 areas and 40) but was not significantly altered in the two frontal areas (Brodmann areas 9 and 10). The distribution of low somatostatin levels, in contrast to the distribution of low CAT activity, thus paralleled the distribution of PET-FDG changes.

Loss of somatostatin-mediated synaptic function could well contribute to the cognitive decline in AD. Like others (51,52), we found consistently low CSF somatostatin levels in patients with this disorder, and this reduction correlated with performance on neuropsychological tests. The somatostatin deficit may occur early in AD, since we were unable to establish any relation between CSF concentrations and the duration of dementia. There could be a threshold for the degeneration of somatostatin-containing neurons before which no symptoms appear; thereafter, a small additional loss of these neurons might result in a significant loss of cognitive function.

Combined analysis of the PET-FDG and CSF somatostatin results lent further support to the suggestion that a loss of cortical neurons containing this neuropeptide may be related to Alzheimer dementia. Spinal fluid somatostatin levels correlated with overall cortical glucose utilization rates. This association was due to the close relation between CSF somatostatin concentrations and glucose metabolism in the posterior parietal area, the region suggested by the PET-FDG technique as being first and most profoundly affected in AD. Postmortem results showing a somatostatin reduction in posterior parietal, but not in anterior frontal, areas also that CSF somatostatin depletion may be due to principally changes in the parietal cortex. The pattern of somatostatin loss was consistent with some (53,54), but not all (20,21), previous studies. Beal *et al.* found loss of somatostatin-like immunoreactivity in frontal and temporal cortex using an assay that quantified somatostatin-14 and somatostatin-28 equally (55). Speculatively, somatostatin-14, the form we studied, may persist in cortical tissues even if the extended forms of somatostatin such as somatostatin-28 are depleted. Somatostatin has been identified both in neuritic plaques and in neurons that contain neurofibrillary tangles (56); other histopathological observations (14) suggest that the cortical changes in AD may occur most prominently in the parietal association area. These considerations thus support the view that a somatostatin system deficit may be closely linked both to the pathophysiology of the parietal cortex hypometabolism identified by PET-FDG changes and to the parietal lobe symptoms which epitomize Alzheimer dementia.

No drugs are yet available for systemic administration to man which act selectively and potently to stimulate central somatostatin-mediated functions. On the other hand, a clinical trial of a somatostatin-depleting drug in patients with Huntington's disease was designed partly to help elucidate the role of this neuropeptide system in the pathogenesis of normal and abnormal cognitive function. In Huntington's disease, concentrations of somatostatin and the density of somatostatin-containing varicose fibers are increased in the basal ganglia (57). The somatostatin system has been linked to the regulation of motor function, since somatostatin injected into rat brain produces hyperknetic and stereotyped movements (58,59). Preclinical studies also tend to link the somatostatin system to cognitive function: intracerebroventricularly administered somatostatin modifies both amnestic responses (60) and avoidance behavior (61).

The clinical effects of cysteamine (2-aminoethanethiol) have been studied in five patients with Huntington's chorea (three men and two women ages 28 to 52 years) in a double-blind, placebo-controlled design (62). This drug, when given systemically to rats, decreases brain somatostatin levels (63) without affecting other cerebral neuropeptides (64). As a result, central somatostatin receptors are upregulated (65), and various behavioral effects occur (66,67) that might be due to a reduction in somatostatin-mediated function. Cysteamine was introduced at a dose of 500 mg/day and, in the absence of clinically significant adverse effects, increased to 4000 mg/day. Three of the five patients tolerated the maximum dose; two others were withdrawn from drug treatment at doses of 1500 and 2500 mg/day because of transient fever, leukocytosis, diarrhea and macular rash. All patients also reported brief episodes of nausea with the higher doses. Cysteamine had no consistent effect on any of the motor or cognitive measures tested. Moreover, ward staff noted no differences in the patients' ability to perform activities of daily living. The administration of cysteamine did, however, increase plasma growth hormone levels from 2.3 ± 0.6 to 5.5 ± 0.9 ng/ml ($p<.0001$). Plasma somatostatin concentrations did not change; the CSF somatostatin levels declined in each patient by 3% to 27%, although this change was not statistically significant.

The apparent failure of cysteamine to influence either extrapyramidal or cognitive performance in Huntingtonian patients might imply the use of doses insufficient to modify cerebral somatostatin concentrations. Although we found no significant alterations in either plasma or CSF somatostatin levels, the radioimmunoassay is sensitive to the portion of the amino acid chain that is biologically active and mainly affected by cysteamine (68,69). On the other hand, few patients completed this study, and it is not clear that plasma or lumbar CSF somatostatin concentrations measure drug-induced cerebral changes. Moreover, the observed cysteamine-induced rise in plasma growth hormone is consistent with preclinical observations (70) as well as with the putative drug action, namely somatostatin reduction at functionally active sites. At least in the hypothalamic-pituitary axis, somatostatin-mediated function was modified by cysteamine treatment. It remains uncertain, however, whether a dose that is sufficient to modify human pituitary function can also influence somatostatin-regulated functions at other cerebral loci. More potent and less toxic pharmaceuticals which selectively augment or attenuate central somatostatin-mediated mechanisms are needed to elucidate the role of the somatostatin system in the pathophysiology and treatment of Alzheimer dementia.

Concluding Speculations

The strategy outlined, which is based on the cortical distribution of neuronal dysfunction suggested by the PET-FDG studies, may facilitate the identification of transmitter system alterations which serve as critical determinants for the dementia of AD. Although applications of this approach remain limited, available results have already drawn attention to cortical somatostatin-containing neurons. Other transmitter systems also deserve further evaluation: recent observations have focused attention on the possible involvement of corticotropin-releasing factor interneurons and glutamatergic efferents from the cerebral cortex. Although unifying hypotheses could be advanced, such as that only neurons which possess a specific type of glutamatergic receptor degenerate in AD it must be conceded that grave uncertainties remain as to whether Alzheimer dementia reflects dysfunction limited to one or at the most a small number of transmitter systems or, on the other hand, involves neuronal aggregates with little or no regard to transmitter specificity. Notwithstanding these pathogenetic considerations, it is still no less uncertain whether transmitter pharmacology approaches directed toward one or more transmitter systems can ever be successful in alleviating the cognitive decline in Alzheimer patients. Future work, especially with appropriate animal models, will ultimately bring the answer. As these investigative efforts proceed, it may be important to note that symptoms of Parkinson's disease, although associated with abnormalities in at least 10 central pathways in addition to the dopamine system, can probably be explained by, and certainly relieved by, an interaction with dopaminergic mechanisms.

References

1. Rossor, M.N., & Iversen, L. L. (1986) *Br. Med. Bull.* **42**, 70-74.
2. Bowen, D.M., Smith, C.B., White, P., & Davidson. A.N., (1976) *Brain* **99**, 459-96.
3. Rossor, M.N., Garrett, N.J., Johson, A.L., Mountjoy, C.Q., Roth, M., & Iversen, L.L. (1982) *Brain* **105**, 313-30.
4. Phelps, M., & Mazziotta, J. (1986) *Science* **228**, 799-809.
5. Sokoloff, L. (1984) *Ann. Neurol.* **15(suppl)**, S1-S11.
6. DiChiro, G., Brooks, R.A., Patronas, N.J., Bairamian, D., Kornblith, P.L., Smith, B.H., Mansi, L. & Barker, J. (1984) *Ann. Neurol.* **15**, 138-146.
7. Chase, T.N., Fedio, P., Foster, N.L., Brooks, R., DiChiro, G. & Mansi, L. (1984) *Arch. Neurol.* **41**, 1244-1247.
8. Mazziotta, J.C. & Phelps, M.E. (1985) *Res. Publ. Assoc. Res. Nerv. Ment. Dis.* **63**, 121-37.
9. Foster, N.L., Chase, T.N., Patronas, N.J., Gillespie, M.M. & Fedio, P. (1986) *Ann. Neurol.* **19**, 139-143.
10. Chase, T.L., Foster, N.L. & Mansi, L. (1983) *Lancet* **2**, 225.
11. Foster, N.L., Chase, T.N., Fedio, P., Patronas, N.J., Brooks, R.A. & DiChiro, G. (1983) *Neurology* **33**, 961-965.

12. Chase, T.N., Foster, N.L., Fedio, P., Brooks, R., Mansi, L. & DiChiro, G. (1984) *Ann. Neurol.* **15 (Suppl)**, S170-4.
13. Foster, N.L., Chase, T.N., Mansi, L., Brooks, R., Fedio, P., Patronas, N.J. & DiChiro, G. (1984) *Ann. Neurol.* **16**, 649-54.
14. Brun, A. & Englund, E. (1981) *Histopathology* **5**, 549-564.
15. Brun, A. (1983) In: *Alzheimer's Disease: The Standard Reference.* cd. Reisberg, B. (Free Press, New York) pp. 37-47.
16. Coyle, J.T., Price, D.L. & DeLong, M.R. (1981) *Science* **219**, 1184-90.
17. Perry, E.K., Tomlinson, B.E., Blessed, G., Bergmann, K., Gibson, P.H. & Perry, R.H. (1978) *Br. Med. J.* 1457-9.
18. Drachman, D.A. (1977) *Neurology* **27**, 783-90.
19. Davis, K.L., Mohs, R.C., Tinklenberg, J.R., Pfefferbaum, A., Hollister, L.E. & Kopell, B.S. (1978) *Science* **201**, 272-74.
20. Foster, N.L., Tamminga, C.A., O'Donohue, T.L., Tanimoto, K., Bird, E.D. & Chase, T.N (1986) *Neurosci. Lett.* **63**, 71-5.
21. Davies, P., Katzman, R. & Terry, R.D. (1980) *Nature* **288**, 279-280.
22. Rossor, M.N., Emson, P.C., Mountjoy, C.Q., Roth, M. & Iversen, L.L. (1980) *Neurosci. Lett.* **20**, 373-377.
23. Thal., L.J., Fuld, P.A., Masur, D.M. & Sharpless, N.S. (1983) *Ann. Neurolo.* **13**, 491-6.
24. Etienne, P., Dastoor, D., Gauthier, S., Ludwig, R. & Collier, B. (1981) *Neurology* **31**, 1552-54.
25. Mohs, R.C., Davis, B.M., Johns, C.A., Mathe, A.A., Greenwald, B.S., Horvath, T.B. & Davis, K.L. (1985) *Am. J. Psychiatr.* **142**, 28-33.
26. Wettstein, A. (1983) *Ann. Neurol.* **13**, 210-12.
27. Christie, J.E., Shering, A., Ferguson, J. & Glen, A.I. (1981) *Br. J. Psychiatr.* **138**, 46-50.
28. Wettstein, A. & Spiegel, R. (1984) *Psychopharmacology* **84**, 572-3.
29. Bruno. G., Mohr, E., Gillespie, M., Fedio, P. & Chase, T.N. (1986) *Arch. Neurol.* In press.
30. Mash, D.O., Flynn, D.D. & Potter, L.T. (1985) *Science* **228**, 1115-7.
31. Rinne, J.O., Laakso, K., Lonnberg, P., Molsa, P., Paljarvi, L., Rinne, J.K., Sako, E. & Rinne, U.K. (1985) *Brain Res.* **336**, 19-25.
32. Manyam, N.V.B., Katz, L., Hare, T.A., Gerber, J.C. & Grossman, M.H. (1980) *Arch. Neurol.* **37**, 352-55.
33. Zimmer, R., Teelken, A.W., Trieling, W.B., Weber, W., Weihmayr, T. & Lauter, H. (1984) *Arch. Neurol.* **41**, 602-4.
34. Mohr, E., Bruno, G., Foster, N., Gillespie, M., Cox, C., Hare, T.A., Tamminga, C., Fedio, P. & Chase, T.N. (1986) *Neuropharmacol.* In press.
35. Perry, E.K., Gibson, P.H., Blessed, G., Perry, R.H. & Tomlinson, B.E. (1977) *J. Neurol.Sci.* **34**, 247-65.

36. Davies, P. (1979) *Brain Res.* **171**, 319-27.
37. Waszczak, B.L., Hruska, R.E. & Walters, J.R. (1980) *Eur. J. Pharmacol.* **65**, 21-9.
38. Tamminga, C.A., Crayton, J.W. & Chase, T.N. (1978) *Am. J. Psychiatr.* **135**, 746-47.
39. Reisine, T.D., Yamamura, H.I., Bird, E.D., Spokes, E. & Enna, S.J. (1978) *Brain Res.* **159**, 477-81.
40. Crow, T.J., Cross, A.J., Cooper, S.J., Deakin, J.F.W., Ferrier, I.N., Johnson, J.A., Joseph, M.H., Owen, F., Poulter, M., Lofthouse, P., Corsellis, J., Chambers, D.R., Blessed, G., Perry, E.K., Perry, R.H. & Tomlinson, B.E. (1984) *Neuropharmacology* **23**, 1561-69.
41. Spillane, J.A., White, P., Goodhardt, M.J., Flack, R.H.A., Bowen, D.M. & Davison, A.N. (1977) *Nature* **266**, 588-59.
42. Spokes, E.G.S. (1979) *Brain* **102**, 333-46.
43. Mountjoy, C.Q., Rossor, M.N., Iversen, L.L. & Roth, M. (1984) *Brain* **107**, 507-18.
44. Adrain. T.E., Allen, J.M., Bloom, S.R., Chatei, M.A., Rossor, M.N., Roberts, G.W., Crow, T.J., Tanimoto, K. & Polas, J.M. (1983) *Nature* **306**, 584-586.
45. Chronwall, B.M., Chase, T.N. & O'Donohue, T.L. (1985) *Neurosci. Lett.* **52**, 213-217.
46. Allen, J.M., Ferrier, I.N., Roberts, G.W., Cross, A.J., Adrain, T.E., Crow, T.J. & Bloom, S.R. (1984) *J. Neurol.Sci.* **64**, 325-331.
47. Foster, N.L., Tamminga, C.A., O'Donohue, T.L. & Chase, T.N. (1984) *Soc. Neurosci. Abstr.* **10**, 173.
48. Tamminga, C.A., Foster, N.L. & Chase, T.N. (1985) *N. Engl. J. Med.* **313**, 1294-1295.
49. Morrison, J.H., Rogers, J., Scherr, S., Benoit, R. & Bloom, F.E. (1985) *Nature* **314**, 90-92.
50. Tamminga, C.A., Foster, N.L., Fredio, P., Bird, E.D. & Chase, T.N. (1986) *Neurology* In press.
51. Wood, P.L., Etienne, P., Lal, S., Gauthier, S., Cajal, S. & Nair, N.P. (1982) *Life Sci.* **31**, 2073-2079.
52. Soininen, H.S., Jolkkonen, J.T., Reinikainen, K.J., Halonen, T.D. & Riekkinen, P.J. (1984) *J. Neurol. Sci.* 1984 **63**, 167-172.
53. Arai, H., Moroji, T. & Kosaka, K. (1984) *Neurosci. Lett.* **52**, 73-78.
54. Crystal, H.A. & Davies, P. (1982) *J. Neurochem.* **38**, 1781-1784.
55. Beal, M.F., Mazurek, M.F., Tran, V.T., Chattha, G., Bird, E.D. & Martin, J.B. (1985) *Science* **229**, 289-291.
56. Roberts, G.W., Crow, T.J. & Polak, J.M. (1985) *Nature* **314**, 92-94.
57. Aronin, N., Cooper, P.R., Lorens, L.F., Bird, E.D., Sugar, S.M., Leeman, S.E. & Martin, J.B. (1983) *Ann. Neurol.* **13**, 519-26.
58. Cohn, M.L., & Cohn, M. (1975) *Brain Res.* **96**, 138-41.

59. Rezek, M., Havlicek, B., Leybin, L., Pinsky, C., Kroeger, E.A., Hughes, K.R. & Friesen, H. (1977) *Can. J. Physiol. Pharmacol.* **55**, 234-42.
60. Vecsei, L., Bollok, I. & Telegdy, G. (1984) *Peptides* **4**, 293-95.
61. Vecsei, L., Kiraly, C., Bollok, I., Nagy, A., Varga, J., Penke, B. & Telegdy G. (1984) *Pharmacol. Biochem. Behav.* **21**, 833-37.
62. Shults, C., Steardo, L., Barone, P., Mohr, E., Juncos, J., Serrati, C., Fedio, P., Tamminga, C.A. & Chase, T.N. (1986) *Neurology*. In press.
63. Sagar, S.M., Landry, D., Millard, W.J., Badger, T.M., Arnold, M.A. & Martin, J.B. (1982) *J. Neurosci.* **2**, 225-31.
64. Palkovits, M., Brownstein, M.J., Eiden, L.S., Bernfield, M.C., Russell, J., Arimura, A. & Szabo, S. (1982) *Brain Res.* **240**, 178-80.
65. Srikant, C.B. & Patel, Y.C. *Endocrinology* **115**, 990-95.
66. Brown, M.R., Fisher, L.A., Sawchenko, P.E., Swanson, L.W. & Vale, W.W. (1983) *Regul. Pep.* **5**, 163-79.
67. Higuchi, T., Sikand, G.S., Kato, N., Wada, J.A. & Friesen, H.G. (1983) *Brain Res.* **288**, 359-62.
68. Bakhit, C., Benoit, R. & Bloom, F.E. (1983) *Regul. Pept.* **6**, 169-77.
69. Patel, Y.C., & Pierzchala, I. (1985) *Endocrinology* **116**, 1699-1702.
70. Millard, W.J., Sagar, S.M., Badger, T.M. & Martin, J.B. (1983) *Endocrinology* **112**, 509-17.

14. Single-Photon Emission Computed Tomography in the Clinical Evaluation of Dementia

WILLIAM J. JAGUST, M.D.*†

Department of Neurology Veterans Administration Medical Center
Martinez, CA 94553

THOMAS F. BUDINGER,† BRUCE R. REED,* MIGUEL COLINA†

ABSTRACT: Physiological imaging using positron emission tomography (PET) has been a useful tool in the investigation of dementia. In particular, patterns of cerebral glucose utilization appear to differentiate various types of dementia, with Alzheimer's disease (AD) demonstrating a propensity for hypometabolism to involve the temporoparietal cortex. Single-photon emission computed tomography (SPECT) using new tracers for the measurement of regional cerebral blood flow is a technique with potentially broader clinical availability than PET and thus may provide a practical method of routinely evaluating patients. We studied eight patients with AD, four healthy elderly controls, and one patient with multi-infarct dementia (MID) using the tracer ^{123}I-N-isopropyl-p-iodoamphetamine with SPECT. We found that blood-flow patterns were significantly different in AD and normal aging and that the patient with MID differed from the AD patients. Although technical factors in SPECT instrumentation and data collection require further modification and issues of sensitivity and specificity need more investigation, SPECT appears to be useful in the diagnosis of dementing illnesses and offers promise as an additional research technique.

Introduction

Clinical imaging studies of patients with dementia have generally been concerned with detecting structural lesions capable of producing the patient's symptoms of cognitive deterioration. The role of x-ray

* Department of Neurology, School of Medicine, University of California, Davis, CA and Veterans Administration Medical Center, Martinez, CA; † Donner Laboratory, University of California, Berkeley, CA.

computed tomography (CT) has therefore been to search for anatomical abnormalities in the hope of finding a treatable or reversible cause of the dementia syndrome. The majority of demented patients have Alzheimer's disease (AD) (1), which is marked by distinctive pathology at the ultrastructural level without any characteristic gross anatomical abnormalities. Although cerebral atrophy is generally more severe in AD patients than in age-matched healthy subjects, there normally is atrophy with aging, and the degree of overlap between normal aging and AD is so great that x-ray CT is of little value in positively diagnosing AD in an individual patient (2).

The advent of new techniques for noninvasive imaging of cerebral physiology *in vivo* has improved our understanding of dementing illnesses, particularly AD. These techniques, through the use of emission computed tomography, image the spatial distribution of injected radiopharmaceutical tracers. Positron emission tomography (PET) utilizes positron emitting tracers and imaging instruments capable of making measurements with spatial resolutions finer than those of X-ray CT or nuclear magnetic resonance (NMR) imaging but with high specificity for such physiological processes as cerebral glucose metabolism, blood flow, neurotransmitter receptors, and blood-brain barrier integrity (3). However, because positron emitting isotopes have short half-lives, they are costly to produce and require an onsite cyclotron or generating system, and as a result, PET technology has not been generally available in the medical community.

This chapter is devoted to recent work in emission tomography using single-photon emission computed tomography (SPECT), a method that can be made more widely available than PET. As will be shown, SPECT is useful in the diagnosis of dementing illnesses.

Whereas PET utilizes nuclei which emit positrons in the process of radioactive decay, SPECT entails the use of radioisotopes which emit gamma radiation. For a more extensive discussion of the physics of these systems, see Chapter 11. Detector systems necessary for the detection of these single-photon emissions are thus different from those used with PET. SPECT detection systems are commercially available, and single-photon emitting isotopes are in routine clinical use in most community hospitals for the evaluation of myocardial, liver and spleen perfusion and bone disease. Recently, compounds labeled with the single-photon emitting isotopes ^{99m}Tc and ^{123}I have been developed which image cerebral blood flow (4,5). The use of these new agents with SPECT camera systems thus promises a readily available technique which will have considerable utility for evaluating cerebral physiology *in vivo*.

PET Studies of Dementia

Most of the work with emission computed tomography in dementia has been accomplished using PET, with particular emphasis on measurements of regional cerebral blood flow (rCBF) and regional cerebral metabolic rates for glucose (rCMRglu) and oxygen ($rCMRO_2$). Blood-flow measurements have primarily utilized ^{15}O-labeled water, glucose metabolic studies have used [^{18}F]-deoxyglucose and oxygen metabolism studies have used $^{15}O\text{-}O_2$. Evaluation of rCMRglu has consistently demonstrated diminished metabolic rates in the cerebral cortex in AD as compared to control subjects. This diminution has generally been most severe and consistent in the temporoparietal cortex (6,8). Previous work in our laboratory calculated the percentage difference between frontal and temporoparietal cortical metabolism and found, on average, a 32% decrease in metabolism in the temporoparietal cortex in AD (9). PET studies of cerebral metabolism have, in some laboratories, demonstrated correlations between the location of regional metabolic deficits and specific cognitive deficits evaluated neuropsychologically (10,11). It has been suggested that the pattern of temporoparietal hypometabolism is sufficiently distinctive that it may be useful in diagnosing AD (12-14).

The potential diagnostic utility of this metabolic pattern is supported by the correlation between basic biological markers of the disease and the metabolic findings. The temporoparietal location of the hypometabolism is similar to the regional distribution of both the cortical histopathology, which tends to predominate in this brain region (15,16), and the regions of loss of cortical choline acetyltransferase (17,18). The mechanism whereby the pathological process involved in AD produces diminished glucose metabolism is not known, since such metabolic changes could reflect an actual abnormality in glucose metabolism or simply normal metabolism occurring in fewer neurons. Although the cause and mechanism of this temporoparietal pattern is of great importance in understanding the etiology and pathophysiology of the disease, it may not be important for the use of physiological imaging in the diagnosis and longitudinal evaluation of patients with dementia.

The finding of different metabolic patterns in other dementias is also relevent to this issue. Pick's disease, for example, is often said to be clinically indistinguishable from AD (19). However, findings of diminished metabolism in the frontal lobes, as opposed to the AD temporoparietal pattern, has now been demonstrated in patients with autopsy-verified Pick's disease (20,21). In addition, the pattern of temporoparietal hypometabolism was not found in patients with normal pressure hydrocephalus who responded to cerebrospinal fluid shunting procedures, suggesting that PET imaging may be useful in selecting demented patients for shunts (13).

Although PET studies using tracers to investigate rCBF in dementia have not been as widely applied as studies of glucose metabolism, the findings are similar. The use of ^{15}O-labeled O_2 and H_2O has enabled the measurement of oxygen metabolism and blood flow in the same patient at one sitting. These studies have confirmed that blood-flow diminution also occurs in regions of diminished metabolism. In addition, since the oxygen extraction ratio is normal, these studies suggest that the diminished flow is secondary to the diminished metabolic demands (22). Since current SPECT brain imaging is related to measurement of cerebral blood flow as opposed to metabolism, the finding that flow is diminished proportionately to metabolism in AD provides further support for the use of SPECT to study rCBF in dementia.

SPECT Instrumentation and Radiochemistry

Simultaneous advances in the development of SPECT imaging systems and single-photon emitting radiotracers are responsible for the current interest in this imaging modality. Several recent reviews have summarized both of these subjects (23-25). An important difference between SPECT cameras and positron cameras is the need of the former for collimation, a process which decreases sensitivity as resolution increases. Thus, as SPECT camera resolution improves, longer periods of imaging are required, with the result that SPECT is incapable of performing rapid dynamic studies of tracer kinetics. Problems of photon scatter and attenuation of photons by surrounding tissues are greater with SPECT than PET and have not been adequately resolved (25). Nevertheless, SPECT images capable of defining most important cerebral anatomical structures are currently being obtained in several centers using clinical imaging protocols which are well tolerated by most patients.

The single-photon emitting isotopes ^{123}I and ^{99m}Tc have the advantages of relatively low patient radiation exposure due to half-lives of 13 and 6 hours, respectively, and of energies appropriate for collimation and good counting efficiency. ^{123}I has been used to label several substituted amphetamine compounds, two of which have been utilized in clinical studies: N-isopropyl-p-iodoamphetamine (IMP), and N,N,N′-trimethyl-N′-[2-hydroxy-3-methyl-5-iodobenzyl]-1,3-propanediamine (HIPDM). These agents are similar in their biological behavior (26) and cross the intact blood-brain barrier to be distributed in brain tissue according to flow. Although retention in brain has been thought to be secondary to occupation of nonspecific binding sites, the exact mechanism has not been elucidated (27).

Most commercially available ^{123}I is synthesized using a (p, 2n) reaction and is therefore contaminated with various amounts of ^{124}I, which degrades image quality and quantitative capability. This factor, along with the greater ease of generation of ^{99m}Tc (from a parent generator rather than a cyclotron), makes ^{99m}Tc a more desirable isotope for the labeling of SPECT tracers. However, difficulties with ^{99m}Tc chemical syntheses have, until recently, impeded the development of radiopharmaceuticals which cross the blood-barrier. Currently, a new tracer, d,l-hexamethyl-propyleneamine oxime (HM-PAO) labeled with ^{99m}Tc effectively images rCBF and is undergoing clinical testing (28,29), and initial reports of the use of this compound in a variety of neurological diseases have been promising (30-32). Other uses of SPECT imaging include blood-brain barrier evaluation and vascular volume determination (33), as well as receptor imaging, which to date has explored only the cholinergic system using the muscarinic antagonist ^{123}I-QNB (34).

Subjects and Methods

We have performed SPECT studies of rCBF in patients with AD or MID and healthy control subjects. All subjects are part of a clinical study investigating both the cerebral physiology and neuropsychology of dementia.

We studied eight AD subjects, all of whom met current research criteria for AD (35,36). All subjects were free of significant medical illnesses including hypertension, were taking no medications, and had an Hachinski ischemia scale score of <4 (37). The mean age of the subjects was 70.8 years (S.D. = 5.26; range = 63-79). The patients were of various disease severities, with a mean score on the Mini Mental Status Questionnaire (MMSQ) (38) of 15.25 (S.D. = 10.2; range = 4-28). There were four men and four women; six of the patients were right handed whereas two were left handed. There were two presenile and six senile patients. All subjects, in addition to laboratory evaluation to rule out treatable causes of dementia, had x-ray CT scans which were normal or revealed only cortical atrophy. Neuropsychological evaluation entailed a battery of tests which included the MMSQ as an index of dementia severity. Other tests evaluated other neuropsychological functions such as verbal and visual memory, constructional ability, language, praxis, visuospatial ability and affect.

Control subjects were free of any significant medical, psychiatric or neurological illnesses, were taking no medications and were functioning at normal intellectual levels. There were four subjects in this group. Their mean age was 78.1 (S.D. = 5.2; range = 67-79), and there were three women and one man. All subjects were right handed. There were no differences between the control and Alzheimer groups in age, sex, handedness, or education.

We also studied one subject with MID. This patient was a 72-year-old right-handed man with a six-year history of progressive dementia with a stepwise course. He had a history of several stokes, and a 20-year history of hypertension which had been treated intermittently. He had mild to moderate dementia (MMSQ of 22), with relatively normal language function except for diminished verbal fluency as measured by a word-list production task. He also demonstrated visuospatial difficulties, memory impairment and severe difficulties with "frontal" tasks, with diminished initiation, poor planning, apathy and disorganization of thought processes. The Hachinski ischemia scale score was 9. In addition, he had extremely brisk reflexes diffusely with bilateral ankle clonus and Babinski signs. There were bilateral forced grasp reflexes and a jaw jerk, with a stiff-legged, spastic shuffling gait.

SPECT imaging is performed on a modified CLEON 810 scanner (39). This instrument has 12 NaI crystals, each with a focal collimator, which tangentially scan the head. The detectors scan a line and then move inward or outward to scan another line. Repetition of this process provides 12 linear scans for each crystal, which are then reconstructed. One tomographic level is scanned at a time, with a resolution of 14 mm full-width at half-maximum (FWHM) in the transverse section, a slice thickness of 13 mm and a sensitivity of 10,000 cts/sec per μCi/ml for ^{123}I (40). Patients are positioned in the scanner and scans obtained at a level parallel to the canthomeatal line. All subjects are studied in a quiet room, in the awake state with eyes and ears unoccluded. IMP is injected as a 5-mCi bolus. Scanning begins 10 min later and continues for 60 min. During this time three to five tomographic levels are obtained. Each level is imaged for either 10 or 20 min.

For the purposes of this study, we quantitatively analyzed data obtained at the midventricular level, usually 7-8 cm above the external auditory meatus (OM + 8). All scans represented 20 minutes of data acquisition. Regions of interest were drawn in anatomical brain regions by an operator trained in neuroanatomy. These regions consisted of left and right frontal cortex (LF and RF), left and right temporoparietal cortex (LTP and RTP), and left and right entire cortex (LE and RE). The system software provided the measurement of activity density in the form of counts/mm^2. We then calculated the percentage difference between frontal and temporoparietal (F-TP) activity using the ratio:

$$\frac{(LF + RF)/2\text{-}(LTP + RTP)/2}{(LF + RF + LTP + RTP)/4} \times 100\%$$

We also evaluated differences between left and right hemispheres by calculating a ratio reflective of right - left percentage difference for each region. Thus, for frontal cortex, the right - left percentage difference was defined as:

$$\frac{(LF - RF)}{(LF + RF)/2} \times 100\%$$

This ratio was calculated for frontal, temporoparietal and entire cortex for patients in the AD and control groups.

Results

Figure 1 shows representative images of an AD patient and a control subject. The Alzheimer subject demonstrates regionally diminished tracer uptake which is localized to the temporoparietal cortex with relative sparing of the frontal cortex. The control image shows symmetrical, even distribution of radiotracer uptake throughout the cortical mantle.

Figure 2 shows images obtained at 10 and 20 min of imaging time with the respective count rates. The quality of the image is acceptable at 10 min but improves considerably at 20 min. We therefore utilized 20-min data for our quantitative analysis of the images. The image shown in this figure was obtained at the basal ganglia level, and subcortical nuclei are clearly seen. For purposes of data analysis, we utilized images obtained only at the midventricular level, as seen in Figure 1.

Images of the MID patient obtained using three modalities are shown in Figure 3. X-ray CT demonstrates significant periventricular lucencies. The NMR study (obtained with a TR of 2000 and TE of 70, second echo) demonstrates increased signal in the periventricular regions as well as basal ganglia lacunar infarcts. The SPECT study demonstrates markedly diminished perfusion of both frontal cortices.

Quantitative analysis of the SPECT data is seen in Figure 4, which demonstrates the F - TP percent difference for each AD and control patient. Since we studied only one MID patient, we excluded him from the statistical analysis. From these data, it is clear that the F - TP ratio is significantly different in the two groups, with AD patients demonstrating a higher value (22% mean) than controls (3%) ($p = 0.003$). The higher value indicates less temporoparietal than frontal activity. There is, however, some overlap between the two groups, as one AD patient with a ratio of 7% clearly falls in the normal range. With the exception of this patient, if we choose a ratio of 12%, there is no overlap between the groups. The MID patient's percent difference ratio was -3. This negative value, demonstrating more severe involvement of frontal than temporoparietal cortex, was well outside the AD group's range.

To evaluate possible asymmetries, single-hemisphere F - TP ratios were calculated. There was no difference between the left- and right-hemisphere F - TP ratio in either group, and the F - TP ratio was significantly different between AD and control groups in both hemispheres. In addition, there was no difference in the asymmetry ratio between groups for either frontal, temporoparietal or entire cortex, suggesting that neither hemisphere was preferentially involved in any of these regions.

We also noted a tendency for the increasing severity of the dementia to be reflected in the severity of the temporoparietal flow diminution. Patients with severe dementia demonstrated large deficiencies in tracer uptake posteriorly, whereas more mildly affected patients did not demonstrate such remarkable changes. This difference is reflected in Figure 5, which shows SPECT images of three patients of different disease severities.

Discussion

These findings demonstrate, most importantly, that the results of metabolic imaging studies in AD using PET are reproducible with the more widely available SPECT technique. Thus, SPECT may be useful in the differential diagnosis of dementing illnesses. This is, however, a preliminary study with respect to answering the question of the utility of SPECT in dementia diagnosis. The small sample size makes conclusions regarding sensitivity and specificity conjectural. Nevertheless, it is clear that the choice of an F - TP ratio of 12% as a cutoff point for our sample produced only one false-negative result and no false positives. Interestingly, the Alzheimer patient who would have been inappropriately classified as a control subjects was only mildly affected, with a MMSQ of 27. The patient's wife had noted slow, gradual cognitive deterioration for three years, but the family physician, who had evaluated him 3 months prior to our study, felt that he was cognitively normal. Nevertheless, performance on neuropsychological testing revealed mild but definite recent memory dysfunction, marked by slow initial learning, a rapid loss of new information after delays and mild problems with intrusion errors on recall. Other cognitive functions appeared intact. Indeed, because of this limitation of cognitive deficits to only one realm (memory), he might be better classified as possible rather than probable AD (35). While an exhaustive clinical neuropsychological evaluation thus suggests a mild stage of the disease, the SPECT results were in the normal range.

Similar findings regarding the sensitivity of SPECT in AD have been reported by other investigators. A recent SPECT study utilizing IMP (41) found that the parietal-to-cerebellar ratio correctly discriminated all patients with severe dementia from controls and incorrectly classified only 2 of 10 patients with mild to moderate dementia. The ratios of frontal, temporal and visual cortex to cerebellum produced considerable overlap between AD and control groups. Two other studies using qualitative observer ratings of SPECT images in dementia demonstrated similar results, finding marked involvement of temporoparietal cortex which discriminated most (not all) of the AD subjects from control subjects and MID patients (42,43). At this point, SPECT seems to be sensitive to most moderate and severe cases of AD but may not discriminate all early cases of the disease. However, only a small number of patients have been studied to date.

Some limitations of SPECT may be attributed in part to the resolution of current instruments. Increased resolution will result in more accurate measurements of radioactivity distribution in structures such as cerebral cortex which are surrounded by structures with relatively less tracer uptake such as scalp and white matter. Improvement in resolution comes at the expense of sensitivity, however. For example, if an instrument with a current resolution of 14 mm FWHM is improved to a resolution of 7 mm FWHM, sensitivity will be reduced by a factor of 4. The use of ^{99m}Tc imaging agents can overcome this problem, as more favorable patient dosimetry will allow injections of up to four times the dose given in ^{123}I studies.

Previous experience using PET in AD is also relevent to the issue of sensitivity of disease detection. One serial PET study of a patient with familial AD demonstrated normal glucose metabolism at a stage when clinical memory deficits were mild but definite (44), suggesting that PET metabolic imaging may not be sensitive in very early stages of the disease. Nevertheless, several studies have included patients in early dementia stages (10,45) and have found metabolic defects. Some of these patients have had clinical neuropsychological deficits limited to memory loss. Whether the presence or absence of these regional abnormalities in a given patient is useful in diagnosis, however, has not been established, since both issues of sensitivity and specificity must be addressed in greater detail.

One potential criticism of SPECT studies is that problems of sensitivity in diagnosis may result from the use of regional brain ratios of radioactivity rather than direct quantitative measurements of absolute regional cerebral blood flow. The current quantitative limitations of SPECT systems due to problems with scatter, attenuation correction, and resolution have resulted in the use of ratios of regional radioactivity which reflect relative CBF, rather than the use of physiological models to measure absolute rCBF. It may be argued that such ratios are less sensitive than absolute measurements of rCBF, since, for example, a F - TP ratio such as the one we used in this study would not show a difference between AD and control patients if both F and TP regions had equally diminished absolute rCBF values in an AD as compared to a control subject. Nevertheless, even PET studies of absolute metabolic rates have been marked by large coefficients of variation (46,47), necessitating the use of regional brain ratios of absolute metabolic values to demonstrate significant differences between groups. Maximum sensitivity may well result from the use of the correct brain ratio which is most sensitive to group and individual differences, rather than from abandoning the use of ratios altogether.

In order to be useful diagnostically, SPECT blood-flow measurements must not only be able to differentiate mildly affected AD patients from healthy controls but must also be able to discriminate different types of dementia. Our findings in the case of MID are interesting in this regard. Clinically and radiologically, our MID patient had a syndrome of multiple lacunar infarcts rather than several large cortical infarcts. In addition, periventricular lucencies were seen on x-ray CT, and increased signal was noted in periventricular regions on NMR. Frontal-lobe signs are a well-described characteristic of lacunar dementia (48), and our patient's symptoms of gait disorder, urinary incontinence, and primitive reflexes are consistent with this neuroanatomical localization. Recently, the neuropathological substrate of these clinical findings has been suggested to consist of lacunar lesions which predominate in white matter, mixed with the incomplete softening in frontal white matter characteristic of Binswanger's disease, or subcortical arteriosclerotic encephalopathy (SAE) (49). In view of the clinical and radiographic findings, our patient thus appears to have a lacunar dementia with possible subcortical arteriosclerotic encephalopathy. Although our SPECT resolution does not allow accurate imaging of white matter, the findings of diminished blood flow bifrontally demonstrate an important pathophysiological concomitant of this syndrome which may be responsible for symptom production. This pattern is not the only one seen in this disease, as a recent report of a patient with biopsy-proved SAE imaged with PET and [^{18}F]-deoxyglucose noted multiple cortical regions of hypometabolism with no frontal predominance (50). These studies may not be directly comparable, however, since the relation between flow (as measured with SPECT) and metabolism (as measured with PET) in vascular dementias is not as clear-cut as in AD.

Nevertheless, other SPECT studies of patients with MID have demonstrated a pattern of multiple cortical perfusion defects (43). Other investigators have suggested that there is no pattern typical of MID (42), a reasonable conjecture given the clinical and pathological heterogeneity of this entity.

The evaluation of other dementia syndromes using SPECT has so far been limited. It appears, for example, that patients with alcohol-related dementia and alcohol-related Korsakoff's syndrome demonstrate no specific cortical abnormalities (42). A frequently important clinical consideration, the differentiation of depression from dementia, has not been rigorously evaluated using SPECT. Nevertheless, the perfusion patterns obtained in AD patients seem to be different from those seen in depressed patients, who show either normal patterns or abnormalities in the frontal lobe of the dominant hemisphere (51).

Our finding of a lack of significant differences between hemispheres is consistent with the results of PET studies, which have demonstrated that overall AD does not have a tendency to predominantly affect one hemisphere more than another (9). These PET studies have shown however that an individual patient may demonstrate significant lateral asymmetry. In addition, it appears that patients with presenile onset more frequently demonstrate right-sided metabolic abnormalities (52). Because of our small subject group, we did not evaluate either of these issues, nor did we explore the relationship between cognitive deficits and particular imaging patterns. The tendency for disease severity to parallel the SPECT image is consistent with some PET studies (22), although others have not demonstrated strong correlations between metabolic data and dementia severity. The ability to study a wider range of patients with SPECT (as more severely demented patients may tolerate the shorter SPECT procedure better than PET) may help in the detection of relationships between severity and these *in vivo* physiological variables.

These preliminary data thus suggest the utility of SPECT in the diagnosis of dementia. The problem of sensitivity must be addressed through the study of mildly affected patients who can then be followed longitudinally. Autopsy correlation is also important in verifying the diagnosis. In addition, it will be important to investigate different patterns in different dementias as well as in depression. SPECT also has promise as a research tool, since it may provide a physiological method of following the progression of degenerative changes in the living patient. Finally, the future use of SPECT with tracers capable of evaluating neurotransmitter receptors may provide specific insights into pathophysiologic processes in dementia.

Acknowledgments

The authors thank the staff of the Northern California Alzheimer's Disease Center and Kay Bristol for assistance and technical support, and Dr. Robert Friedland for encouragement and advice. Photon Diagnostics, Inc. provided the basic SPECT instrumentation through Mr. Peter DeLuca. This work was supported by NIH grant AG05890-02 from the National Institute on Aging, by the Medical Research Service of the United States Veterans Administration, and by the Director, Office of Energy Research, Office of Health and Environmental Research of the United States Department of Energy under contract DE-AC03-76SF00098.

References

1. Tomlinson, B.E., Blessed, G. & Roth, M. (1970) *J. Neurol. Sci.* **11**, 205-242.
2. Gado, M., Hughes, C.P., Danziger, W. *et al.* (1982) *Radiology* **144**, 535-538.
3. Phelps, M.E. & Mazziotta, J.C. (1985) *Science* **228**, 799-809.
4. Kuhl, D.E., Barrio, J.R., Huang, S-C. *et al.* (1982) *J. Nucl. Med.* **23**, 196-203.
5. Ell, P.J., Hockness, J.M.L., Jarritt, P.H. *et al.* (1985) *Nucl. Med. Commun.* **6**, 437-441.
6. Benson, D.F., Kuhl, D.E., Hawkins, R.A. *et al.* (1983) *Arch. Neurol.* **40**, 711-714.
7. Friedland, R.P., Budinger, T.F., Ganz, E. *et al.* (1983) *J. Comput. Assist. Tomogr.* **7**, 590-598.
8. Chase, T.N., Foster, N.L., Fedio, P., Brooks, R., Mansi, L. & DiChiro, G. (1984) *Ann. Neurol.* **15** (suppl), S170-S174.
9. Friedland, R.P., Budinger, T.F., Koss, E. *et al.* (1985) *Neurosci. Lett.* **53**, 235-240.
10. Haxby, J.V., Duara, R., Grady, C.L., Cutler, N.R. & Rapoport, S.I. (1985) *J. Cereb. Blood Flow Metab.* **5**, 193-200.
11. Foster, N.L., Chase, T.N., Fedio, P., Patronas, N.J., Brooks, R.A. & DiChiro, G. (1983) *Neurology* **33**, 961-965.
12. Friedland, R.P., Budinger, T.F., Brant-Zawadzki, M. & Jagust, W.J. (1984) *JAMA* **252**, 2750-2752.
13. Jagust, W.J., Friedland, R.P. & Budinger, T.F. (1985) *J. Neurol. Neurosurg. & Psychiatr.* **48**, 1091-1096.
14. Ferris, S.H., deLeon, M.J., Wolf, A.P. *et al.* (1983) In: *The Dementias,* eds. Mayeus, R. & Rosen, W.G. (Raven Press, New York) pp. 123-129.

15. Friedland, R.P., Brun, A. & Budinger, T.F. (1985) *Lancet* **1**, 228.
16. Brun, A. & Englund, E. (1981) *Histopathology* **5**, 549-564.
17. Davies, P. (1979) *Brain Res.* **171**, 319-327.
18. Rossor, M.N., Garrett, N.J., Johnson, A.L., Mountjoy, C.Q., Rothe, M. & Iverson, L.L. (1982) *Brain* **105**, 313-330.
19. Karp, H. (1983) In: *Clinical Neurology*, eds. Baker, A.B. & Baker, L.H. (Harper & Row, Philadelphia) pp. 1-31.
20. Friedland, R.P., Jagust, W.J., Ober, B.A. *et al.* (1986) *Neurology* **36 (suppl 1)**, 268 (abstract).
21. Kamo, H., McGeer, P.L., Harrop, R., McGeer, E.G., Pate, B.D., Martin, W.R.W. & Li, D.K.B. (1986) *Neurology* **36 (suppl 1)**, 266 (abstract).
22. Frackowiak, R.S.J., Pozzilli, C., Legg, N.J., DuBoulay, G.H., Marshall, J., Lenzi, G.L. & Jones, T. (1981) *Brain* **104**, 753-778.
23. Jaszczak, R.J. & Coleman, R.E. (1985) *Invest. Radiol.* **20**, 897-910.
24. Coleman, R.E., Blinder, R.A. & Jaszcak, R.J. (1986) *Invest. Radiol.* **21**, 1-11.
25. Budinger, T.F. (1985) In: *Positron Emission Tomography,* eds. Reivich, M. & Alavi, A. (Alan R. Liss, New York) pp. 227-240.
26. Holman, B.L., Lee, R.G., Hill, T.C., Lovett, R.D. & Lister-James, T. (1984) *J. Nucl. Med.* **25**, 25-30.
27. Loberg, M.D. (1980) *J. Nucl. Med.* **21**, 183-196.
28. Neirinckx, R.D., Nowotnik, D.P., Canning, L., Harrison, R.C., Pickett, R.D., Volkert, W.A., Troutner, D. & Chaplin, S. (1986) *J. Nucl. Med.* **27**, 905 (abstract).
29. Volkert, W.A., Hoffman, T.J., McKenzie, E.H., Chaplin, S.B. & Holmes, R.A. (1986) *J. Nucl. Med.* **27**, 905 (abstract).
30. Podreka, I., Suess, E., Goldenberg, G., Steiner, M., Brucke, Th., Muller, Ch. & Deecke, L. (1986) *J. Nucl. Med.* **27**, 887 (abstract).
31. Yeh, S.H., Liu, R.S., Hu, H.H. *et al.* (1986) *J. Nucl. Med.* **27**, 888 (abstract).
32. Berberich, A., Buell, U., Eilles, A. *et al.* (1986) *J. Nucl. Med.* **27**, 888 (abstract).
33. Kuhl, D.E., Reivich, M., Alavi, A., Nyary, M. & Staum, M. (1975) *Circ. Res.* **36**, 610.
34. Eckelman, W.C., Reba, R.C., Rzeszotarski, W.J. *et al.* (1984) *Science* **223**, 291-293.
35. McKhann, G., Drachman, D., Folstein, M., Katzman, R., Price, D. & Stadlan, E. (1984) *Neurology* **34**, 939-944.
36. American Psychiatric Association. (1980) *Diagnostic and Statistical Manual of Mental Disorders.* Third Ed., pp. 124-146.
37. Hachinski, V.C., Iliff, L.D., Zilkha, E., DuBoulay, G.H., McAllister,

V.L., Marshall, J., Russell, R.W.R. & Lindsay, S. (1975) *Arch. Neurol.* **32**, 632-637.

38. Folstein, M.F., Folstein, S.E. & McHugh, P.R. (1975) *J. Psychiatr. Res.* **12**, 189-198.
39. Kirsch, C-M., Moore, S.C., Zimmerman, R.E., English, R.J. & Holman, B.L. (1981) *J. Nucl. Med.* **22**, 726-731.
40. Hill, T.C., Holman, L., Lovett, R. *et al.* (1982) *J. Nucl. Med.* **23**, 191-195.
41. Mueller, S.P., Johnson, K.A., Hamil, D., English, R.J., Nagel, S.J., Ichise, M. & Holman, B.L. (1986) *J. Nucl. Med.* **27**, 889 (abstract).
42. Sharp, P., Gemmell, H., Cherryman, G., Besson, J., Crawford, J. & Smith, F. (1986) *J. Nucl. Med.* **27**, 761-768.
43. Cohen, M.B., Graham, L.S., Lake, R. *et al.* (1986) *J. Nucl. Med.* **27**, 769-774.
44. Cutler, N.R., Haxby, J.V., Duara, R. *et al.* (1985) *Neurology* **35**, 1556-1561.
45. Duara, R., Grady, C., Haxby, J. *et al.* (1986) *Neurology* **36**, 879-887.
46. Duara, R., Grady, C., Haxby, J. *et al.* (1984) *Ann. Neurol.* **16**, 702-713.
47. Reivich, M., Rosen, A.D., Kushner, M., Gur, R.C. & Alavi, A. (1983) In: *Functional Radionuclide Imaging of the Brain,* ed. Magistretti, P.L. (Raven Press, New York) pp. 311-318.
48. Roman, G.C. (1985) In: *Senile Dementia of the Alzheimer Type,* eds. Hutton, J.T. & Kenny, A.D. (Alan R. Liss, New York) pp. 131-151.
49. Ishii, N., Nishihara, Y. & Imamura, T. (1986) *Neurology* **36**, 340-345.
50. Friedland, R.P., Koss, E., Jagust, W.J. & Borcich, J. (1986) *Neurology* **36 (suppl 1)**, 102 (abstract).
51. Holman, B.L. (1986) *J. Nucl. Med.* **27**, 855-860.
52. Koss, E., Friedland, R.P., Ober, B.A. & Jagust, W.J. (1985) *Am. J. Psychiatr.* **142**, 638-640.

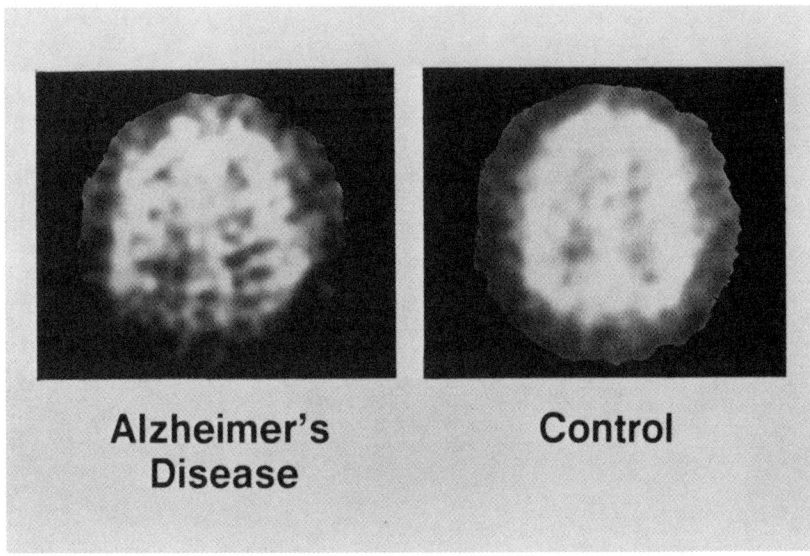

Fig. 1. Representative SPECT-IMP images from a patient with Alzheimer's disease and a healthy control subject.

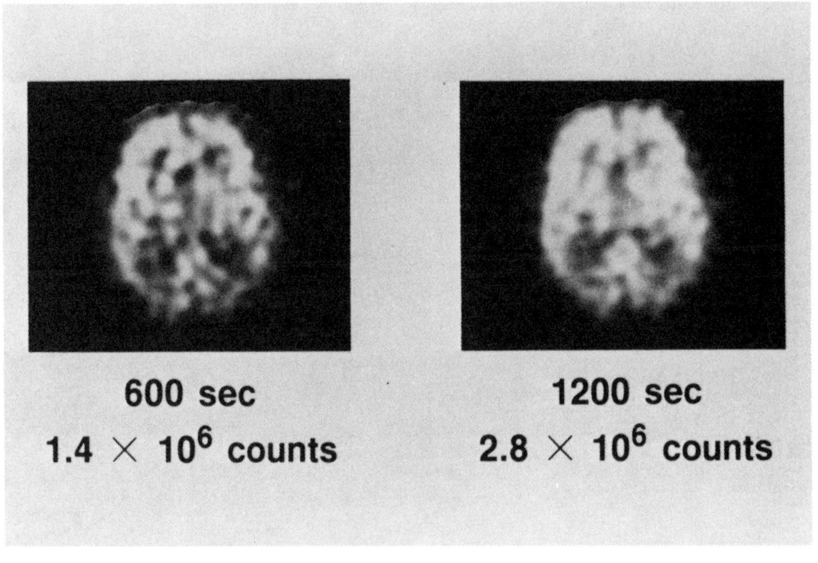

Fig. 2. An example of the effect of imaging time on the quality of data. The image on the left was obtained after 10 minutes of data collection at one level, while the image on the right includes an additional 10 minutes of imaging time. Total number of counts in the slice is shown beneath each image. Imaging was begun 10 minutes following the injection of 5 mCi of IMP.

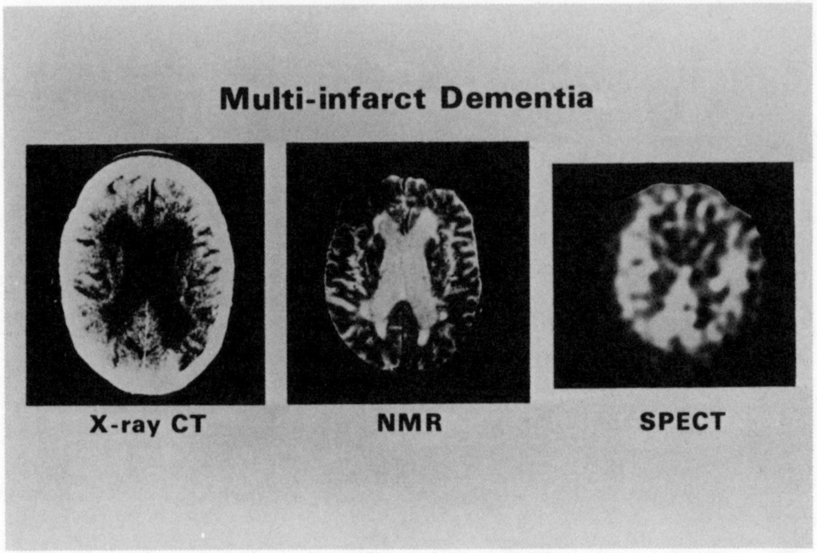

Fig. 3. X-ray CT, NMR (TR 2000, TE 70), and SPECT-IMP images of the patient with multi-infarct dementia demonstrating periventricular lucencies on CT and increased signal on NMR, with deep subcortical infarction. The SPECT image demonstrates diminished flow in bilateral frontal cortex.

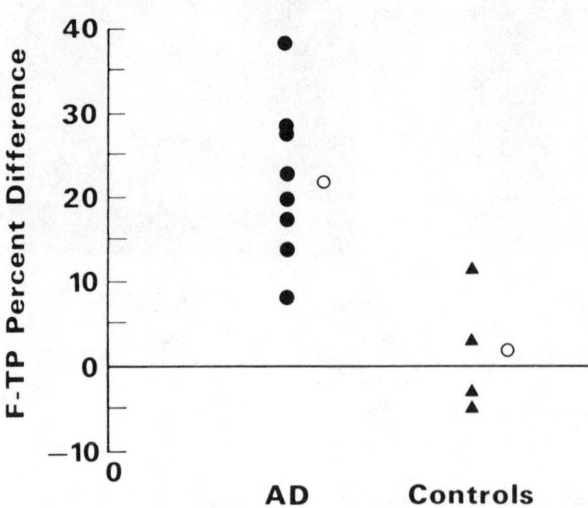

Fig. 4. The frontal-temporoparietal (F-TP) percentage difference for Alzheimer's disease (AD) and control subjects. Means for the two groups (represented by open circles) are significantly different, p=0.003.

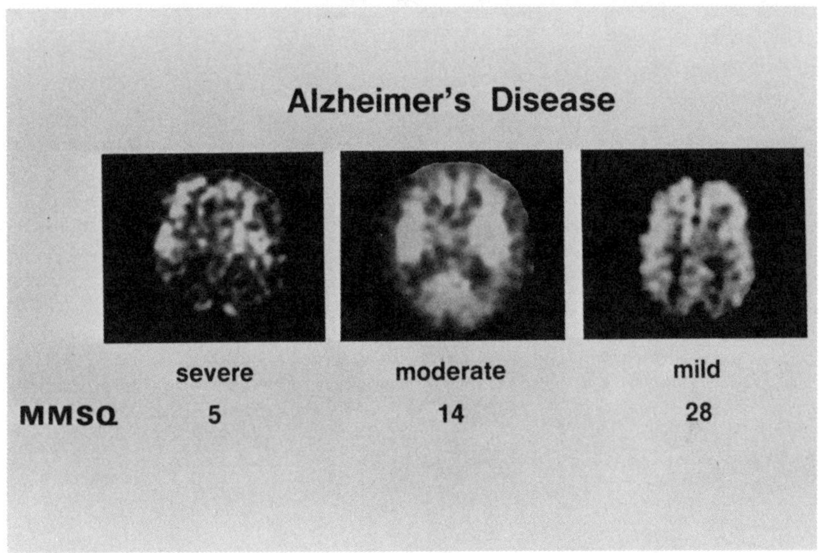

Fig. 5. SPECT-IMP scans for patients of varying disease severities, demonstrating more pronounced temporoparietal blood flow deficits with increasing dementia severity (measured by mini mental status questionnaire, MMSQ).

15. Clinical Diagnosis of Alzheimer's Disease

D. FRANK BENSON, M.D.

The Augustus S. Rose Professor of Neurology
Department of Neurology UCLA School of Medicine
Los Angeles, California 90024

ABSTRACT: An assured diagnosis of Alzheimer's disease is difficult in the living subject, a serious dilemma since inaccurate diagnoses lead to mismanagement of the demented patient and produce erroneous and/or inconclusive results in Alzheimer research. Various sets of clinical criteria, minimal neuropathological criteria and a myriad of "markers" for the disease have been devised. All fall short but together they have produced a consistent improvement in diagnostic accuracy. Current clinical criteria for diagnosis of Alzheimer's disease will be reviewed and a number of the better confirmatory tests will be outlined.

Introduction

With the sharp increase in research on Alzheimer's disease (AD) in the past decade, a serious dilemma has been highlighted. In the living patient, an assured diagnosis of AD has proved difficult; and inaccurate diagnoses, particularly the inclusion in AD research protocols of individuals with causes of dementia other than AD, has produced both inconclusive studies and erroneous research outcomes. In addition, incorrect diagnoses continue to lead to mismanagement and inappropriate or inadequate treatment of patients with dementia.

For a number of reasons, this absence of ready accurate diagnosis of AD was not a problem in prior decades. Originally, the diagnostic criteria for AD were restrictive and the disorder was thus rare; in addition, the population at risk for the disorder was not large. Both of these features have changed. The current definitions of dementia of the Alzheimer type (DAT) and senile dementia of the Alzheimer type (SDAT) have been greatly broadened, and the population at risk has grown immensely. As a result, AD has become a significant public health problem.

In the past decade, the problem of providing a working diagnosis of dementia, particularly of AD, has been faced, and considerable progress has been made. Lipowski published a series of essays concerning psychiatric diagnoses with particular emphasis on what was then called chronic brain syndrome (1,2). He refused to accept the then-current definition of dementia as a permanent and irreversible defect of intellectual function. Because of this influence, the third edition of the *Diagnostic and Statistical Manual of Mental Diseases (DSM-III)* of the American Psychiatric Association presented an operational definition for dementia (3) (Table 1). As an addendum to this definition, a disorder that became known as primary degenerative dementia (PDD) was introduced (Table 2). Many workers consider PDD a euphemism for AD, and at best it is a loose diagnosis.

More recently, the National Institute of Neurologic and Communicative Disorders and Stroke (NINCDS) and the Alzheimer's Disease and Related Disorders Association (ADRDA) combined forces to present criteria for the clinical diagnosis of dementia of the Alzheimer's type (4). A blue-ribbon committee agreed on practical, clinical observations and suggested diagnostic criteria for determining probable AD, possible AD, and probable exclusion of AD. As in DSM-III, the principal criteria for the diagnosis of "probable" AD were progressive worsening of memory and other cognitive functions and the absence of other known causes for the mental deficits. Separate criteria were suggested for neuropsychological testing to confirm the diagnosis.

Even more recently, a number of neuropathologists have jointly presented criteria that will allow the neuropathologist to diagnose probable AD on the basis of histologic changes only; i.e., when no history is available (Table 3).

Unfortunately, each of these sets of criteria has significant defects. For example, the criteria used in DSM-III are far too broad, although they represent a significant forward step: far too many non-AD causes of dementia fit the PDD classification. One important step is the inclusion of a clause demanding that a diagnosis of PDD be made only after excluding other causes of dementia. This concept is correct, but exclusion is entirely dependent on the energy and clinical acumen of the investigator. When an evaluation is incomplete or incompetent, many individuals with a cause of dementia not of the Alzheimer type will legitimately be said to have PDD. Despite these weaknesses, the DSM-III criteria have been the principal guidelines for research in dementia in the past five to six years, so much of this research must be considered tainted by the inclusion of non-DAT subjects.

The criteria set up by NINCDS/ADRDA are better but are sufficiently broad to include other recognized causes of dementia and, as is also true of the DSM-III criteria, suffer from being cross-sectional. The early stage of AD cannot be classified with the NINCDS/ADRDA criteria: only when the disease has become pronounced can a diagnosis of probable AD be entertained. Moreover, as the disease progresses toward an end-stage dementia, these criteria no longer prove valid. It is a well-known fact that dementias with a wide variety of causes produce similar end-stage clinical states. Thus, although a useful and necessary step, the NINCDS/ADRDA criteria have not proved instrumental in improving AD research.

Finally, the proposed neuropathological criteria appear of value but are of such recent origin that they are not yet in use in any institution. Almost no neuropathological confirmation of AD in the current literature meets these criteria. It will be some years before they have been validated and are in use for research confirmation.

Difficulties in Diagnostic Research

A number of problems stemming from the style of the disorder deserve consideration. First, DAT is insidious; rarely does an individual present with an ictal onset of the symptom picture. Moreover, the timing of the initial suspicion of the presence of Alzheimer dementia usually depends on the sensitivity of the patient's family and friends. Only rarely is a personal physician sufficiently knowledgeable about the patient to suspect the diagnosis until the disease is fairly well established. Thus, early cases are rarely available for research activities.

A second problem lies in the fact that DAT is progressive, and this longitudinal course must be recognized if Alzheimer research is to be valid. The symptoms and signs change slowly but continuously during the course of the disease; each patient's disorder therefore must be viewed in separate states: as many as seven, although a more manageable three states appears sufficient (5,6) (Table 4). In other words, to make a diagnosis of AD, testing must be performed on a longitudinal basis, and the disorder cannot be described adequately by any single cross-sectional set of criteria such as those of DSM-III or NINCDS/ADRDA. Although the variations in the clinical picture in the different stages are well known, rarely are these variations taken into consideration in protocols for research.

Another problem facing the investigator concerns the variability of DAT. In particular, the presentation may vary, with distinctly different prime features. For instance, it is consistently stated that memory disorder must be present and may be the only problem noted early; but cases have been recorded in which a progressive aphasia was present for many months before other findings could be discerned (7), and some cases record a serious apraxia without evidence of other disorder until later in the course. One of the most common findings prompting medical evaluation is visuospatial disturbance, a disorientation in a familiar environment, suggesting yet another type of onset. Clinically, it is common for mild memory and language defects to be ignored by the family, but when the patient gets lost, medical advice is sought. Although any of these disorders may be present as the prime feature, careful testing usually demonstrates the presence of some problem with the other cognitive functions also. Unfortunately, most physicians are not skilled at behavioral examination, and pertinent features therefore are overlooked.

Yet another problem stems from the type of patients at risk for AD. Although classically the disorder occurs in the presenile years, it is far more common in the later years; and this group, the elderly patients, almost always have some other medical disorders that may compromise mental efficiency so that a complex clinical picture is often present. The exclusion criteria of DSM-III, if rigidly applied, would reject many cases of primary AD.

Finally, as noted, the end-stages of the dementias produced by many different disorders tend to be similar. A diagnosis of AD suspected at one stage may not be confidently confirmed by longitudinal evaluation. Demonstration of end-stage dementia may appear to confirm a diagnosis of DAT when, in fact, it is the end-stage of another cause of dementia.

Correct diagnosis and confirmation of AD is crucial for both clinical and research purposes. Nevertheless, currently, many clinicians find it difficult to distinguish DAT from the hundreds of other causes of dementia.

Differential Diagnosis of Dementia

At present, the chief means of diagnosing dementia revolve about the clinical examination, so a review of this process is indicated. First, an operational definition of dementia is needed. Table 5 presents one suggested definition. When the clinician suspects dementia, crude confirmation may be obtained from one of the many short tests for dementia currently in use; these include the Mini-Mental State examination (8), the Blessed examination (9) and the Washington University examination (10) among others. Each has significant limitations, but such tools can be useful in confirming and monitoring the progression of dementia. They are far less successful as diagnostic tools, as many patients with disabling mental impairment score well on these tests.

Following determination of the presence of dementia, various causes of the problem must be considered. For this step, we suggest use of a differential diagnostic inventory (Table 6). Interpretation of results with this inventory usually separates cortical degenerative dementia from other types. The criteria outlined in the diagnostic inventory provide a positive approach to the diagnosis of AD, eliminating the exclusion criterion.

Once the probable causes of AD and Pick's disease have been identified, other causes of dementia must be sought. Figure 1 contains a diagnostic flowsheet suggested for this process. Each entity in this flowsheet—degenerative dementia, vascular dementia, the dementia of movement disorders, the dementia of depression, hydrocephalic dementia, and the chronic confusional states—can be suspected on the basis of specific symptomatology plus, in most cases, specific confirmatory laboratory studies. Thus, in addition to mental impairment, individuals with vascular dementia almost always show some degree of basic neurologic defect; e.g., spasticity or visual field defect; and a simple guide list, the Hachinski test (11), almost always produces an elevated score when vascular dementia is present. Movement disorders are routinely diagnosed by noting the obvious abnormalities of movement. A slowing of thought processing, bradyphrenia, is the basic mental impairment in these disorders. At present, the most common cause of dementia of movement disorders are the drugs used for the treatment of psychiatric disorders, a helpful medical clue.

The dementia of depression can prove difficult to diagnose. Questionnaires such as the Beck (12) or Zung (13) can provide helpful confirming information. Unfortunately, the results can also be misleading. Depression is extremely common in the elderly but is not a common cause of dementia. Hydrocephalic dementia can be suspected from the presence of the triad of movement problem, dementia and incontinence and can be confirmed by computed tomography (CT) or isotope cisternography. Finally, a huge group of causes of dementia, the chronic confusional states, deserve careful attention (Table 7). Clinical suspicion plus many laboratory studies are needed, and even then these entities can be difficult to demonstrate. The chronic confusional states are frequently misdiagnosed, most often as AD. This is unfortunate, as many of the disorders producing a chronic confusional state will respond to appropriate treatment.

The abundance of different disorders that can produce dementia that resembles DAT at least superficially creates a significant diagnostic problem for the clinician and, as would be anticipated, misdiagnosis is common. Table 8 presents the figures compiled in one year at various UCLA-operated clinics showing the final diagnosis of patients referred for management of AD (or euphemisms such as chronic brain syndrome, senile dementia or PDD). In fewer than 25% of the patients was a diagnosis of AD confirmed. The frequency of erroneous diagnoses, particularly false-positive ones, of AD must certainly concern any investigator attempting to carry out research on the disorder.

Laboratory Examinations

To aid the diagnosis of AD, a number of laboratory examinations have been recommended. Without exception, these tests have significant defects.

Neuropsychological testing is frequently used in the evaluation of dementia and does provide useful information. Most specifically, the presence and severity of dementia (intellectual impairment) can be demonstrated, and serial testing readily demonstrates the worsening, or lack thereof, of a dementing condition. Most currently used psychological tests focus on the higher cortical functions, and dementia featuring psychomotor retardation may be overlooked because the patient appears to function far better in the test situation than in real life. Also, current neuropsychological tests do not provide etiologic diagnoses; none can either suggest or confirm a diagnosis of AD.

The clinical laboratory provides many tests of great value for the evaluation of dementia, but none is useful for the diagnosis of AD. Thus, although tests such as blood counts, electrolyte levels, endocrine assays, heavy-metal screening and tissue studies may provide diagnostic information for some disorders causing dementia, these tests only aid in exclusion of these disorders in a workup for AD.

Both electroencephalography and various measures of evoked response have been suggested as tests for AD. However, both have failed to provide useful information. Much research on the use of P300 or other late-occurring wave forms in evoked-response studies continues, but to date, none of these measures has proved sufficiently specific to confirm a diagnosis of AD.

Many means of imaging the brain have likewise failed to provide specific information in patients with AD. Both CT and magnetic resonance imaging are valuable in the workup of dementia but do not provide definitive information in AD (Fig. 2). Isotope emission studies appear promising but do not yet provide data that confidently distinguish AD from other causes of dementia. Positron emission tomography (PET) scans, both blood flow and metabolic, are distinctly abnormal in patients with AD but are also abnormal in other dementias. The possibility that cerebral activation studies with isotope techniques may provide diagnostic information can be considered but there is no evidence at present to support their usefulness.

A number of cerebrospinal fluid (CSF) metabolites have been looked at in the hope that they would indicate the presence of AD. These substances include cholinergic, monoaminergic and peptidergic neurotransmitters. Alterations are noted in the CSF in cases of AD, but unfortunately they are not unique to this disorder. Additional studies have looked at somatostatin and opiate concentrations in the CSF but have yet to prove conclusive. Peripheral-blood abnormalities have been studied as diagnostic markers, with considerable work having been done on acetylcholine metabolism in erythrocytes and the presence of abnormal amyloid deposits or an altered thermophilic reaction of lymphocytes. To date, none has proved specific for AD.

In the past several years, an old technique, brain biopsy, has been resurrected as a means of providing positive confirmation of an AD diagnosis. In recently reported studies, Neary and colleagues demonstrated that brain tissue from patients with AD shows both chemical (neurotransmitter) and anatomical abnormalities that appear specific (14). Unfortunately, cerebral biopsy is a mutilating surgical procedure with a risk of significant residuals and is used only as an experimental procedure. Nonetheless, biopsy appears to be the most promising confirmatory test for AD and may become essential as a tool for designating individuals for research.

Finally, autopsy is the "gold standard" of diagnostic procedures for confirmation of suspected AD. As noted earlier, stringent histopathologic criteria are now available, but they have not yet been validated and are not in use in most laboratories. The suggested criteria demand exacting evaluations but if successful may represent a basic standard to confirm the diagnosis of AD in subjects utilized for investigation.

Conclusion

The making of a confident diagnosis of AD in the living patient is difficult, and errors create a serious problem for research into the disorder. Better diagnostic methods are needed for antemortem diagnosis.

References

1. Lipowski, Z.J. (1975) In: *Psychiatric Aspects of Neurologic Disease*, eds. Benson, D.F. & Blumer, D. (Grune & Stratton, New York), pp 11-34.
2. Lipowski, Z.J. (1980) *Am. J. Psychiatr.* **137**, 674-678.
3. *Diagnostic and Statistical Manual of Mental Disorders, Third Edition* (1980) (American Psychiatric Association, Washington, D.C.).

4. McKhann, G., Drachman, D., Folstein, M., Katzman, R., Price, D. & Stadlan, E.M. (1984) *Neurology* **34**, 939-944.
5. Berg., L., Hughes, C.P., Cuben, L.A., Danziger, W.L., Martin, R.L. & Knesevich, J. (1982) *J. Neurol. Neurosurg. Psychiatr.* **45**, 926-968.
6. Cummings, J.L. & Benson, D.F. (1983) *Dementia - A Clinical Approach* (Butterworths, Boston).
7. Chawluk, J.B., Mesulam, M-M., Hurtig, H., Kushner, M., Weintraub, S., Saykin, A., Rubin, N., Alavi, A. & Reivich, M. (1986) *Ann. Neurol.* **19**, 68-74.
8. Folstein, M.F., Folstein, S.E. & McHugh, P.R. (1975) *J. Psychiatr. Res.* **12**, 189-198.
9. Blessed, G., Tomlinson, B.E. & Roth, M. (1968) *Br. J. Psychiatr.* **114**, 797-811.
10. Storandt, M., Botwinick, J., Danziger, W.L., Berg, L. & Hughes C.P. (1984) *Arch. Neurol.* **41**, 497-499.
11. Hachinksi, V.C., Illiff, L.D., Zilkha, E., Duboulay, G.H., McAllister, V.C., Marshall, J., Russell, R.W.R. & Symon, L. (1975) *Arch. Neurol.* **32**, 632-637.
12. Beck, A.T., Ward, C.H., Mendelson, M., Mack, T. & Erbaugh, J. (1961) *Arch. Gen. Psychiatr.* **4**, 561-571.
13. Zung, W.W.K. (1965) *Arch. Gen. Psychiatr.* **12**, 63-70.
14. Neary, D., Snowden, J.S., Mann, D.M.A., Bowen, D.M., Sims, N.R., Northen, B., Yates, P.O. & Davison, A.N. (1986) *J. Neurol. Neurosurg. Psychiatr.* **49**, 229-237.

TABLE 1. Diagnostic criteria for dementia according to DSM-III

A. A loss of intellectual abilities of sufficient severity to interfere with social or occupational functioning.

B. Memory impairment.

C. At least one of the following:

(1) Impairment of abstract thinking, as manifested by concrete interpretation of proverbs, inability to find similarities and differences between related words, difficulty in defining words and concepts, and other similar tasks;
(2) Impaired judgment;
(3) Other disturbances of higher cortical function, such as aphasia (disorder of language due to brain dysfunction), apraxia (inability to carry out motor activities despite intact comprehension and motor function), agnosia (failure to recognize or identify objects despite intact sensory function), "constructional difficulty" (*e.g.*, inability to copy three-dimensional figures, assemble blocks, or arrange sticks in specific designs);
(4) Personality change; *i.e.*, alteration or accentuation of premorbid traits.

D. State of consciousness not clouded (*i.e.*, does not meet the criteria for Delirium or Intoxication, although these may be superimposed).

E. Either (1) or (2):

(1) Evidence from the history, physical examination or laboratory tests of a specific organic factor that is judged to be etiologically related to the disturbance;
(2) In the absence of such evidence, an organic factor necessary for the development of the syndrome can be presumed if conditions other than Organic Mental Disorders have been reasonably excluded and if the behavioral change represents cognitive impairment in a variety of areas.

TABLE 2. Diagnostic criteria for primary degenerative dementia according to DSM-III

A. Dementia (see Table 1).

B. Insidious onset with uniformly progressive deteriorating course.

C. Exclusion of all other specific causes of dementia by the history, physical examination and laboratory tests.

TABLE 3. Neuropathology of Alzheimer's disease

Age (years)	*Minimal microscopic criteria**
<50	≥2–5 plaques or tangles anywhere in neocortex
50 – 65	≥8 plaques/field
60 – 75	≥10 plaques/field
>75	≥15 plaques/field

* Slice thickness: 5–15 m; magnification: 200×.

TABLE 4. Stages of Alzheimer's disease*

Characteristic	*Stage I* (*1 - 3 years*)	*Stage II* (*2 - 10 years*)
Memory	New learning defective; mild impairment of retrieval	Both recent and remote memory defective
Language	Poor word list generation; anomia	Fluent aphasia
Cognition	Alterations of judgment, calculation and abstraction	Significantly impaired
Visuospatial skills	Topographic disorientation; poor construction	Significantly impaired
Personality	Occasional irritability; possible sadness	Indifference, unconcern, disinhibition
Motor	Normal	Normal, restless
Laboratory	CT and EEG normal	EEG - slight slowing; CT - mild atrophy

* Modified from reference 6.

TABLE 5. Definition of dementia*

Dementia is an acquired, persistent impairment of intellectual function with compromise affecting at least three of the following spheres of mental activity:

Speech and/or language

Memory

Cognition

Visuospatial skills

Personality

*Adapted from reference 6.

Stage III (8 - 12 years)
Severely impaired
Severely impaired
Severely impaired
Severely impaired
Total unawareness
Increasing limb rigidity and flexion posture
EEG - diffusely slow CT - atrophy

TABLE 6. Differential diagnosis inventory

Characteristic	*Cortical dementia*	*Subcortical dementia*
Language	Aphasic	Normal
Speech	Normal	Hypophonic, dysarthric, mute
Memory	Amnesia (learning defect)	Forgetful (retrieval defect)
Cognition	Impaired calculation, judgment, abstraction	Slow and dilapidated
Visuospatial skill	Disturbed	Messy and dilapidated
Personality	Unconcerned, disinhibited	Apathetic, depressed
Tone	Normal (until late)	Increased
Posture	Erect (until late)	Stooped, extended
Gait	Normal (until late)	Unsteady
Movements	Quick, nimble (until late), slowed	Tremor, dystonia, chorea

TABLE 7. Classification of chronic confusional states

Category	*Abnormality*
1. Systemic diseases	Pulmonary insufficiency, cardiac insufficiency, anemia
2. Endocrine diseases	Panhypopituitarism, myxedema, Cushing's disease, steroid therapy
3. Vascular diseases	Systemic lupus erythematosus, temporal arteritis, periarteritis nodosa
4. Infectious diseases	Syphilis, Creutzfeldt-Jakob disease, cysticercosis, tuberculosis
5. Chemical poisonings	Organophosphates, anilines, mercury, lead, arsenic
6. Drug poisonings	Haloperidol, lithium, phenothiazines, belladonna, phenytoin
7. Deficiency states	Pellagra, B_{12} deficiency
8. Intracranial masses	Glioma, meningioma, hematoma, metastasis, pituitary adenoma
9. Chronic neurologic disorders	Epilepsy, multiple sclerosis, Parkinson's disease, Machado's disease
10. Miscellaneous	Trauma, dementia pugilistica, hydrocephalus, basilar impression

TABLE 8. Ultimate diagnosis of 90 patients referred with diagnosis of Alzheimer's disease

Diagnosis	*No.*
Alzheimer's disease	22
Pick's disease	2
Multi-infarct dementia	31
Depression	6
Brain tumor	2
Hydrocephalus	4
Chronic confusional state (alcohol, trauma, syphilis)	15
Subcortical dementia (Huntington's disease, parkinsonism)	5
Amnesia	2
Undetermined	1

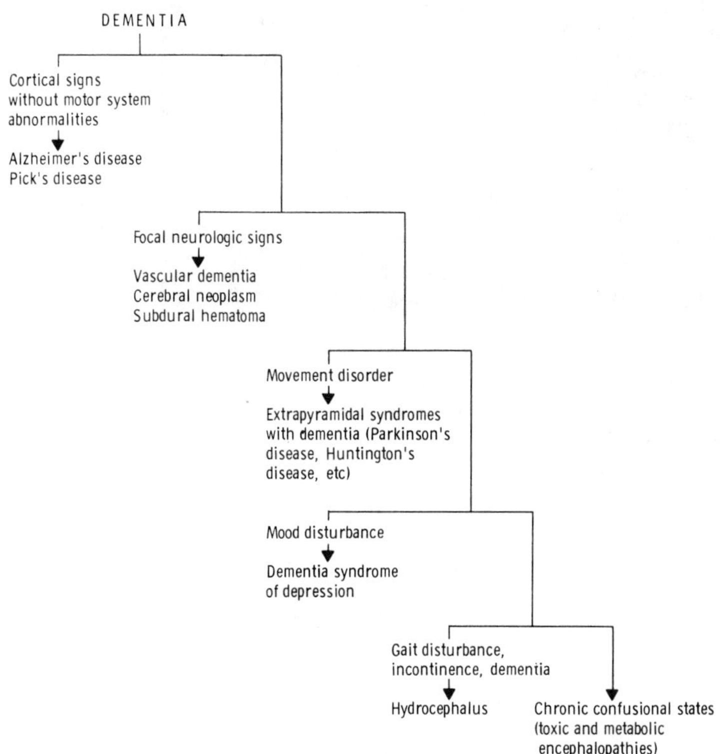

Fig. 1. Diagnostic flowsheet of suggested systematic evaluation of dementia.

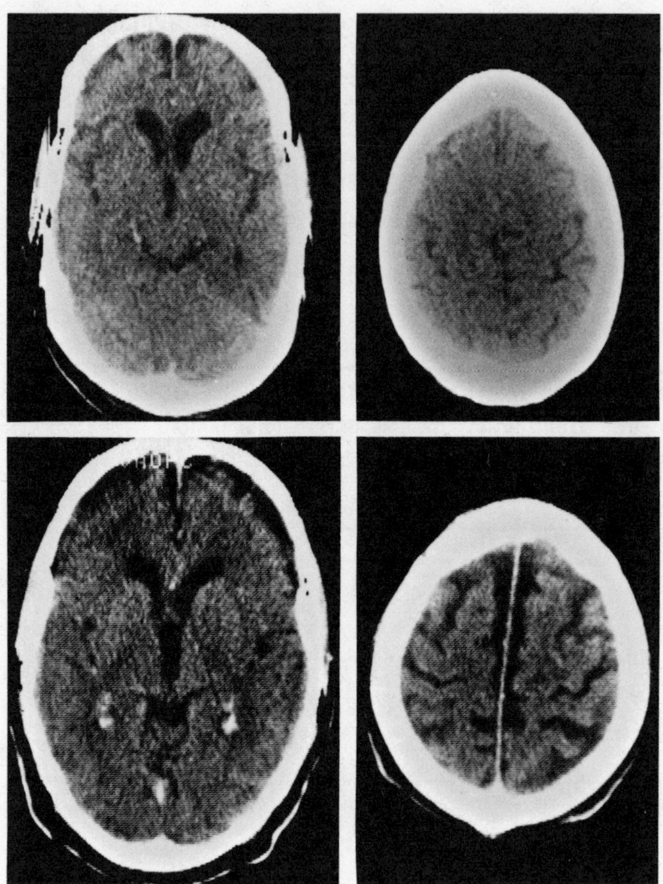

Fig. 2. CT scans on two individuals referred for evaluation of dementia. (Top) Scans were considered within the limits of normal for the patient's age; patient had advanced AD. (Below) Scans show marked central and cortical atrophy. Individual was not demented (IQ 137) but did abuse alcohol. (Reprinted from Benson, D.F. [1982] In: Psychiatric Aspects of Neurologic Disease, Vol. 2. ed. Benson, D.F. & Blumer, D. [Grune & Stratton, New York]).

16. Toward a Psychobiological Taxonomy of Cognitive Impairments

HERBERT WEINGARTNER, Ph.D.*

George Washington University Department of Psychology
Washington, D.C. 20052

JORDAN GRAFMAN,† PAUL NEWHOUSE*

ABSTRACT: Cognitive functions are not unitary but are comprised of psychobiologically distinct component processes. These processes can be identified through systematic studies which contrast how cognition fails in neuropathologically different clinical syndromes as well as through studies in which different classes of drugs are used to model different forms of cognitive dysfunction. An outline of some of those component processes is presented, along with a rationale and strategies for demonstrating that two cognitive domains are psychobiologically distinct. This approach has implications for the diagnosis of cognitive dysfunctions as well as for the development of effective therapies for attenuating impairments in higher mental functions.

Introduction

Neuroscientists have turned to the study of neurological disorders such as Alzheimer's disease (AD), not merely because of clinical or public health (epidemiological) concerns, but also because they see such research as an opportunity to explore the biological basis of cognition and memory. On the basis of such research and of studies in lower animals, structures such as the hippocampus and the ventromedial temporal lobe and neurochemical systems such as the cholinergic nervous system have been shown to play a role in learning and memory processes (1). Our understanding of the underlying neuroanatomy and neurochemistry of cognitive failures has matured to the point where it is possible to describe the neurobiology of the memory system in differentiated detail. The hippocampus, association cortex, basal

*Cognitive Studies Laboratory of the National Institute of Mental Health and National Institute of Drug Abuse; †National Institute of Neurological Disease and Stroke, National Institute of Mental Health, Bethesda, MD.

forebrain, thalamus, and hypothalmus are just a few of the structures that have been identified as warranting detailed study in severely memory-impaired patients with AD.

It has become increasingly obvious that we must consider the possibility that memory impairments, including those seen in patients presumed to have AD, can take various forms and may be determined by different mechanisms (2). For example, some memory-impaired patients demonstrate recent-memory failures linked to disturbances in accessing their previously acquired knowledge, whereas in others, dysfunctions in recent memory are unrelated to problems in accessing knowledge. Moreover, some memory-impaired patients can learn and later perform procedures although they cannot recall having learned the procedure (3). Yet other patients demonstrate memory impairments only on tests that require effort and sustained concentration (2,4). Still other memory impairments are due to retrieval failures, not failure of acquisition. In fact, it is a retrieval failure, rather than a disruption in the acquisition and retention of new learning, that may account for the preservation in memory of skills and procedures which cannot be freely recalled by amnestic individuals.

If we are to define a psychobiology of cognition, we must be prepared to obtain a systematic and differentiated picture of the cognitive structure of memory impairments and to relate these data to the rich yield of neurobiological findings. Not only can cognitive impairments appear quite different in different central nervous system diseases, they can also appear with considerable variation in the same disease, as in the case in senile dementia of the Alzheimer type (SDAT). In order to understand the nature and mechanisms of cognitive impairments, and also to appreciate the effects of treatments for attenuating cognitive impairments, careful evaluation of multiple cognitive and noncognitive domains is required. The resultant maps of the islands of impaired and spared higher mental functions can then be used in defining aspects of the neurobiology of cognitive processes and for clinical application.

The study of preserved learning functions in memory-impaired patients is, by its very nature, concerned with the neurobiological specificity of memory (cognitive) processes. The empirical foundation for demonstrating such biological specificity is studies that show that various factors, such as diseases or drug manipulation, that alter cognitive functions do not result in ubiquitous cognitive changes but rather cause factor-specific responses in different cognitive domains. This paper is intended to provide a general framework for the analysis of such discrete changes in memory processes.

There are a number of ways to explore the specificity of cognitive functions and dysfunctions in terms of impaired and spared memory. A classical approach has been to examine changes that result from destruction of a specific brain structure, such as the hippocampus and amygdala, in primates (reviewed in refs. 1 and 5). Other researchers have pursued a similar strategy, attempting to relate memory function (failure) to discrete histologic lesions in man. A similar but less precise strategy has been to examine the progressive patterns of cognitive decay seen in more diffuse forms of neuropathology such as AD or Huntington's disease. More recently, neuroscientists have also begun to use neuropharmacological tools to produce reversible but reproducible central nervous system changes and to relate such biological changes to specific forms of memory impairment (2).

From these types of research, and from the convergent evidence that can be derived from these efforts, it is becoming clear that memory is not a single entity, nor is it mediated by a single unitary biological process. It would follow that no single measure of memory can index the cognitive response to some treatment. Instead, it would be of value to diversify and contrast the memory-impairing effects of a given central nervous system treatment across several systematically chosen cognitive measures representing potentially different cognitive processes.

Research and Clinical Problems in Defining Cognitive Dysfunctions

Problems with recent memory are experienced by many individuals and are common to many syndromes and situations. Forgetting recent events may first be noticed by significant others or by the affected individual. It is a change in recent memory that is seen as central to the mental changes in AD; indeed, to the disorder itself. However, as will be explained in this paper, recent-memory failure is not specific to aging or AD but rather is common to many disorders, situational or environmental conditions and drug states. Thus, recent-memory failure should be seen as a common final-target cognitive response that can be the result of "failures" in a variety of cognitive determinants and domains. These cognitive domains appear to be psychobiologically distinct and susceptible to disruptions in different aspects of central nervous system functioning.

Relatively little research has reflected this differentiated nature of cognitive impairments. Instead, both researchers and clinicians have overemphasized documentation of the severity of recent-memory loss, in large part because this aspect of memory performance is the most obvious and, more important, because it is the easiest to measure. However, that does not imply that it will be the most useful aspect of cognitive functioning for research or diagnostic purposes.

An explosion of biological data are now available to characterize neuropsychiatric patients. Data from computed tomography (CT) scans, various neurochemical assays, positron emission tomography (PET), genetics, and neuropathological examinations are being used for presumptive definition of the neuropathologies of central nervous system disorders. However, these data are likely to be of value only to the extent that clinically defined classificatory schemes used to label the patients are appropriate. The principal feature of these schemes remains a description of changes in higher mental functions or cognitive performance. Only to the extent that our methods and interpretation of such data are accurate and appropriate can we learn about the neurobiology of disorders such as AD. Obviously, we depend on an appropriate system for identifying who has what syndrome or subtype of a syndrome.

Noncognitive aspects of behavior are often viewed as having nothing to do with cognitive changes that are apparent in a patient or a study group. In fact, aspects of mood can have highly specific effects on cognitive functioning. Likewise, motivation, arousal and sensitivity to rewarding stimuli can play a significant role in mediating and modulating facets of cognitive processing. Therefore, thorough appreciation and assessment of noncognitive factors is essential if we are to make sense of a profile of cognitive functioning in neuropsychiatric disorders (6).

Since many disorders are likely to result in failures in aspects of memory and related cognitive functions, it is important to compare cognitive dysfunction seen in a single patient or in groups of patients with cognitive changes seen in various types of neuropsychiatric disorders. That is, cognitive impairments can be appreciated and evaluated only when contrasting types of dysfunctions, with known neuropathological determinants, represent the system of comparison. Too often, memory impairments are defined exclusively with respect to a normative control group, and this practice is likely to lead to errors in diagnosis, particularly if we choose measures of memory pathology that are nonspecific for a particular neuropsychiatric disease.

It is instructive to attempt to model or mimic how different facets of cognition alone fail. Such an exercise is one way of developing convergent findings which can validate our understanding of the contrasting mechanisms of cognitive failures. Modeling of impaired cognitive functioning can be accomplished using drugs that reversibly alter central nervous system functioning or through behavioral manipulations; *e.g.*, stimulus presentation, response constraints and environmental contingencies.

Regardless of the strategy used in clinical assessment or research, the use of multivariate (multidependent measure) designs are crucial. Performance in various cognitive domains in response to the same treatment; *e.g.*, a form of neuropathology, is essential to assess cognitive functioning adequately.

Criteria for Concluding That Two Cognitive Processes Are Distinct

A number of criteria are important in testing whether some cognitive function is partially or completely spared while another is disrupted. Most important, such a comparison requires evidence from studies that permit direct comparisons of changes in identifiable and distinct cognitive processes in contrasting types of neurological and neuropsychiatric syndromes. Also, the measures should be reasonable indices of the dependent memory processes of interest. Other important features are reliability and comparable elasticity or sensitivity to changes in cognition in response to changes and disruptions in brain function.

If one considered this issue of comparability in terms of a model of psychophysical scaling, it would mean having two measures representing cognitive domains that were equally sensitive to threshold levels of changes in brain function produced by some disease or some drug treatment that might mimic a neurological disorder. That is, the measures should be comparable in identifying a just-noticeable, reliable measure of memory change in response to some drug treatment or change in brain state. Further, such measures should be equally useful in reflecting changes in some aspect of cognition as a function of progressive deterioration of brain function. This might also be reflected in comparable changes in cognition as a function of increasing doses of some drug that, when administered to normal volunteers, temporarily models a cognitive dysfunction. If one relates changes in stimulus intensity-for example, as indexed by various doses of drugs—to the cognitive response in different domains, then comparable sensitivity of measurement would be indicated if the slopes of the dose—response functions were similar, although their intercept need not be the same.

Changes in various aspects of cognitive functioning should be expressed along the same metric if direct comparison between measures and processes is to be possible. Comparable metrics might include t or z transformations of cognitive changes resulting from drug treatment. This normalization of measures of different types of memory, and of changes in these measures, allows direct, meaningful comparisons of changes in different domains.

If two neuropathologically different diseases were to impair memory processes but to do so by affecting two distinct component processes, then this would provide one form of support for arguing that these two processes may have different psychobiological mechanisms. If, in addition, two other forms of neuropsychiatric disease could be demonstrated to alter these same two component cognitive processes in a distinct manner but in the opposite direction, then these findings would lend further, convergent, support for the psychobiological distinctiveness of these processes. Such data could be seen as a double dissociation between these component processes. In directly measuring and comparing performance in two domains; *e.g.*, domain 1 (recent memory) and domain 2 (access to previously acquired knowledge in long-term memory), several outcomes are possible. The first is that two types of progressive neurological disorders, at some point in their courses, produce equally severe cognitive impairments on measures appropriate to each domain. It is also possible that with continued progression of the disease, performance in one domain may fall off more rapidly than performance in another. However, this finding may simply reflect unequal cognitive demands or sensitivity of the tasks used to assess functions 1 and 2. That is, apparent dissociations in the performance of type-1 tasks and type-2 tasks are confounded with the severity of the generalized cognitive impairment associated with the two hypothetical different neurological disorders. If, however, this differential sensitivity can be ruled out, then an uneven pattern of increasing impairment in function for tasks 1 and 2 can be presumed (Fig. 1).

Characterizing Distinct Cognitive Processes on the Bases of Detailed Laboratory Testing

Possible candidates for distinct cognitive processes come from several types of research. Models of memory processing in normal volunteers forms a classical and obvious basis for identifying distinct cognitive processes. For example, the effects of manipulating the processing conditions, stimulus material (pictures vs words) and retrieval conditions (recall vs recognition vs partial information and priming) have been used to argue for differences in some types of memory processes and representations of events in memory. Systematic clinical neuropsychological observations have also served as an important source of evidence pointing to distinctive features of memory functions (see ref. 5 for a review of current theories about the differentiated nature of memory pathology). Research in memory processes in animals has similarly led to the proposal of different types of memory (1,5).

On the basis of the results of these research strategies, the following cognitive processes appear most likely to be distinguishable in terms of the underlying psychobiological mechanisms:

1. Cognitive processes with and cognitive processes without conscious awareness. The role of consciousness (the subjective experience of knowing) and metacognitive (self-monitoring) operations is increasingly seen as an important determinant in the differentiated characteristics of various types of memory processes. Are memories for events in which subjects are "consciously" aware of what they know and appreciate the circumstances in which the memories were formed the same as memories about which subjects have no such awareness or appreciation (7)?

2. Context-dependent and context-specific retrieval processes; i.e., state-dependent learning. The importance of retrieval context to the likelihood of retrieving events from memory has been clear for some time and, in fact, has increasingly been used in accounting for various types of forgetting. The link between the encoding context and the retrieval context has also been important in accounting for learning and memory in the unimpaired normal subject and in patients in various psychiatric and mood-altered states as well as for drug-state-dependent learning and memory (8-10).

3. Reward-related and reward-independent learning. Most studies of cognitive processes in normal subjects are designed either to eliminate or to randomize and minimize reinforcing consequences. Neuroscientists have recently shown that brain structures and systems involved in the mediation of reward and reinforcement overlap to a considerable degree those systems important in learning and memory (11). The cognitive disturbances in depression and perhaps in some amnesias may well be determined by disruptions in the sensitivity of the reward system.

4. Respondent (conditioned) learning vs. operant or instrumental cognitive processes. The extent to which patients are able to form conditioned responses and maintain a "record" of such conditioning (learning) may involve brain systems different from those involved in "knowing" that learning has occurred and being able to encode in memory information about such learning, as would be the case for most instrumentally conditioned cognitive responses. Although classical conditioning techniques are rarely used in neuropsychiatric studies, we would view these as providing valuable data about aspects of central nervous system functioning that may be distinct from those tested by other procedures such as measures of effort demanding episodic memory.

5. *Acquisition, retention and retrieval process.* The reason a patient does not remember some previous event can be failure in any of these three broadly defined cognitive systems. Too often, the clinician attributes an inability to remember an event to acquisition failure. However, many clinical examples demonstrate that altering retrieval conditions, such as by recreating the context in which the event was originally experienced, can result in successful recall. Cognitive failures associated with disturbances in mood or with drug-altered states are examples in which apparent memory failure may be related more to difficulties in accessing or retrieving information that was acquired in some other state. Likewise, conditions that follow successful acquisition and storage of information (retention-consolidation processes) can affect the probability that some event will be remembered. Whether some event is reinforced, or whether some subsequent event interferes with previous learning, as well as changes in alertness or brain activity can alter the relative long-term viability of events represented in an unconsolidated form of memory.

6. *Passive memory consolidation vs working memory.* Psychobiological studies of memory processes in lower animals have often showed that postacquisition processing is necessary for forming a relatively permanent trace of recent and therefore "plastic" memory representations of events (12). This processing may involve multiple steps, including active, conscious reworking and updating of information already in memory. Similar processes may also account for the establishment of stable memory traces in humans (13).

7. *Attention, working memory and elaborative transformational processes.* The boundaries between attention and memory have always been unclear. However, it is apparent that some learning and memory impairments are directly attributable to attentional failures. For example, in hyperactive children (minimal brain dysfunction), alterations in attention, and particularly in sustained attention, account for information-processing failures. One aspect of this "attentional dysfunction" is that these children do not elaborate, encode or transform and enrich the stimulus material in terms of their previously acquired knowledge and so provide an interactive context for new learning.

8. *Short-term (working memory) vs long-term memory.* This distinction is a classic dichotomy that has been redefined during the past decade in terms of "single memory trace" theories of information processing. Some memory theorists view this distinction as useful, particularly in bridging lower animal and human learning-memory phenomena. Clinicians describing

memory failure, especially those whose roots are in medicine rather than psychology, are most likely to consider this distinction useful.

9. Elaborate vs superficial processing operations. Distinctions between memory-learning processes are defined along a continuum in terms of the operations subjects perform at the time of information input and when retrieving acquired experience from memory. Memory for past events is a function of the degree to which subjects have effectively processed, rehearsed and elaborated input information (14,15). The likelihood of remembering also depends on the similarity between processing conditions and retrieval conditions, particularly in terms of contextual factors which determine how information is encoded and the nature of the strategies used to search memory (16).

10. Automatic vs effort-demanding processes. The role of capacity-demanding cognitive processes (those requiring sustained attention and concentration) as opposed to those that require little cognitive capacity or mental work has received increasing attention during the last decade (17). Some drugs and some changes in brain structure and activity appear to affect either automatic or effort-demanding processes selectively (13,18). Many clinical examples come to mind in support of the distinctiveness of these various cognitive processes: patients who are depressed may have selective impairments in cognition in situations that require sustained concentration and cognitive effort but be unimpaired in using processes that can be accomplished automatically, including even some tasks that are complex (19). Parkinson's disease patients demonstrate such a pattern of dysfunction. Conversely, some patients demonstrate selective impairments in automatic processing but not in effort-demanding processes, whereas patients with AD, Korsakoff's disease or Huntington's disease generally are comparably impaired in both of these domains (20). In assessing cognitive changes in the elderly, distinguishing between levels of functioning in effort-demanding vs automatic processing is therefore particularly important for both diagnosis and assessment of treatment.

11. Language vs pattern processing. Neuropsychological investigations have provided strong evidence for a neuroanatomic differentiation between the processing and retention of language and of pattern information. Comparisons of the relative effectiveness of processing and production of information that involves language mediation as opposed to information have been used for decades to determine the neuroanatomical systems involved in some forms of cognitive failure.

12. Procedural vs declarative memory. The distinction between learning-memory processes involved in learning skills, rules and procedures and those involved in knowing that such learning has occurred is important in the study of congnitive domains (3), and much recent attention has been given to the distinction between these two types. Some memory-impaired amnestic patients are able to learn a procedure and accurately perform it later without remembering the circumstances in which they learned it. This dissociation between procedural and declarative memory effects can also be associated with some commonly prescribed sedative drugs such as the benzodiazepines (21). Whether this dichotomy has diagnostic significance in individual patients remains to be seen.

13. Episodic vs knowledge memory. Some memory representations are linked to the unique context and sequence in which those events have been processed, whereas other memories represent a knowledge base that is dissociated from the circumstances under which that information was learned. It is this knowledge that is largely the basis for encoding and organization of input. Impairment that results in an inability to access previously acquired knowledge is often the major determinant of recentmemory failure in patients suffering SDAT (22). The degree to which such patients are unable to bring to awareness, or working memory, knowledge that is related and therefore pertinent to encoding ongoing events can determine whether those events can be remembered later (23). Treating unimpaired subjects with cholinergic antagonists reproduces this distinctive pattern of cognitive failure (2,24). On the other hand, many memory-impaired patients, such as those with Korsakoff's disease, exhibit marked disturbances in recent memory without any impairment in access to the knowledge in long-term memory. Several types of drugs also mimic this latter form of cognitive failure in unimpaired subjects. These clinical and pharmacological findings provide convergent evidence that these two cognitive systems are at least partially independent and driven by different psychobiological mechanisms. Assessment of these functions is of considerable importance in establishing an appropriate diagnosis in subjects presenting with a disturbance in memory.

Listed here in tabular form is an as yet crudely conceived classification scheme for contrasting unique patterns of cognitive dysfunctions expressed in different neuropsychiatric disorders (Table 1). This compilation, although incomplete, does provide an outline of how our knowledge of the differentiated nature of the psychobiology of cognitive functions can be put to use in the diagnosis and evaluation of patients. A parallel scheme summarizes how different classes of drugs that affect distinct neurochemical systems can be expressed in highly specific changes in cognition (Table 2). The rationale and evidence for clustering cognitive dysfunctions in this manner only outlined in this paper, is presented in detail elsewhere (2,6,25,26). In fact, drug manipulations model common neuropsychiatric disorders and so provide us with tools for understanding those disorders and for developing effective therapies for cognitive dysfunction.

Conclusions

Simply measuring the presence or severity of memory impairments in man or beast will no longer, by itself, teach us a great deal about the neurobiological complexity of the memory. Systematic examination of preserved memory-learning functioning in the face of clearly evident disturbances in some aspects of memory provides an appreciation of that complexity. It forces us to grapple with issues that include the explanatory utility of some type of memory process that may be linked to a given model or heuristic. Studies of islands of preserved learning in memory-impaired patients demand that some of our attention be addressed to neurophysiological comparative equivalence of types of cognitive processes. At the same time, considering preserved learning-memory processes represents an appropriate challenge to cognitive theorists who are building solely on the basis of findings from unimpaired young subjects. Defining aspects of preserved learning in cognitively impaired patients is also important for neuro-pharmacologists interested in the biology of cognition who for so long have simply used a single memory assay to characterize response to some treatment. Initially, for clinicians interested in the diagnosis and treatment of memory-learning dysfunctions, an appreciation of the memory-learning tasks that the patient is able to accomplish is crucial in appropriately defining their deficits and in appreciating the value of our interventions.

References

1. Olton, D.S., Gamzu, E. & Corkin, S., eds. (1985) Memory dysfunctions: an integration of animal and human research from preclinical and clinical perspectives. *Ann. NY Acad. Sci.* **444**.
2. Weingartner, H. (1985) *Ann. NY Acad. Sci.* **444**, 359-369.
3. Cohen, N.J. & Squire, L.R. (1980) *Science* **210**, 207-210.
4. Weingartner, H., Burns, S., Diebel, R., & Lewitt, P. (1984) *Psychiatr. Res.* **11**, 223-235.

5. Squire, L.R. & Butter, N., eds. (1984) *Neuropsychology of Memory* (Guilford Press, New York).
6. Tariot, P. & Weingartner, H. (1986) A psychobiological analysis of cognitive failures. *Arch. Gen. Psychiatr.* (in press).
7. Jacoby, L.L. & Witherspoon, D. (1982) *Can. J. Psychol.* **36**, 300-324.
8. Reus, V.I., Weingartner, H. & Post, R.M. (1979) *Am. J. Psychiatr.* **136**, 927-931.
9. Leight, K.A. & Ellis, H.C. (1981) *J. Verb. Learn. Verb. Behav.* **20**, 251-275.
10. Eich, J.E. (1980) *Mem. Cognit.* **8**, 157-173.
11. Esposito, R.U., Parker, E.S. & Weingartner, H. (1984) *Subst. Alcohol Act. Misuse* **5**, 111-119.
12. McGaugh, J.L. & Herz, M.J. (1972) *Memory Consolidation.* (Albion, San Francisco).
13. Weingartner, H. & Parker, E.S. (1984) *Memory Consolidation: Psychobiology of Cognition.* eds. Weingartner, H. & Parker, E.S. (LEA Press)
14. Eysenck, M.W. & Eysenck, M.C. (1979) *J. Exp. Psychol. (Hum. Learn. Mem.)* **5**, 472-484.
15. Craik, F.I.M. (1979) *Annu. Rev. Psychol.* **30**, 63-102.
16. Tulving, E. & Thomson, D.M. (1973) *Psychol. Rev.* **80**, 352-373.
17. Hasher, L. & Zacks, R.T. (1979) *J. Exp. Psychol. (Gen.)* **108**, 356-388.
18. Newman, R.P., Weingartner, H., Smallberg, S. & Calne D. (1984) *Neurology* **34**, 805-807.
19. Roy-Bourne, P., Weingartner, H. & Birer, L. (1985) *Arch. Gen. Psychiatr.* **43**, 265-267.
20. Strauss, M.E., Weingartner, H. & Thompson, K. (1985) *Mem. Cognit.* **13**, 507-510.
21. Wolkowitz, O., Tinklenberg, J. & Weingartner, H. (1985) *Neuropsychobiology* **14**, 88-96.
22. Weingartner, H., Grafman, J., Boutelle, W., Kaye, W. & Martin, P. (1983) *Science* **221**, 380-382.
23. Weingartner, H., Kaye, W., Smallberg, S., Ebert, H., Gillin, J.C. & Sitaram, N. (1981) *J. Abn. Psychol.* **90**, 187-196.
24. Sitaram, N., Weingartner, H. & Gillin, J.C. (1978) *Science* **201**, 274-276.
25. Wolkowitz, O., Tinklenberg, J. & Weingartner, H. (1985) *Neuropsychobiology* **14**, 133-156.
26. Wolkowitz, O.M., Weingartner, H. Hommer, D., Thompson, K. & Pickar, D. (1986) Diazapam-induced amnesia: modeling amnestic disorders. *Am. J. Psychiatr.* (in press).

TABLE 1. Dysfunctions in specific cognitive processes or domains in neuropsychiatric disorders

	Examples of types of cognitive domains			
Examples of disorders	*Effort demanding episodic and attentional processes*	*Knowledge memory*	*Rules and procedures*	*"Automatic" cognitive opeartions*
SDAT	Decr.*	Decr.*	Decr.	Decr.
Depression; Parkinson's Disease	Decr.*	=	?	=
Amnesia; *e.g.*, of Korsakoff's type	Decr.*	=	=	Decr.
Forms of learning disabilities in children	Decr.	?	?	=

Dysfunctions are coded through the use of Decr. with an * indicating processes that are particularly likely to be impaired. = indicates domains in which cognitive performance is generally within normal limits. ? indicates additional data needed.

TABLE 2. Dose-dependent changes in specific cognitive processes or domains in response to different classes of psychoactive drug treatments

	Examples of types of cognitive domains			
Example of drug class	*Effort demanding attentional processes*	*Knowledge memory*	*Rules and procedures*	*"Automatic" cognitive operations*
Cholinergic antagonists	Decr.*	Decr.*	?	Decr.*
Benzodiazepines	Decr.*	=	=	?
Serotinergic drugs	Decr.	?	?	Decr.*
Drugs that attentuate catecholamine activity	Decr.*	=	?	=
Neuropeptides	Decr.	?	?	=

Symbol Key: See Table 1.

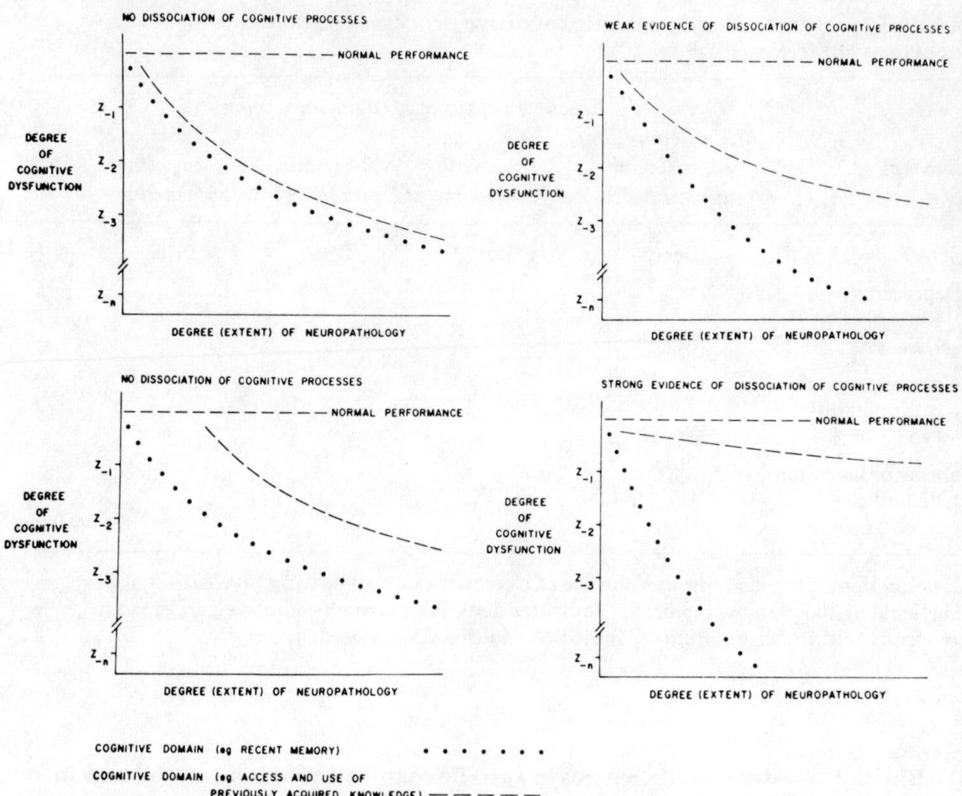

Fig. 1. Distinguishing between forms of cognitive pathology.

Index